# SERIOUSLY SILLY

Robert Ross is Britain's comedy historian, whose books include biographies of Marty Feldman, Sid James and Peter Sellers, as well as the *Monty Python Encyclopedia*. He has toured a number of comedy history shows including *Oh, What A Carry On!*, *Christmas Crackers* and *Forgotten Heroes of Comedy*. He was a close personal friend of Terry Jones and is very proud to have written his authorised biography.

# SERIOUSLY SILLY

## THE LIFE OF TERRY JONES

R O B E R T   R O S S

Foreword by Sir Michael Palin

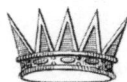

CORONET

First published in Great Britain in 2025 by Coronet
An imprint of Hodder & Stoughton Limited
An Hachette UK company

The authorised representative in the EEA is Hachette Ireland, 8 Castlecourt
Centre, Dublin 15, D15 XTP3, Ireland (email: info@hbgi.ie)

1

Hardback ISBN 9781399742917
Trade Paperback ISBN 9781399742924
ebook ISBN 9781399742948

Typeset in Minion Pro by Hewer Text UK Ltd, Edinburgh
Printed and bound in Great Britain by Clays Ltd, Elcograf S.p.A.

Hodder & Stoughton policy is to use papers that are natural, renewable
and recyclable products and made from wood grown in sustainable
forests. The logging and manufacturing processes are expected to conform
to the environmental regulations of the country of origin.

Hodder & Stoughton Limited
Carmelite House
50 Victoria Embankment
London EC4Y 0DZ

www.hodder.co.uk

*For my wife, Gemma.*

*Terry would have loved you and your cooking . . . but would never have been quick enough to pinch something from your plate!*

# CONTENTS

Foreword by Sir Michael Palin     ix

Introduction     1
1   From Colwyn Bay to Claygate     6
2   Oxford     20
3   Frost Over the Fringe     38
4   Inside the British Broadcasting Corporation     52
5   The Two of Us     71
6   1969 and All That     95
7   Python! Python! Python!     120
8   Once a Knight's Enough for Anyone . . .     141
    A Middle Word by Eric Idle     165
9   Tall Tales and Real Ales     167
9¾   Sitting Comfortably? Terry the Children's Author     201
10   Calling the Shots – Terry as a Film Director     228
11   Albatross? Python Reunited     262
12   Is No One Interested in History?! Presented
    by Terry Jones     287
13   Fantasy and Reality     303
14   Pressing the Reset Button     325
15   The Silent World of Terry Jones     347
    The Epilogue: The Brain of Terry Jones     362

    Afterword by Terry Gilliam     369
    Acknowledgements     370
    Picture Acknowledgements     372
    Terryography     373

# TERRY: AN APPRECIATION

## A FOREWORD BY SIR MICHAEL PALIN

TERRY knew me better than anyone, apart from my long-suffering wife. We'd sat together over a desk for day after day, and, when we weren't sitting over a desk, we were sitting over a pint, and when we weren't sitting over a pint we were sitting over a menu. So we got to know each other outside the bounds of success and celebrity (though both helped us get a good table). In fact, neither of us was particularly good at success and celebrity.

The most important thing Terry knew about me was that I could get quite cross if I didn't get regular meals. If I turned a little petulant at five past one, Terry would explain that 'Michael gets very grumpy if he doesn't get lunch'. He was, of course, absolutely right and my worst nightmare was, and still is, having to work with someone who doesn't care about lunch.

I in turn knew that what made Terry grumpy was being served beer in a tankard – 'Straight glass, please!' – and being taken by taxis on their preferred route rather than his.

These are the sort of things I miss most about Terry, who was the most steadfast friend for fifty-odd years. And they were some odd years. In 1971 he and I drove around the States together. We found ourselves in a bar south of New Orleans, helping the owner shell peas. Only when she showed us the waterbed and invited her two friends round did Terry and I understand what shelling peas really meant.

Terry was no prude, far from it, but I once saw him shocked to silence when a be-gowned lady at an Oxford college ball shouted in an impeccable upper-class accent, 'Show us your cock then!'

I was with Terry in Central Park in New York when one of the horses waiting to pull a tourist carriage around took a bite out of his thick, rather stylish fur coat. Terry didn't see the funny side at all and rebuked the horse in the tone of high-pitched indignation only he was capable of. 'That was a new coat!' he protested, in a voice that could have registered on the Richter scale, whereupon it bit him again.

Apart from everything else he did so well, Terry was a seriously well-informed scholar, whose favourite period of history was the Middle Ages. As a consequence, he was drawn to the authoritarian kings of the period and disdainful of anything that followed them. Mere mention of the word 'democracy' would have Terry thumping the dinner table. In fact, he would regularly thump the dinner table if he felt his point of view was not being heard. The irony was that Terry had just laid out the most superb meal on that same table.

Terry was a man of so many talents and so little ego. This, I think, must be why he was never given the level of appreciation he deserves. Which is why this book is timely. I hope it will send people back to his work, whether it be films he's directed, roles he's played, scripts he's written, the opinion pieces he wrote for the *Guardian*, the children's books he's written, the history he's rewritten, the Crusades he revisited and everything else that made him everybody's favourite polymath.

Now it's lunchtime and, as Terry knew all too well, I have to go.

Michael Palin
Gospel Oak, May 2025

# INTRODUCTION

*If dead leaves were money I'd never be broke*
*And if troubles were funny we'd all share the joke*

I N the spring of 1983, I snuck into my local cinema via an emergency exit. That it was always half ajar was a well-known fact swapped around the corners of the school playground like doublers in a collection of Panini football stickers. It wasn't that I didn't want to pay, although the sneaking in did mean I had a little bit of pocket money to spend on pick 'n' mix from Woolworths. The problem was that there was a film I was desperate to see but it was an 18 certificate and I was only twelve. The poster for it was so intriguing: a caricature of God weighing up the pros and cons of a round world and a square world.

*Monty Python's The Meaning of Life* was a revelation, of course. Something of the true meaning of comedy for me, to this very day. My prized film magazines had already alerted me to the fact that Terry Jones played the grossly overweight Mr Creosote in that body-horror restaurant moment – something right up my street at the time and also one of the reasons that I shouldn't really be seeing it at that tender age. Not only that but I had noted that the film – that naughty, far-too-old-for-me film – was also directed by the same Terry Jones. The Terry Jones I knew off of the telly, when my dad allowed me to stay up late with him and watch repeats of *Monty Python's Flying Circus*. The Terry Jones who was the naked organist and the screaming women with curlers in their hair.

1

A little over a year after I had discovered the meaning of life, in more ways than one, that self-same Terry Jones was on television again. And not in some old repeat from when my dad wore a younger man's clothes. Terry appeared – albeit fleetingly – in a new comedy, a pioneering comedy, my comedy. *The Young Ones*. He was in the horror-themed episode, 'Nasty'. The same Terry as I had seen on that illicit jaunt to the cinema was now doing his comedy business alongside my generation's funny characters: Rick and Vyvyan and Neil and Mike the Cool Person. I didn't know then of course that Terry's 42-year-old comedy brain was as active and as interested as ever, and he'd even phoned his friend Michael Palin to alert him to the brilliant comedy writing of *The Young Ones*, singling out Ben Elton as a talent to watch. For me, now fourteen and watching on our Baird TV set, on the never-never from Radio Rentals, this was Terry playing in the sandpit of today's comedy, bringing a sense of history and gravitas to his blink-and-you'll-miss-it comic cameo as a very drunk vicar at a graveside. The meeting of the comic generations was seamless. And irresistible.

So irresistible was it that, as a result of that episode of *The Young Ones*, I wrote Terry Jones a fan letter. And being the lovely bloke that I would find out he was, Terry wrote back, including a 7x5 signed photograph. It was inscribed 'To Robert', and the image was a rather stern-faced Terry sat in what I could only guess was his study, and wearing a Groucho Marx fake nose and glasses.

Fast forward fifteen years. The year is 1998. I am now a published comedy historian, with my second book, the *Monty Python Encyclopedia*, an exhaustive and exhausting overview of the output of all the Pythons, together and apart. Eventually, the five surviving team members contributed to the book, but Terry Jones was the first. Terry was always enthusiastic, always helpful. Even before we met, in frantic, handwritten correspondence in his trademark brown ink he had eagerly endorsed my endeavour. He wrote, and would repeat verbally to anybody who cared to ask him about the encyclopaedia, that: 'I have learnt more about the Pythons from reading this book than from being one!' That level of generosity was very typical of Terry.

The following year, I was invited to the thirtieth-anniversary celebration of Python with a twentieth-anniversary screening of *Monty Python's Life of Brian*, at the (Roman) Empire cinema, in London's Leicester Square. Four of the Pythons took to the stage, to be interviewed or, as it turned out, refereed by Jonathan Ross. The chat, without Eric, or Graham, naturally, swiftly and typically turned into those four comic behemoths talking very loudly and very animatedly and all at the same time. It was a blast.

Afterwards, I took myself off to a favourite public house, the Hand & Racquet. It's long gone now but it was a comedy mecca. Tommy Cooper used to drink there; *Hancock's Half Hour* writers Ray Galton and Alan Simpson frequented it so often with Tony Hancock and Sid James that they would mention it in the show for an assured free pint. Immediately after the Python bash, who should walk into the Hand & Racquet but Terry Jones. Nervously, I approached, introduced myself and offered to buy him a drink. Instead, Terry grabbed hold of me, insisted on buying me a drink and gushed about how grateful he was for the *Monty Python Encyclopedia*: 'You saved me a job!' he chuckled. Although, he rather gleefully informed me that I had forgotten to include one of his books. It wasn't so much a criticism; he was mostly just relieved that I was human after all. The book in question was *Attacks of Opinion* – a collection of his gloriously opinionated articles for the *Guardian*. 'Oh no, a letter A entry!' I said. 'I forgot aardvark as well!' Terry beamed. He got the reference. It was a Ben Elton joke from *Blackadder III*. 'If only it was *The Young Ones*. You could have added it at the end,' he replied. And my comedy life came full circle at that moment. I was in comedy heaven. And, most excitingly of all, I left that potent, albeit brief encounter with Terry's home number, his newfangled email address and an insistence that I get in touch. As would soon become crystal clear, Terry not only embraced the fresh and the innovative, he was also very insistent on cultivating brand new friendships.

Grasping this opportunity to hang out with absolute comedy royalty, I duly did get in touch with Terry. And, bless his brilliant heart and soul, he seemed to remember me. And that's how nigh-on twenty-five years of friendship and fun and funny and unforgettable encounters began. I was lucky enough to enjoy many, many conversations with him – spiralling chats and inspirational flights of fancy, the tallest of tales and rarefied recollections of the most fantastic achievements – that usually took place within rustic public houses. I have used my memories of these happiest of times throughout the book, weaving in and out of anecdotes from those who knew Terry best. People who even, on many levels, knew Terry better than he knew himself.

When I spoke to many of those closest to Terry, who enjoyed that same twenty-five years, or forty-five years, even sixty-five years of friendship, two phrases have kept coming up. One is 'polymath', in simple and perfect summation of his great, pretty much all-encompassing talent. 'He did so much!' I blathered to his first wife, Alison, one day, to which she replied, 'You don't have to tell me!' His second wife, Anna, remembers: 'Terry would wake up at 7 a.m. every morning and go straight to his study to write. He would often have six incredible ideas before breakfast!'

The other recurring word is 'passion': a perfect description for this Toad of Toad Hall kind of chap, who fell in love with a project or a person completely and utterly. In a way, Terry lived his life all at once. He seemed to be able to do everything and do everything well, and, at times, do everything all at the same time. It was never an ordinary life. Very much an extraordinary one. Almost from the very beginning.

Sir Michael Palin was the first person I contacted when I was commissioned to write this biography of his dearest friend, frequent writing partner and even more frequent drinking buddy. Without Michael's input the story of Terry Jones just would not compute. With an 'anything for Terry' attitude, a meeting was arranged at Michael's home in Gospel Oak and, after a fruitful and, at times, fruity chat about his old mate, I left with his cheery but portentous words ringing in my ears: 'Good luck with the book. Terry wasn't easy!'

And so it has proved. I knew Terry was a complex man. A glorious mess of passions and projects intertwined throughout his life. Once Terry found a subject or an interest that fascinated him, it was part of his very psyche for good, be it Buster Keaton, Geoffrey Chaucer, real ale or the Welsh countryside, although, again like Mr Toad, a new idea could swiftly dull interest in an old idea he had conquered and achieved. While there was often a desire to do something completely different, Terry also couldn't resist or avoid going back to doing something exactly the same.

Here, then, is the story of an extraordinary man who, yes, may not have been easy, or indeed often not easy to understand, but was always very easy to love and extremely easy to admire.

This is the life of Terry Jones.

# CHAPTER ONE

## FROM COLWYN BAY TO CLAYGATE

*My childhood was like a secret life. Something*
*just told me that I was going to be a poet. Sort of*
*Dylan Thomas . . . with more jokes, I suppose.*

He was born Terence Graham Parry Jones, in Colwyn Bay, a quaint North Wales seaside resort with bracing breezes from the Irish Sea. The date was right bang centre in the middle of the Second World War, on 1 February 1942, to be precise. A Sunday. Ironic for the man who would direct, co-write and act in *Monty Python's Life of Brian*. This particular Sabbath Day child would indeed be happy and wise, and good and gay. And, like any good Aquarian, he would be self-contained, apt to swim on his own. Terry would be clever, undoubtedly, and innovative. Moreover, he would be truthful. Truthful to himself, and truthful to other people. Painfully, obsessively, often destructively truthful. But enough of the traits that fit the star sign, for Terry Jones was not a child who would grow up to conformities. He would actively and gleefully tear down conformities and put them back together again, in a different, challenging, funnier way.

He was decidedly Welsh though. Through and through, and for ever. He would become wistful and rueful when talking about Wales – his idyllic first home that would be taken away from him when he was aged only five. Although he did see the funny side when pondering the country's unofficial national anthem, 'Land of My Fathers'. For the land of Terry's dad was in actual fact

Streatham, south London. Even so, Alick George Parry Jones was, according to Terry, 'Welsh, and very proud of the fact'. His English birthplace was presumably something of which he was less proud.

In the years immediately before the outbreak of the Second World War, Alick had moved to Ruthin, a picturesque market town in the southern section of the Vale of Clwyd. Nearby Denbigh, the historic heart of Denbighshire, had a bank, its own little financial fortress, and in that bank young Alick had secured employment as a clerk. A little less than twenty miles north of Denbigh, in Colwyn Bay, a certain Dilys Louisa Newnes was living with her parents. Although Terry didn't have a clue how Alick and Dilys met. 'That was the kind of thing that wasn't really talked about in those days,' he said. 'A bit like being born in Streatham.'

Dilys' parents were big music fans, involved in the running of the local Colwyn Bay Amateur Operatic Society, a fun and friendly group of like-minded singers who specialised in staging productions of Gilbert and Sullivan comic operas.

Terry emerged, mewing and wailing, to be greeted by his loving, stagestruck grandmother, his exhausted but relieved mother, and his two-year-old brother, Nigel. Not his father, though. By that point, Alick was serving in the Royal Air Force, in Scotland. In later years, Terry made a joke out of it. He would do that a lot, reasoning that his father must have been 'guarding the grouse', although, in more candid moments, he would hint at something much more important. The wilds of the Highlands were ideal for concealing secret tests of a revolutionary new system that used radio waves to detect enemy aircraft and ships, known as RADAR. Alick got compassionate leave to visit his wife and new, one-week-old son, before being sent to a base in India with the rank of Flight Lieutenant (Temporary). Young Terry would be four years old before he saw his father again.

The family home was Bodchwil, sometimes spelt Bodhwyl, or, as Terry's mum used to translate it, 'House-in-a-Whirl', which sums up rather well the chaotic family life of a husband-less wife, two kids and an entertaining grandparent, all under the same roof. As a result of this wartime upheaval, Terry's maternal grandmother, Sarah Ann Newnes, née Pilkington, who Terry knew as La-La, became pivotal to his upbringing. And, despite the cliché of the Valley of Song, this Welsh household was a very musical one. As well as all that Gilbert and Sullivan, La-La taught music. Family legend also insisted that Terry's maternal grandfather had been a musical conductor in the Australian navy. It's one of those 'facts' that Terry just accepted as a child because his grandfather, who became a schoolmaster in Colwyn Bay, had died in 1941, the year before Terry was born, although, in later years, he would often question the feasibility of his grandfather having served in the navy of a country on the other side of the world. 'To be honest with you, I started not to believe it at all!' he said once.

The whole story appeared to rest on one particular photograph of his grandfather standing on the deck of a ship: 'He was in full dress uniform,' recalled Terry. 'What's more, he was stood in front of this military orchestra. So perhaps it was true after all.' Truth being stranger than fiction is nothing new, and the physical proof was in that item of warfare that could excite any small child: his grandfather's ceremonial sword. This had to be the clincher. An elaborate dress sword for special occasions, with 'W.G. Newnes' engraved upon it. As if to fire the young imagination to breaking point, young Terry was occasionally allowed to slip the sword out of its sheath and gaze at the elaborately engraved blade. Terry said that his grandmother would talk of William, and take great glee in pointing out the huge groove down one side of the sword. La-La would explain that William had said the groove was 'for the blood to run out'.

Terry's mum was a homemaker and fiercely protective of the home she had made. Even when her choice of interior decor failed to impress young Terry. He vividly remembered being in his pram 'and Mum had bought this horrible alabaster bust of a shepherd-ess. She put this figurine in the pram with me and for some stupid reason I got really cross with this lady's face staring at me. So cross that I picked up a pot of marmalade from Mum's shopping and hit the shepherdess with it! I chipped off its nose even before Mum had got it home. I think I was trying to defend Mum from this stranger. She wasn't grateful though. She was absolutely furious!'

Terry didn't seem to mind the absence of his dad in these years. To him, it was normal, after all. 'He wasn't there long enough to miss, really,' he observed, pragmatically. Indeed, for a small child born during the time of a faraway war it was thrilling to have a heroic dad serving somewhere that must have seemed pretty exotic compared to North Wales. Terry was perfectly content with his reality, his version of a family life. And there was always Nigel, his big brother. A stoic sort of chap who would try to control, start the fun and invariably take the blame. Terry had a clear memory of himself and his brother getting up very early one day to go into the field opposite to collect mushrooms. Terry guessed they must have had a combined age of six years – Terry two and Nigel four. Terry was pretty scared. They got across the road (in those days roads had very little traffic on them) and ventured into the field carrying their baskets. Terry was already quaking in his little white socks when his brother – who always had an eye for the dramatic – pointed to the brook at the far end of the field and told him about the bear that lived there. That was it. Terry was out of that field, across the road and safe back in La-La's kitchen before that bear had a chance to roar. Here was the stuff of nightmares – or, more pertinently, the stuff of children's books, of storytelling. A vivid imagination was already beginning to form. And at the epicentre of this imagination were the colourful and carefree and almost other-worldly delights of Colwyn Bay.

Even though he was so young when the family lived at Bodchwil, Terry always insisted that the recollections of his Welsh first home remained vivid for the rest of his days. Even when, late in life, the clouds descended on his imagination, his mental pictures of a Wales coastline would gently and reassuringly linger. Terry would half-joke that those Colwyn Bay memories 'are often more vivid to me than what happened to me yesterday!' Those almost fairy-tale days of riding in the charabanc, changing into his bathing suit on the beach, the mystery and wonder of Eirias Park – a council-owned playing fields, opened in September 1923 and known as 'the park by the sea'.

Three-year-old Terry was cheeky, playful and ever-smiling, but he seemed already to have a fledgling brain for abstract comedy and, yes, silly comedy. He could actually remember his first joke. As he told it, he and his family were sitting round the table in their home. They'd just had pudding and La-La asked if anyone wanted seconds of custard. Suddenly, Terry's three-year-old mind saw the opportunity for a bit of humour. Instead of passing up his bowl, he passed up his table mat. He watched with bated breath and then delighted disbelief as the joke went like clockwork. He had expected someone who passed his mat along the table to notice, but no one did. La-La plunged the ladle into the custard and – bliss! – ladled out a good dollop of custard onto the mat. Terry sat back and waited for the laughter and the applause. But then it all seemed to go wrong. Instead of the laughter and the applause, all he heard was a chorus of recrimination: 'You stupid boy! What did you do that for? Look what you've done!' Nobody turned on his gran and said, 'Why didn't you look where you're pouring the custard?!' or blamed the people in between who'd passed the mat along, 'Why don't you look what you are doing?' The injustice of it all stuck with Terry for decades after, but that notion of the joke that upsets and offends ... now, that was interesting. That was worth pursuing. That, my boy, was the pathway to destructive, convulsive laughter!

By May 1945, the sound of laughter and the craft of comedy had begun to infiltrate Terry's consciousness as well. Apart from the funnies in the newspapers and children's comics, typically it had been the wireless that would bring a daily burst of humour into the home. And these radio shows reassuringly broadcast from the BBC would invariably have great swathes of military chit-chat – nothing so careless as to cost lives, of course. *Welsh Rarebit*, a pioneering comedy variety show produced in Wales for the Welsh but quickly gaining nationwide popularity, had showcased the comic antics of Wyn Calvin, Gladys Morgan and Harry Secombe. Alongside the comedy, *Welsh Rarebit* also featured sentimental extracts of 'Dai's Letter to the Forces', performed by Lyn Joshua. Concurrently Kenneth Horne, serving as a flight lieutenant in the Royal Air Force, starred in *Much-Binding-in-the-Marsh*, set on a fictional and farcical RAF station; and Tommy Handley had kept the home fires burning with his satirical and silly sketch show *It's That Man Again* – or *I.T.M.A.* for short. The comedy was slick and cheerful; loud and optimistic, with great gales of live studio audience laughter mixing with the shared laughter of Terry's family. The young lad liked that sound of laughter. He liked it a lot.

Even in rural North Wales, the impact of war was felt in many ways. Colwyn Bay, in particular, had seen a huge increase in its population thanks to the relocation of the staff of the Ministry of Food from London to the relative safety of the Welsh coast. These personnel were billeted cheek-by-jowl with American servicemen, Liverpool evacuees and Belgian refugees. Terry's view of the actual conflict itself was mostly restricted to a quick peek in his grandmother's newspaper or his mother's periodical, but these lodged themselves in the highly fertile brain of the fledgling film director. In that embryonic visual eye. Then one day an army tank came rumbling up the dusty road between the high hedgerows to his home. This very real, very three-dimensional spectre of war came seemingly straight from the front line to the home front. Another vivid memory for Terry was his mum coming into the boys' bedroom one night and drawing back the curtains to show them the sight of shafts of artificial light playing across the sky. Terry remained convinced that these were the searchlights from Liverpool celebrating VE Day and his mum wanted to share this momentous occasion with her children. 'It was absolutely magical. The searchlights were like vast, long fingers striding across the sky.'

VE Day in May was followed by the surrender of Japan in August 1945, marking the end of the war. Still, though, Terry's father remained in India. Eventually, word came that he was expected home in February 1946. Just after his fourth birthday, Terry was taken, along with his brother Nigel, to Colwyn Bay train station to meet his dad from the train. That awkward, rather haunting first encounter since he was an unaware infant would be etched onto Terry's consciousness for the rest of his life. He could even remember walking up the stairwell to the station concourse: 'every step boasted a blue enamel sign advertising destinations for such exotic places as Brighton and Lulworth Cove!'

Levels of anticipation were high. Terry saw that his mum was getting anxious and didn't understand why. Of course, in retrospect he realised his mum was fearful in case her husband was not on the train after all. And perhaps even nervous about being reunited with him after such a long absence. After all those years it must have been a real mix of emotions for her. The train arrived and the railway platform was suddenly flooded with people. As the crowd dispersed, Dilys spotted at the far end of the platform a man in RAF uniform with a forage cap on his head and a kitbag slung over his shoulder: 'That's him!' They ran up to him and it was hugs and kisses all round. Terry remembered feeling discombobulated, even a bit scared – he just wasn't sure. When his dad finally picked him up, all Terry could recall was the sensation of being kissed by this strange man. Suddenly, Terry went off the whole idea of having this 'dad' back in their lives. Terry was used to being kissed by women. Moustaches weren't his cup of tea at all.

Interestingly, Terry wrote about this experience in an essay for school when he was seven years old. By then, all that remained from that pivotal scene was his father's 'strange and prickly moustache'. He was grateful to his seven-year-old self for recording this stark first memory of his dad, ambivalent though it was.

Four-year-old Terry's little universe certainly changed when the absent father returned from war. A certain amount of tension entered family life and Terry started to hear stern words for the first time. He realised later that it must have been terrible for Alick: he'd been shipped off to India and missed his family growing up at the most important stage. He'd left behind a one-week-old baby and a two-year-old and arrived back to find a four-year-old and a six-year-old. And his youngest son didn't really want much to do with this stranger. Terry supposed that, subconsciously, he regarded his father as a bit of an intruder – or an outsider. Terry had bonded with his mum so strongly that, for him, no relationship could ever be as real as that. He supposed Alick also knew – deep down – that he couldn't reach Terry at all, except that Terry felt sorry for him. Terry learned later in life that his dad was a caring, gentle, humorous man, just like he appeared in those family photos that his mum treasured so much, but something was wrong when he came home. Maybe Terry's parents couldn't re-find whatever it was they had in the first place. Maybe Terry's mum resented his return. Maybe his experiences away at war had changed him. Terry didn't really know. But whatever it was it turned his dad into something of a tyrant, who could only communicate with his sons by telling them off or yelling at them. Luckily, as was the case throughout most of his life, Terry's sense of humour and sense of community were more than enough to counterbalance this early confusion and disorientation. However, this was about to be shattered.

As if the expected but rather mysterious reappearance of his dad was not enough of a shock to the system, the removal of the family from home to horrible Home Counties, as necessitated by his dad's work, just a few months later proved a much more seismic upheaval. Claygate, a well-to-do suburban village just outside Esher in Surrey, certainly was not Colwyn Bay. It was, in fact, a small disaster. The home in Colwyn was the only one Terry had known, and now where was he? Where had the seaside gone? The pier? The prom? Where was fairy glen? Furthermore, beloved La-La had declined to go with them.

For Terry, real life was, and would remain, Wales, and the few bright spots as the wide-eyed five-year-old became a six-year-old and then, with alarming inevitability, a seven-year-old, were trips back home, back to Colwyn Bay, to visit his beloved grandmother. His born and bred Welshness was and is crucial to understanding Terry's passion and drive. It was the source of his Celtic charm and hot temper; he always retained his pride in his Colwyn Bay roots and an anger that it had been ripped away from his young grip. Michael Palin detected it throughout their working life together: 'Terry was always very strong-willed, and I think his Welshness gave him that feeling of being right. All the time!' While, typically, Terry Gilliam talks in the prose of a broken fairy tale: 'as if he was a kid taken away from this beautiful kingdom and dragged off to horrible England.'

Terry spent the next twenty years insisting that he was Welsh and that he didn't fit in with where he now found himself. He never felt he belonged there. The whole period of living in Claygate, from five to nineteen, was like an interruption. Wales was the source of the ruggedness and truthfulness and humanity in his writing. It was the fire in his belly in debate and that stoic quality that ignited the lightning determination and quiet bravery displayed throughout his life. All this passion and intensity just couldn't be content in, of all places, the heart of stockbroker Surrey, just fourteen miles out of London as the crow flies, but not as the Python slithers.

Typically of Terry, it was the juvenilia he had penned while at school that served as his memory for his flashbacks to sorrow in Surrey. Again, at the age of seven, a school essay reflecting upon Christmas revealed that his planned gift for his dad was to be some new underwear because, as he wrote, 'his was all in tatters'. Terry would shudder slightly at the recollection, claiming it must have been an expression he had picked up off his poor mum, who probably never lived down the public humiliations of her son's shock-horror revelations in his schoolwork. And there was another school essay that asked the students to ponder on what they would like to do when they grew up. Terry's future ambitions were clear, albeit misspelt: He wrote 'I am hopping to be an actor.' He would later joke, 'Well, I'm still hopping. And I've hopped quite a bit while fulfilling that early hope to be an actor. However, whatever the misspelled word I wrote in my essay, I really knew, deep down, that I wanted to write.'

Despite an early, albeit disapproved of, display of silly pranks, Terry had never had any particular interest in comedy. Humour was just something that came with everything in life as far as he and his brother were concerned. Something in home life and from the radio. However, that radio comedy was more strongly seeping into Terry's imagination. Those *Crazy People* the Goons started broadcasting in May 1951, when Terry was nine. He was bewitched and coaxed into the surreal universe created by Spike Milligan. And *Welsh Rarebit* comedian Harry Secombe was in the nutty mix as Neddie Seagoon, a kind of everyman representative within the mad asylum of military buffoons, pimply youths and aged crones. That it was someone familiar and Welsh made all the difference. For Terry, Secombe was his tangible portal to *The Goon Show*. His way to identify and interact with the characters. Why not endeavour to see the funny side in absolutely everything?

And why not follow your older, cooler brother and all his touchstones of popular culture and learning? Nigel was Terry's guru in all things cultural. He formed Terry's tastes. Told him what he should listen to and what he should not listen to. Nigel taught Terry about the wonders of blues and traditional jazz as well as the evil snares of modern big band music, which, he told his brother, lacked any sort of improvisation. Nigel also scorned popular songs with a deep and sincere disrespect. Ten-year-old Terry didn't dare let Nigel catch him humming '(How Much Is) That Doggie in the Window' or 'You Belong to Me', with its evocative opening line 'See the pyramids along the Nile . . .' The only time Nigel cracked was when he took a liking to Kay Starr, and then suddenly Terry was allowed a certain limited repertoire of pop music. This was clearly lust rather than musical integrity, but Kay Starr passed the Nigel test and, as a result, that of Terry too. But other than that, Terry was to stick to Bessie Smith, Ottilie Patterson and Muddy Waters.

Nigel was instrumental too in Terry's lifelong love of reading, the unquenchable kick he got out of books and his voracious appetite for absorbing knowledge on all sorts of subjects. Terry was rather late getting off children's books, and the love of *Rupert Bear* never left him, but he went straight from Rupert to Ray Bradbury, which was quite the leap of faith. However, there was one area of his literary passion that, as a schoolboy, he was keen to keep under his hat. In those days, he supposed he had a secret life. His gran had got him reading poetry, 'The Brook', by the mysteriously named Alfred Lord Tennyson. And he was into writing poetry. A more self-contained, achievable ambition than being an actor, just so long as he could do 'something creative'. Terry would hear that phrase 'make something of yourself' from grown-ups all the time. Like we all did. Parents; teachers; everyone in authority; all those people Terry would later mock and undermine in his comedy. Terry himself would embrace and adapt that phrase. All he wanted to do when he grew up was to 'make something'.

Still, even his big brother had to exercise all his powers of persuasion to introduce Terry to certain worthy literature. One day, Nigel announced, to Terry's consternation, that he was going to listen to a radio drama that was being broadcast that very night and would last for an hour and a half. That there was a heavy Welsh overtone to this radio drama won Terry over. So that evening they sat in the dining room – well, Terry crawled under the dining-room table – to listen to the first performance of Dylan Thomas's *Under Milk Wood*, narrated by Richard Burton. 'A Play for Voices', as it was billed in the *Radio Times*, was first heard on the BBC Third Programme, on 25 January 1954. One can imagine the young Terry, just a week shy of his twelfth birthday, held enraptured on that Monday evening, although he admitted that he didn't think he'd realised at the time what a tremendous influence Dylan Thomas was going to have on him and on his whole attitude to poetry. Terry was by turns inspired and dispirited, reasoning: 'How could I ever write stuff as magical as he had?' He did though. And would see his poetry published. Magical, and, yes, with more jokes.

Moreover, Terry received encouragement in his poetical aspirations from his teachers at Esher Church of England Primary School. Indeed, despite the slight embarrassment that his headmistress was called Miss Terry, which did lead to some teasing from his peers, Terry remembered with fondness that: 'my primary school really took an interest in my poetry. That was all I needed. A nod of approval, and I was away.' In fact, Terry was showing an aptitude for schoolwork in general, even if his parents might have preferred his autobiographical essays to be a little less revealing about the state of his father's underclothes. He seemed to take the 11-plus grammar school entrance exam in his stride, although he thought he had failed because he didn't get into his first choice: King's College School, Wimbledon. That was a public school and his parents and teachers had been hoping Terry would win a scholarship there, but he didn't. So he found himself going to the Royal Grammar School, Guildford.

At school he was exceptional at everything, academic and sporting. He was captain of the rugby team. He was captain of boxing. He won a prize for shooting. He was skilled at archery and he found a talent for gymnastics. A supple body and fearless mind saw Terry perform backflips and somersaults with alacrity. Unsurprisingly, Terry soon found himself head boy. But his burning ambition was undimmed by academic success and educational prowess – Terry still really wanted to write, but in those days that wasn't at all the sort of thing a grammar school could encourage. He missed the days of primary school. There they had an active interest in his poetry, but at the grammar school they took the very negative and discouraging attitude that you can't ever make a living out of writing. Rather than that lovely nod of approval, his teachers simply said: 'It can't be done, so stop thinking about it. The best you can hope for is to become a teacher!' However, there was one master, Mr Martin, who did encourage Terry. He used to read Terry's essays out to the class, and that really boosted the pupil's confidence. Mr Martin gave Terry a feeling that somebody appreciated the kind of things he was writing, but otherwise he had a restrictive impression that grammar school was like being fitted out with a straitjacket. It certainly fitted Terry and he could see it was very practical, but, with the best will in the world, you couldn't expect to do anything in it. Certainly Terry couldn't, at any rate.

It is tempting to see this top performance at school as the display of a brilliant scholar but, really, it was more a distraction against the circumstances that had moved him out of Wales. His mum was forever reluctant to even consider moving back, despite Terry's clear unhappiness, particularly after the death of La-La in 1952. A hard-working housewife, Dilys herself was very ill for a long time, and prone to phantom heart attacks and breakdowns. So Terry's record at school is all the more remarkable when one considers that he was forced to miss a lot of education in order to care for her. Alick was out, working at the bank. Brother Nigel proved reticent. Still, those four years without a father present; those schooldays of looking after his sick mother; those magical shared memories of Colwyn Bay. All of it engrained a tight closeness between Dilys and her youngest son.

Nevertheless, Terry's ambitions became geared to just one thing: to get away from Surrey. As solace against this frustration he turned to comedy and, crucially, comedy he created himself. He would make his own stop-motion home movies in and around the Jones abode. These, the first films Terry directed, were short and silly and often brought his mother's precious furniture to life. Mucking about with a camera didn't quite keep him sane but it gave him a purpose. Something to do when he pined for Colwyn Bay. This drive and motivation and talent was all channelled as a means to achieve his ends. Whether his parents approved or not was irrelevant.

Terry loved his mother deeply; his father he found rather stiff and awkward, but he would always remain a loyal son. Even when he had moved on and was reluctant to leave Oxford or south London, he would jump into his clapped-out motor car and drive back for a visit to the place he had been so keen to get away from. The vehicle would invariably break down en route to Claygate and again on the way back home, but he would always, always make time for his mum.

# CHAPTER TWO

## OXFORD

*If I had never gone to Oxford I wouldn't have met either
Mike Palin or Geoffrey Chaucer! And without those two,
the rest of my life would have been very different indeed.*

I F Colwyn Bay gave Terry his identity and Claygate gave him a
chip on his shoulder, then Oxford made him the man he was
destined to be. Often, over a pint and a packet of pork scratchings,
Terry would recall his time in 'that sweet city with her dreaming
spires'. Even though the spires were a little grimy in Terry's day, his
eye for beauty took in the sweep of Oxford's architecture and his
heart beat faster to the pulse of excitement in discovery and cerebral gathering. When, as he often did, Terry would admit to
himself and me that he never felt he was particularly funny, I
would joke that perhaps he would have been happier if his life had
taken a more academic turn. He could have stayed in Oxford and
become a respected don, with plush, book-lined rooms in college,
and an eternal, circular existence of learned lectures and fulsome
feasts. Sharing knowledge with keen students and dining on fine
food in the hall every night would be very Terry. At this thought,
Terry's brow would crease slightly. He could see that. It was a life
that appealed. For the briefest of moments. Then he would snatch
up his beer, take a big gulp, and say: 'No, no, no. I wouldn't change
a thing. I've had the loveliest, most lucky of lives.'

Lucky or not, it cannot be doubted that without the Oxford
experience all that loveliness would never have happened. Terry

knew that. Terry also knew that this vital step in his life and in his education was not a foregone conclusion at all. He applied to Oxford and Cambridge and by a stroke of good luck that, at the time, he took as bad luck, he was eventually offered places at both universities. This was not only slightly annoying, it was also a total shock. Indeed, Terry had done so badly at his A levels that none of the provincial universities would consider him. In his own defence, Terry explained that he had been in such a rush or such a haze or such a something that he didn't read the exam paper properly. He just wrote what he knew he could write about and not what he was asked to write about. Terry was convinced the only reason he got into university at all was that in those far-off days both Oxford and Cambridge were their own, self-contained oases of education with their own entrance exams and interviews. In passing these, he crept under the wire somehow, he felt.

Still, a talent to creep under the wire at both Oxford and Cambridge was no mean feat. Terry decided that he really wanted to study modern poetry at Cambridge. Looking back, he didn't think he would have joined the Cambridge Footlights there. It sounded far too organised for his liking. Certainly, that avenue in which to perform wasn't the reason for his favouring Cambridge. It was simply that the university and the modern poetry course had captured his imagination, harking back to his early passion for Tennyson and Dylan Thomas. But he initially heard nothing from that venerable institution, while St Edmund Hall, Oxford, offered him a place to read English. He accepted rather reluctantly, out of sheer desperation. The fates were being playful that week though. A few days after opting for the opportunity at Oxford, Terry received notification from Gonville & Caius, in Cambridge. The college had put his name on the waiting list and had now decided to offer him a place. The Royal Grammar School firmly told him that, having accepted the Oxford offer, he could not go back on his word. They said that it would put them in bad favour with Oxford, and that would never do. As far as he remembered he put up absolutely no fight at all. That was that. With a philosophical shrug of acceptance, Terry reasoned, 'What do I know about it?' He thought he wanted to go to Cambridge. He *did* want to go to Cambridge, but who really knows what they want to do at that age? So, Oxford it was. It was educational bureaucracy and 'good form' that sealed Terry's future. Lucky, really. If Cambridge had been in touch a week earlier his entire life would have changed.

Terry was reading English. Typically, he dismissed this as 'tantamount to reading nothing, really'. St Edmund Hall College, Oxford, or Teddy Hall, as everybody knew it, had taken its name from Edmund Rich, St Edmund of Abingdon, a devout and decidedly dull sort who, having studied and taught in Paris, returned to Oxford, at the close of the twelfth century, as administrator, priest and, eventually, Archbishop of Canterbury. Despite being one of the oldest educational institutions in the city, St Edmund had only been made a college of the university in 1957, four years before Terry's arrival in 1961. A relatively small and thus intimate place, with just over two hundred undergraduates in residence at one time, it was a historic place too, with a minute chapel, a dining room – in use for evening meals since the late 1600s – and the even older occupants of the St-Peter-in-the-East graveyard as immediate neighbours.

Despite this attractive combination of the ancient and the fresh, and the fact notwithstanding that, had he been just a year older, he would have been called up for national service (the horror of an 18-month conscription for 17–21-year-old-men was abolished in 1960), Terry was initially unenthusiastic about Oxford. He went up ready to be intimidated by everything and everybody. He expected everyone to be incredibly clever and incredibly highfalutin. And, sure enough, on arrival Terry felt rather overwhelmed. His son, Bill, recalls his dad reflecting upon 'turning up at Oxford with full impostor syndrome. He really didn't think he should be there. He was from a working-class family, and this place was full of people from the upper classes. In particular, he was really scared of this one guy who had a beard and smoked a pipe. He seemed so intelligent and every time Dad saw him he was standing, pondering and smoking and stroking his beard, looking like he was about to drop some wonderful pearls of wisdom. Then one day, this guy shaved his beard off, and Dad was like: "Oh, he's no more intelligent than me. He's no different to me really!"'

The other thing that really struck Terry was the sheer, unbridled ambition of his fellow students. They all seemed so determined to succeed. He had never met a bunch of people who were so single-mindedly competitive. Terry was pretty competitive too, though. After all, he had been school captain, captain of the rugby team, captain of boxing. The men-only St Edmund Hall was a bit more renowned for its students' sporting prowess than their academic prowess and would have looked favourably on Terry's athletic achievements. Even today, tournament triumphs remain chalked up upon the walls, invariably joined by the chough, the black bird with fire-bright legs and beak that is the college's emblem. And yet, despite his early ambivalence, which lasted most of his first year, when he vaguely and unenthusiastically thought his future career may be teaching, St Edmund Hall, and the University of Oxford, would go on to shape Terry's views, doubts and opinions about everything, not least himself.

Uniquely, at the time St Edmund had not one but three dons. These three wise men would shape Terry too. Immeasurably. Graham Midgley, an affable Yorkshireman, brought wit and wonder to his lectures. His most popular was 'Minor Poets of the 18th Century', with its follow-up '18th-Century Poets More Minor Still!' Bruce Mitchell, an ebullient Australian, was the language expert, as well as the doyen of Anglo-Saxon literature. Reggie Alton, by contrast, published very little, but had a vast knowledge of nineteenth-century watercolours and Elizabethan handwriting.

He had also served with distinction during the Second World War and was brilliant at cricket. Terry loved him. Indeed, this excellent 'English Trifecta' appealed to Terry enormously and, through this, moulded his linguistic understanding – and no doubt, inadvertently, his comic dexterity.

One of Terry's contemporaries at Oxford, who became a lifelong friend, was Annabel Leventon. Annabel was reading English too, albeit at St Anne's, one of the five women's colleges, but she and Terry would go to lectures together. Annabel says that her memories of her first year at Oxford are 'all a bit vague', yet she remembers with crystal clarity that there was definitely something about Terry. A quiet, brooding something. He was cool, though without really knowing it, which just made him all the more cool. Annabel also remembers Terry as being very attractive. They would see each other around Oxford and discuss their reading lists, though it wasn't until their second term that their friendship bloomed.

Oxford was putting on a drama festival for one-act plays. Despite a love of theatre and an interest in acting, Annabel didn't even dare to go and watch performances, because she felt so terrified she wouldn't pass her first-year exams: the dreaded 'preliminaries', sat at the end of the second term (known within the college as the Hilary term). Terry, however, couldn't resist getting involved straight away – exams or not. Annabel believes he had an insatiable passion for performing: 'Terry jumped in with the theatre stuff right away. And he was recognised pretty quickly as the brilliant talent he was.' Terry might have been expecting to go into something like teaching, but it seems that he had not completely stopped 'hopping' to be an actor.

Terry's school hadn't had a drama society – the boys' grammar was too keen on cadet corps and shooting teams and things. So the opportunity for extracurricular thespianism was both new and enthusiastically seized – degree be damned. In the spring of 1962, once those second-term exams were behind them, Terry and

Annabel joined the drama workshop run by Texas-born Michael Rudman, who was also at Teddy Hall, reading English, and president of the Oxford University Dramatic Society. Under Rudman's direction, Oxford had already been presenting major plays to national acclaim, and places within his workshop groups were hotly competed for. Terry and Annabel were soon learning to improvise and finding out about Stanislavski. It was utterly thrilling for them – now this, Terry thought, was an education! Then, the following term, under the auspices of the John Oldham Society of Teddy Hall, Michael Rudman staged a production of *A Month in the Country* by Ivan Turgenev. A Russian writer, working in France in the 1850s, Turgenev pre-dates Chekov and developed the intimate, domestic style of theatre that his more famous successor became revered for. Terry was fascinated by him. Annabel was given the part of Vera, the seventeen-year-old ward who is being married off to an elderly peasant landowner – played by Terry.

'He was very brilliant,' recalls Annabel fondly. Terry provided his own padding – a few clothes stuffed up his jumper alongside the natural padding of his student days. On stage, hot and sweating, he would mop his brow with his handkerchief a lot. He would 'harrumph' a lot too. Terry was prone to doing this anyway, already tending to get a little irritated if things weren't done his way, and he utilised this on stage, which was perfect for the part. Seeing as he had just turned twenty, this was a display of extraordinary character acting. Terry was wonderful and he, and the production, got phenomenal reviews.

Such great reviews, indeed, that Terry came to the attention of Frank Hauser, who ran the Playhouse, situated on Beaumont Street, one of two proper theatres in Oxford, the other being the New Theatre. Twice or thrice a term, Hauser would encourage the students of the Experimental Theatre Club to take the Playhouse for a limited run of two weeks and put on a show. The club was founded by Chaucerian scholar Nevill Coghill, in 1936, as an alternative to the Oxford University Dramatic Society. Its members called themselves the Etceteras, after its initials. But the very name wallows in the knowledge of being an addition to the main event – something frivolous, almost something taken for granted, in which the audience could perhaps fill in the gaps themselves.

This Playhouse run was a living, breathing and, above all, professional opportunity for Oxford students to experience proper theatre. As with his poetry at primary school, Terry swelled as a result of this encouragement and freedom. Indeed, Hauser had heard such good things about *A Month in the Country* that he invited Rudman to stage the production, as part of the professional company at the Playhouse, in the summer term of Terry's first year, from Thursday through to Saturday, 14 to 16 June: 'a unique event,' believes Annabel Leventon.

On returning to Oxford for the start of their second year, Terry and Annabel were cast in Rudman's production of *The Good Person of Setzuan*, a gender-non-specific retitling of Bertolt Brecht's original play, first staged in 1943 and presented in English translation, in 1953, as *The Good Woman of Setzuan*. In the 1962 production Annabel was cast as the Good Woman, with Terry as one of the play's three gods. These gods would descend from the heavens and land in Setzuan in search of the good woman of the title, to whom they gifted a lot of cash as a test to see if she could remain good while also being fabulously wealthy. The other gods were played by Doug Fisher (who would go on to have an acting career, being best-loved now as Larry in the Thames Television sitcom *Man About the House*) and Joe Durant-Smith (who later became a renowned documentary film-maker). Terry was, by Annabel's account, dark and wonderful in the role. She gleefully remembers the three gods as collectively one of the most joyous things she was ever on a stage with.

Terry clearly impressed Doug Fisher. Another pivotal figure in his Oxford days, and beyond, was Ian Davidson – who had also been in *The Good Person of Setzuan*, playing the role of the water seller. Doug and Ian were the leading lights of Oxford drama, a year ahead of Terry, and were pulling together the theatre revue for their final year. Ian Davidson, as well as starring, was writing, producing and directing the show, and, rather against tradition, invited Terry to take part. The show was, rather provocatively, called ****. That's four asterisks. Serving as both a potential four-star review and a redacted four-letter word. As Annabel remembers, the fact that Ian was so impressed with Terry said a lot. Terry's acting and comic delivery were considered so brilliant that the performing group of the year above embraced him. He was allowed to do comedy with the 'Big Boys'! It was a huge honour. (Terry would never forget Ian's confidence in him and would go on to give him several supporting roles within Monty Python on television.)

Performed under the auspices of the Oxford Theatre Group, **** was written by, along with Ian Davidson, Jane Brayshaw, Doug Fisher, Robin Grove-White and Paul McDowell. It was more satirical than silly, more *Beyond the Fringe* than Monty Python. There was even a pastiche of the outgoing prime minister Harold Macmillan, who, rocked by the Profumo scandal, and claiming ill health, would resign in October 1963.

Terry's real break came with the departure of McDowell, who accepted an offer to join The Temperance Seven, a successful novelty pop combo who specialised in the 1920s sound, and whose single 'You're Driving Me Crazy' had reached number one in the British hit parade in May 1961. And so McDowell became a full-time pop star (although those heights were never reached again) and Ian Davidson recruited Terry to write and, most importantly of all, perform in the revue for the Edinburgh Festival Fringe of August 1963.

And so it was that Terry, already noted as a superb mime and an able mimic, brought his brooding intensity and elegantly scruffy affability to play in Edinburgh for the first time, performing nightly at 10 p.m. at the Cranston Street Hall from 20 August through to 7 September 1963. Although satire was still the spearhead of the comedy, including an attack on Labour Members of Parliament accepting life peerages, the revue was tweaked and tailored towards the Fringe audience – there was, for example, a skit on how the Edinburgh Tattoo was created – while silliness in everyday life was addressed in a conversational sketch around scoring a tennis match. There were, too, undoubtedly foreshadows of Terry's future. He donned women's clothes on stage for the first time, in order to poke fun at middle-Englander Tory voters; while, the tight, proper Fringe hour also included a light-hearted documentary section on what a modern English Civil War would be like. Very Terry, that. A sketch called 'You Too Can Be the Life of the Party' was an early version of the kind of thing Terry would write for *The Frost Report* and, subsequently, *The Two Ronnies*. The *Glasgow Herald* praised the 'visual knockabout [that] makes a memorable hour' and said that the five performers 'are all quite brilliant in this effervescent nocturnal whoop-up'. Well, quite.

Terry was twenty-one and performing at what was essentially a playground for young and talented artistes, a showcase in which to be discovered. **** was the primeval quagmire for the next generation of comedy. It was also very, very funny. So hilarious that, off the back of the Fringe, **** was picked up for a two-week stint at the Phoenix, in London's glittering West End, which was packed out every night with an audience receptive to the group's satire and silliness.

Their laughter was a drug. Terry had found his passion for comedy and, as with everything, he took to the art with dedication and perception: 'comedy is a dangerous business,' he would say. He believed that if people find something funny you're OK. But the moment you do something that's meant to be funny and someone doesn't find it funny, they become angry. It's almost as if they resent the fact that you tried to make them laugh and failed. Terry felt that there was a unique kind of pressure put on the comic: nobody came out of a mediocre performance of *Hamlet* seething with rage because it didn't make them cry, he would argue, but you just have to listen to people coming out of a comedy that didn't make them laugh!

The reception of **** was no doubt a pivotal moment in Terry's life. But perhaps an even more important development still had come with the arrival of a nineteen-year-old chap from Sheffield by the name of Michael Edward Palin. This was a true light-the-blue-touchpaper moment and it was comedy love at first sight. Michael's first Oxford friendship was formed with Robert Hewison. They met on Michael's first day at Oxford. They got on straight away, mainly because they liked Sellers and Spike and all the Goon stuff.

In fact, the first time Michael saw Terry was on a theatre poster – for a production of Arthur Adamov's absurdist comedy *Professor Taranne*. The poster featured Terry in a huge coat with a cigarette hanging out of the corner of his mouth. He was crouched in the corner looking weird and cool, Michael recalls: 'Like an alien from another planet!'

Terry had been doing all that serious Turgenev and Brecht stuff. Michael admits: 'Terry was a brilliant actor, actually.' And he was 'a warm, open, and very honest critic.' Terry was of course a year older than Michael – quite a lot when you are that age. Terry was already a rather influential English student.

And the first time Terry saw Michael, he was in the audience for Mike's serious debut, as Petruchio in Shakespeare's *The Taming of the Shrew*. He felt Michael came across as very warm and very engaging on stage, though he would later guiltily admit to laughing heartily at Mike's performance. After the play, they met in person for the first time. Michael's pal, Robert Hewison, knew Nigel Walmsley, a contemporary of Terry's. The bridge between

Terry and Mike was completed. Michael remembers that Terry was wearing 'that coat!' The huge, hairy, checked coat he had been wearing on the poster for *Professor Taranne*. Once Michael got to know Terry, he soon discovered that he wore this coat everywhere. It was Terry's unique look and his trademark, although he was far too cool to think of it as such. This coat just seemed to be his wrapping. It kept all that Welsh intensity tight and vital.

But it was a love of comedy that kept on proving the cement of these friendships. Michael and Robert began doing a cabaret at the Oxford Union Cellars. Terry thought it was very funny, original stuff, and he particularly liked what Michael was doing. He felt Michael 'just seemed to have a gift'. In Terry's opinion, Hewison was rather alienating on stage, whereas Mike was simply loveable. Terry instinctively knew that it was this contrast between Palin and Hewison that gave them their on-stage chemistry. It was the very essence of the good double act. Whether Terry consciously had strong realistic ambitions to write and perform comedy for a living at this early stage is unlikely, but the Jones and Palin dynamic had been planted in his head.

The feeling was mutual and built on Michael's respect for Terry's talent: 'Terry was a very good actor. I don't think that's ever been credited as much as it should be.' Terry quickly became a good friend. An acting friend, really. Michael remembers Terry being a very impressive man, even aged twenty-one: 'His looks, first and foremost, were arresting. That mop of dark hair. Those dark, good looks he had.' Michael also echoes Annabel Leventon's sentiment that 'he was very good looking. And he was very brooding on stage. The audience couldn't take their eyes off him.' However, Michael could also see that Terry took it all very seriously. The acting wasn't a university lark for him. He was extremely dedicated in everything he did.

Terry, Michael and Annabel became great mates, a real unit of companionship and camaraderie. Together with a mutual friend,

Michael Wynn-Jones, Michael and Annabel began actively encouraging Terry to go into cabaret and feed that fledgling comedy performing bug. Not big things . . . but good things. High-profile – although it must be said it was only Oxford high-prolife. Big fishes in a little pond. But an important little pond nonetheless. And, most importantly, Terry Jones and Michael Palin had started writing material together.

Certainly, Terry's love of writing was overtaking his love of reading. His studies were pushed to an even more remote back burner when he became involved in what he called 'the student rag'. That was the *Isis*, the University of Oxford magazine that had been established in 1892. Terry would design the covers. He was a very good graphic designer, which Michael Palin sees as just another facet to this multifaceted man. Whatever the role, Michael saw that Terry was a real creative force: 'There was a real energy about Terry. A feeling that things would get done while he was around.'

In turn, Terry was inspired by the careful precision of Michael's comedy. A quality he had spotted immediately. It was often tediously dull in its detail, delivered ironically for comic effect, but delivered with such calm, and such schoolboy-like dedication to facts and figures. So earnest, in fact, that it was funny. Relentlessly funny. And relentlessly funny exactly describes the very first sketch Terry and Michael wrote together. To say it has had comedy legs is an understatement.

Then one day came a breakthrough – for both Terry and Michael personally as much as for the Experimental Theatre Club. It was an invitation from Chris Braden. The son of respected Canadian-born actors and broadcasters Barbara Kelly and Bernard Braden, Chris was producing the Oxford revue for the end of the summer term. The revue was entitled *Loitering with Intent* and was to be staged in a tent for dramatic irony and comical relevance. Chris drafted in Terry and Mike to rewrite a sketch that has become alternatively known as 'Slapstick', 'Comedy Lecture', 'The Custard Pie Sketch' or simply 'Hey, Vance!' Regardless of what you call it, it was the perfect first building block for what became the Jones and Palin style. The ultimate meta joke for the joker. The joke about joke-making. About the DNA of comedy itself. Indeed, it stemmed very much from that rather dull, detailed, monotonous lecturing style of Palin's that Terry had found so funny. The sketch was simple: a lecturer laboriously and, totally without humour, discusses and dissects various slapstick tropes while three students, in laboratory white coats, enact the classic physical comedy moments: from whacks with a plank of wood to the best way to deliver and receive a custard pie to the face, to the groin, to anywhere!

It was the makings of something special, as later it would be embraced by Python, the root of that comedy tree, performed, and witnessed by millions, at the Hollywood Bowl in 1982. After its success in *Loitering with Intent*, the sketch, the ultimate deconstruction of humour, was happily passed round like the latest hit song. Everybody was doing it. Including Terry, alongside Doug Fisher and Ian Davidson; and Graham Chapman and John Cleese, who had struck a deal in order to perform it in the *Cambridge Circus* show Edinburgh Festival Fringe presentation for 1963. It would be reworked and resurrected at Oxford for years afterwards. A fellow student and friend, David Wood, would perform it, several times, in later Oxford revues and in Oxford cabaret, well after Terry had left the university. It was a perennial for quite a few years.

David Wood was instrumental in Terry's last and arguably greatest straight role on stage. While the Etceteras and Oxford Theatre mob had been playing it for laughs, concurrently directors Braham Murray and David Wright were pulling together their socially conscious piece *Hang Down Your Head and Die*, or 'Oh, What a Lovely Hanging!', as more than one journalist put it. Indeed, the shade of Joan Littlewood loomed large over the basic premise – *Oh! What a Lovely War* had first been performed in

London in March 1963. *Hang Down Your Head and Die* was a serious, immersive theatrical experience piece on the inhumanity of capital punishment, wrapped up in a brightly coloured circus presentation, with clowns and acrobats. At its core, it was a piece about injustice. Something that meant and would always mean a great deal to Terry.

Annabel Leventon was on the committee for the show, and it was the Oxford breakthrough of David Wood, who penned several original songs and won critical plaudits as the principal clown. For David, though, this was the one where he really got to work with Terry. Terry was in his third year and David in his first year. There was an unwritten rule at Oxford that third-year students weren't really supposed to be taking on plays. But Terry ignored that.

Terry would often, modestly, remember the show as something that was 'basically just me droning on!' Although it would prove a landmark in his career and a source of fond memory for many decades afterwards, Terry was not initially convinced about the project. A week before they were supposed to be doing the dress rehearsal, it was still so cumbersome that Robert Hewison, Michael and Terry stayed up late in someone's room going through the script, desperately trying to put some shape on to the show. Terry's concern would have been compounded because he was playing the condemned man, the character at the very centre of it. Hewison and Palin were safely out of the glare of the limelight, playing lots of supporting characters including, as Terry remembered, 'a couple of policemen who came in and took me away at the end'. Although it was an ensemble piece, nobody could deny that Terry was pretty much the star of it. *Hang Down Your Head* was a showcase for Terry at his most dramatic – as a brilliant mime. His handyman, a general dogsbody figure, was a clown, in white face, whose expression hardly changed. Every emotion was told through body movement.

David Wood explained that Terry played his role perfectly straight, feeling that the best comedians – in the widest possible sense – were often the best actors. People like Max Wall and Jimmy Jewel – and David would bracket Terry with those great talents. Critics too were queuing up to praise the production in general and Terry in particular, with Don Chapman in the *Oxford Mail* of 12 February 1964 picking out:

the white-faced auguste, an exquisite mime in the form of Terry Jones, who is destined to play the part of the victim and to be carried screaming to the gallows as the rest of the company belt breezily down to the footlights to take their final bow. It is this figure . . . which gives the evening its dramatic unity.

The rather more hip reviewer for *Cherwell*, the Oxford University newspaper, opined that:

the quiet authority and graceful talent of Terry Jones gives the show a core of sympathy that no audience can fail to dig.

Regardless of the plaudits ladled upon him from college cohorts and distinguished press alike, Terry was acutely aware of his own perceived limitations as a singer. He made a positive out of his passionate renewed commitment to the piece, enriching his performance of the number 'I'll Have Gas' with an earnestness and a gravitas that, by all accounts, left audiences spellbound. It was truly a show-stopping moment. Written by David Wood as a sort of blues-rock pastiche on the theme of the various methods a convicted criminal could be put to death, the lyrics are powerful indeed. Even more so with a thumping anthem behind: '*When I was first convicted on a gloomy, faithful day . . . the judge he said to me, "have you anything to say . . .?" Give me gas!*' Terry did it full out; he wasn't the greatest singer in the world and he would always admit that, but he was passionate and vivid.

David Wood noticed that, by this point, it was clear that Terry and Michael were forming a double act, certainly in terms of writing, but also in terms of performing. It was during *Hang* that 'Mike and Terry really started', David thought. When they'd thought that things weren't going quite right with the play, they'd worked together to fix the problems. The programme for the West End run would credit them with writing 'additional material' for the production. This was crucial in their development as a writing team. Not least because *Hang* wasn't just funny songs and sketches – it was a proper theatre piece, with a message. The interest in long narrative storytelling would niggle at the edges of their three-minute bursts of comedy business for a decade.

The show's West End transfer, to the Comedy Theatre, lasted for six weeks. It was an extraordinary success. Cambridge student Eric Idle saw it and was greatly impressed. The topic of hanging was a powerful one. As Eric jokes: 'there was a lot of it about!'; and it knowingly and concisely splits the difference between the universities' senses of humour: 'Oxford took it seriously. Cambridge would have sent it up!' Bernard Levin's glowing critique of *Hang* basically said that these *'young people do honour to the theatre and themselves'*.

The show also helped change – perhaps by just a little bit – the legal system in Great Britain. In August 1964, the House of Commons passed a decree for a five-year trial period in which committed criminals would not hang. Just months after *Hang*. This issue was obviously in the air when they chose the subject, and all involved were anti-capital punishment, of course. However, at the same time they were all people interested in being on stage doing a show rather than saying, '*We are waving a banner for a cause.*' Still, the many theatregoers who saw *Hang Down Your Head*, and were particularly moved by Terry's performance, wouldn't have been able to help thinking about the issue. It is often the way that people will listen to and take heed of how they are made to feel by, say, a theatre revue rather than a politician pontificating in the House of Commons.

In the audience for a performance of *Hang Down Your Head and Die* at the newly reopened Oxford Playhouse was a botany student by the name of Alison Telfer. She had arrived at Oxford as a fresher in 1963 and thus her time at the university overlapped with Terry's by just one year. Alison didn't get involved with the drama groups at Oxford, but she adored theatre.

Alison says that she was gobsmacked by the play. She thought all the actors in it were absolutely marvellous. Particularly Terry. Somehow, she ended up backstage after the performance, but she didn't meet Terry. It was to prove just one of a few sliding-doors moments in their lives, one that was to set the tone for the next couple of years.

Theatre obviously meant a great deal to Terry too. It was an oft-returned-to topic of conversation. Indeed, as well as his own room at Oxford and those of his chums, Terry discovered another place to debate and discuss: the pub. The British pub would quickly become God's gift to Terry, if one believes in such generosity, and of course Michael Palin was there with him. Despite spending so much time in the pub they didn't actually do a lot of drinking while at Oxford, although as Michael cheekily recalls, 'We made up for it post-Oxford, I can tell you!' The Oxford pub conversation would always be about theatre. Terry was always very enthused, very fizzy about trying new things. The conversation often centred around ideas for the future – not pie-in-the sky student fantasy, though. It was more practical stuff like: 'Can we hire this hall?', and 'Maybe we could do a show there?' Politics came into the discussion a bit, those who were there remember, but mainly it was show business.

Michael Palin and his first Oxford friend, Robert Hewison, would also join Terry on cabaret tours during college breaks. One such tour took in Devon and Cornwall. There was the gang, with silly props and high hopes, careering round the West Country in a little van. Michael recalls one particular booking, a three-night residency at a hotel in Newquay: 'We were shown our stage – in the grill room restaurant. The stage wasn't much and the food was even worse. And the audience! Two or three courting couples who were there to hold hands and gaze at each other lovingly and, suddenly, the romantic moment was broken by one of the management shouting: '. . . and now it's comedy time! Direct from Oxford University . . .' and we would go on and do some sketches about the financial system at our colleges or something. I can just remember looking at this poor audience and thinking, "They don't want to sit through this . . ."'

At the end of a third year that saw Terry take the West End, if not the West Country, by storm, he returned to Oxford to earn his degree in English language and English literature. After nine three-hour exams, he became a Bachelor of Arts with Honours. And, although his love of words and, in particular, his love of Geoffrey Chaucer's literary ability to make the Middle Ages live for him, would burn bright, it was still those show business dreams he spent hours down the pub talking about. That was by now his true vocation. Having tasted West End success and proved himself as an actor with serious integrity, it was back to Oxford for his third and final year. And one last Oxford revue. This was *the* Oxford revue. Simply and unforgettably called *The Oxford Revue*.

# CHAPTER THREE

## FROST OVER THE FRINGE

*The shops are full of cobweb pies. The buses
have bad feet. They've Homes For Eaten
Sandwiches, Dead-ends to every street.*

THERE was to be another near-miss, almost-meet-cute moment for Alison Telfer and Terry at the Lady Margaret Hall Summer Ball. *The Oxford Revue* was scheduled to be the entertainment at the event, with Annabel Leventon and the Four Beats singing the songs, including 'A Newspaper Sky', which Annabel had written for herself, and Terry and the boys doing the sketches.

It was summer of 1964, still Alison's first year at Oxford. She was at the ball with a date, who had bought a bottle of champagne, which they drank in her room before the ball got going. To Alison, the occasion felt all terribly proper. She remembers she was wearing a sort of off-pink dress, with flowers all over it, and laughs now that it was 'the most hideous dress! Really awful.' Unfortunately, she hadn't eaten anything since lunchtime, and it was common at these Oxford balls to get food at about one o'clock in the morning . . . so, naturally, she consumed a plateful of food after half a bottle of champagne. Following the meal, the cabaret in the hall commenced. Alison went into this hall, with its raised dais, and seated herself on the floor next to the gentleman she was attending with. During the cabaret, she began to feel unwell, really unwell. All of a sudden she knew what was about to happen.

She was violently sick. She recalls now: 'Thank heavens I didn't like the dress.'

At the time, of course, Alison was mortified. Her gentleman companion, being slightly older and, as she says, 'probably more used to dealing with drunks', hustled her out of the hall. He managed to get her back to her room and, when she woke up the next morning, 'he had somehow managed to get the dress off me and put me to bed!' She still had to deal with the dress, though, and the shame of having to get it dry-cleaned.

Fifteen years later, by which point she was married to Terry, Alison finally decided to confess to him that it had been her causing a disturbance during his performance at the ball. 'Yeah! I remember that', he said. 'There I was doing this cabaret and suddenly there was this awful sound and this awful smell!' That was the first time Terry was aware of Alison – as some poor misfortunate, vomiting while he was on stage. If he had been distracted enough to break the fourth wall of performance, he would not have seen a huge Pythonesque finger with a neon sign reading 'One Day You Will Marry This Girl!', but he would have seen his future wife, in a dress covered in her own sick, being carried out of the room . . . as he persevered with the funny sketch he was performing.

And it was a good sketch too. Michael Palin asserts that: '*The Oxford Revue* was more bizarre, for sure. One had the feeling one was doing something new and slightly different. Completely different, you could say!' And as far as Terry was concerned *The Oxford Revue* was the production that really achieved something fresh, that was most like what he thought they should be doing. Critics were calling it '*zany*'. Suddenly, they were the new Marx Brothers . . . they were the new Goons . . . all impossible people to be compared to . . . but people Terry greatly admired and *wanted* to be compared to. Although the programme notes for *The Oxford Revue* screamed that '*Terry is merely 22*', he was certainly displaying sophistication in his structuring and pacing of a sketch. One of his favourites to perform was with Annabel Leventon, concerning a couple of would-be lovers who could only talk in clichés. 'But it was so touching', recalls Annabel. She was the young woman on a train and Terry was the nervous suitor on the platform, waiting for the train to leave and take her away from him. And they simply cannot speak to each other and express their real emotions. It was all:

'*Well, bye bye then. Don't do anything I wouldn't do!*'
'*No, if I can think of anything, I won't!*'

As Annabel recalls, it was: 'Classic Terry! It was just cliché after cliché after cliché, and so clever. Eventually, the train moved off, and they would be waving their hankies, and you just knew they were never going to get it together. It was a really lovely little sketch.'

Sketches like this had a sweetness and poignancy that stands in contrast to the rather more assured and cynical sketches by the Cambridge Footlights. It is interesting to compare the two styles. The Cambridge Footlights was well established – they had been going since the 1880s, and, certainly as far as Michael and Terry were concerned, since Peter Cook in the late Fifties the Footlights had been a recognised breeding ground for fresh comedy talent. Almost manufactured. A boy band of satire and silliness, if you will. But, to Michael at least, the Oxford comedy was more real, somehow. Everything 'just felt more organic at Oxford,' he said. For Terry too the Footlights felt very slick, like there was a formula. At Oxford, there was no organisation to speak of. How they decided who did the revue, Terry just didn't know, but he liked that. That sort of creative freedom for all worked for him. That Cambridge took the organisation of their comedy a little more rigidly was very indicative of the difference between the two universities. There seemed to be more stress about everything at Cambridge, and you can witness it in the comedy that emerged. The comedy of John Cleese and Graham Chapman is very uptight, very repressed; Terry and Michael just really enjoyed themselves.

By this point, Terry had already been privy to the alchemy of John Cleese. While Terry didn't meet John, he certainly saw him in Edinburgh, in 1963. The Oxford crew weren't doing matinees, so one Wednesday afternoon they had all gone off to inspect the opposition. Terry was a little miffed to see how well the Cambridge show was doing. It was packing them in, and Terry and co. were not. John came on stage. He loomed over the audience, being terribly funny as this stiff-upper-lipped Brit in India, slapping his neck all the time to kill the mosquitoes, and being frightfully awkward with his leading lady, Jo Kendall. There was something within that dynamic that was both funny and a little old-fash-ioned. Deliberately so. A pastiche of the passé. Whereas Terry's style was different. For example, that train station sketch with Annabel channelled a sense of awkwardness into a mini love story. It was a skit of unrequited love that was as touching as it was clever in its layering of cliché. As knowing a poke at the pedestrian prose of the past as the Cambridge lot, but a poke with a pillow.

By the summer of 1964, it was a foregone conclusion that *The Oxford Revue* was destined for the Edinburgh Festival Fringe. What was more, this would be Terry's last hurrah with the university company. And that inevitable transfer would indeed make everything different. The show they took comprised mainly silly songs, with the pairing of Terry with Michael Palin very much to the fore, although it was the individual numbers that seemed to stick in the memory. For Annabel Leventon, *The Oxford Revue* was a joy. Terry even wrote a song for her. A wonderful and ridic-ulous song. It was called 'Song About a Toad' and Terry wrote it for her simply because he thought she 'didn't have enough to do. They were fitting me in.' The song was gifted to Annabel. And it was so very Terry. A toad! A toad who belched. A toad who smelt.

A toad who picked his nose. The song was touched with the silly surrealism Terry would perpetuate throughout his comedy career.

Terry's stand-out song that he wrote for himself concerned a Miss World competition from long ago, which he would perform as a ragged old tramp, wistfully recalling his glory days when he had been crowned Miss World and was as 'proud as a peacock and as proud as the Queen!'

Terry also wrote the amusingly mournful lyrics to 'Forgive Me' – '*Forgive me for being such a crashing bore last night. Forgive me for doing all that on the floor last night!*' – which he gifted to Nigel Pegram for *The Oxford Revue*. There was a real sense of community and camaraderie among the Oxford students. 'Edinburgh was a joy,' remembered Nigel Pegram. It was an adventure. They all stayed at Roman Eagle Lodge, with its boys' floor and its girls' floor. Meals were a pound a week, supplemented by a team trip to a little café on the corner for a bacon bap for sixpence. Nigel Pegram gleefully recalls that: 'we used to go to the public baths once a week, where lurked women in white coats, very stern, amidst the smell of bleach! It sounds awful, but it was wonderful.'

For Michael Palin, the venue in which they performed *The Oxford Revue* was also rather disquieting. The space, within the Cranston Street Hall, 'was very small and very dark', and, when the cast were due to go on for their final curtain call, a required blackout made it seem even smaller and even darker. The Manfred Mann single *5-4-3-2-1* had been a pop sensation earlier in 1964, and inspired the team's comic reworking of it: *R-S-P-C-A*. So, in complete darkness: 'Terry, still with his guitar in hand from the *R-S-P-C-A* number, was halfway up this very steep staircase – our only access to the stage. Suddenly, from out of the darkness, I heard this loud discordant crash. All wood and strings. There was a brief silence and then Terry's high-pitched whine saying: "Oh no! I've broke my sodding guitar!"'

Edinburgh was certainly a bonding experience, and the revue under the direction of Doug Fisher got rave reviews and generated such a buzz that all twenty-two performances were sold out. That was 22 times 228 seats at up to 8/6d each! The most crucial 8/6d, if indeed he didn't grab a complimentary ticket, was from a certain David Frost. Seemingly, like Terry, David Frost had sensed the turning tide in comedy, from satire to silliness. David didn't just like what he saw, he loved it, and Terry was aware that this was a very big deal. The difference between doing a revue in Oxford and doing a revue in Edinburgh was that when you performed in Edinburgh, people noticed you. Really important people. An impressed David Frost would invariably go backstage and talk to the cast, gushingly, and then other people from London would take notice too. Terry got the feeling it was going in their direction. Frost, having seen the group, promised to remember them. And this was no fair-weather, showbiz flimflam.

A little over a year later, true to his word, David Frost got in touch. That was the defining moment. The moment when a career in comedy might, just might, be a possibility. Frost was impressed most of all with Terry and Mike, and with at least one pun-tastic exchange that would resonate from the days of *The Oxford Revue* through television exposure and into the bumper book of classic comedy quotes. For, within eighteen months, a throwaway gag greeting between policemen would go from the mouths of Jones and Palin and into the mouths of the Two Ronnies:

'*Morning Super.*'
'*Morning Wonderful!*'

This was deliciously silly comedy for silliness's sake. As the *Oxford Revue* team were quoted in the *Daily Mail*:

we are against attacking people. We want to build up something that is funny in itself. No satire, no mention of the prime minister. We want to avoid the idea of being clever young men in suits being witty.

The much-anticipated review from the *Scotsman* caught the spirit of the show completely:

> it is much more than a stimulant for culture-sated minds or a pleasant nightcap. It is proof that a new generation of satirists with fresh style is arising fast through the debris of mediocrity left in the wake of those now rather passé sub-culture symbols, Beyond the Fringe.

*Beyond the Fringe* alumni Peter Cook and Dudley Moore would argue the toss about that, with *Not Only . . . But Also* in the works for a television launch in the upcoming January, but even Pete and Dud's comedy was veering away from political point-scoring and onto that silliness for silliness's sake style. The contents of *The Oxford Revue* could and would have a laughter life for decades to come. Not contemporary, simply comic.

It was also pure theatre. In one Jones and Palin item, Michael, playing a seedy entertainer, came onto the stage and started to sing a terrible song. In the middle of the song he would suddenly become conscious of a cardboard box on the side of the stage. Stopping his song to take a look at it, he presumes it is a present from the audience. Palin would turn to the crowd, smile and thank them profusely. He would put the box in the wings and go on with the song. At that moment there would be a huge explosion as bits of shattered box would fly across the stage. End of sketch.

The whole sixty minutes of *The Oxford Revue* had a fevered Spike Milligan madness about it too, with 'Last One Home's a Custard (or, Six Characters in Search of a Song)', 'Song of British Nosh', which hilariously contrasted bland, home-approved snacks with the distrusted but delicious foods of foreign countries, and

'I've Invented a Long-Range Telescope' adding fuel to the sing-song insanity. The Pythonesque pokes at authority were there in embryonic form too, with crazed British eccentrics and lunatics to the fore in the songs and sketches.

Further Cambridge influence on The Oxford Pythons was added to the mix when Terry once again went along to check out the opposition. And vice versa. Performing the *Cambridge Circus* sketches while the original cast were on tour in 1963, and back writing and performing *Stuff What Dreams Are Made Of*, in 1964, was Eric Idle. Cambridge and Oxford did an impromptu show – a 'Rejects Night'. This was performed immediately after the performance of the revue from Oxford, on the same stage with, as often as not, the same audience, but, as Eric explains, 'it wasn't a historic collaboration. Us Cambridge lot were in the audience. After their show they would do this extra show where they would read out sketches that nearly made it and invite comments from the audience.' There was no charge. They all sat round a big dustbin on the stage and got up and read out sketches that they hadn't finished or had rejected for some reason, carrying on as long as they got laughs. When the audience stopped laughing, they just crumpled the sketch up and threw it into the dustbin. For Eric Idle it was a pure form of comedy that was fresh and exciting: 'I rather liked it. I found it interesting. And we joined in, because we were in the audience, but we weren't collaborating, we were watching!'

Graeme Garden, also in the Cambridge show, was there with Eric watching too, and remembers the event as something more than a Reject Night: 'I seem to remember it being a kind of "Best of . . ." show. Maybe their rejects were that good! Anyway, I was very impressed with Terry. He was a jolly kind of fellow, and very, very funny!' Be it aborted ideas or the most popular material, it was as close as Oxford and Cambridge ever got to improvisation. After the show, the united Oxbridge comedians would discuss the discarded material, even the possibility of resurrecting the best bits and working on them. All, Eric and Michael included, maintained that of everyone involved, 'Terry was a stand-out'.

Terry's combined contribution of clever wordplay, silly songs and those mournful, slapstick comedian's facial expressions were qualities that were getting *The Oxford Revue* more and more notice. Often labelled *'this endearing quintet'*, that Oxford team did have an attitude of 'now' about them. Or, at the very least, a youthful difference that journalists eagerly picked up on. An opinion piece published in the *Scottish Daily Express* on 17 August 1964 yelled:

> Guitars, beat music and an attractive girl singer – it could be the latest Liverpool pop group, but, in fact, these rockers are playing strictly for laughs. Hoping to get to the top of the 'Festival Hit Parade' are the Oxford Theatre Group with their 13th Edinburgh Festival Revue.

It ran from 18 August to 5 September:

> The 27 numbers, too many to my mind, range from the good to the ineffectual, the best being the comic songs like the 'Song of British Nosh' and the girl's song about the toad she loved until it turned into a prince, and the worst being the satire of current American politics.

In an echo of many, boring commentators on the patchy quality of Monty Python to come, the *Scottish Daily Express* went on to state that:

> some numbers that begin well (*'Scotland Yard Investigates'*, *'The Great Clog'*) go on until we are tired of them. There are very funny numbers to begin and end with.

Under the heading 'Edinburgh Night-Life', further praise from reporter on the spot B.A. Young was reprinted in the *Financial Times*, thus giving *The Oxford Revue* national attention. It was unsurprising then that the group were offered a transfer to London. Although this was fast becoming the norm for the Oxbridge efforts, this year the Oxford comedians were to play an extended season at the near-legendary Establishment Club, on Greek Street in Soho. Perhaps that should be once-legendary, for by the summer of 1964 the intimate cabaret club established and owned by Peter Cook and Nicholas Luard had already lost its Swinging Sixties razzmatazz.

Terry was blunt when he looked back on the experience at the Establishment, stating that the place was 'horrible'. By that time it was just the front for a gambling place and was run by a fellow called Raymond Nash. Nash could only be described as a very dodgy character who, when he wasn't ostensibly running the Establishment, was allegedly running a gold-smuggling operation. The Gambling Den was on the first floor and they did two shows a night. Terry would recall that there was a croupier with this great scar down his face. He would sit in the front row and clap very loudly, then turn round to make sure that everyone else was clapping. This intimidating situation was hardly eased by the fact that Michael Palin could not honour the Establishment commitment. Dedication to his third-year university work meant his place was taken by David Walsh. Nigel Pegram too was out, having joined the company of *Wait a Minim*, at the Fortune Theatre, so *The Oxford Revue* was now a foursome. To be honest, they could have done with the extra man in more ways than one. The shows were so badly attended that most nights the cast outnumbered the audience – quite the come-down from the packed shows in Edinburgh.

Annabel Leventon also noted how the houses were a bit thin, but they had to stick it out. The flamboyant impresario Willie

47

Donaldson was the producer who took *The Oxford Revue* to the Establishment, and he added to the dodginess of the deal. 'We were all so naive,' says Annabel with a laugh (she was attending the London Academy of Music and Dramatic Art by then and so had to moonlight for the engagement under a different name, in the hope that her school wouldn't notice this transgression of the rules). It was clear none of them knew anything about the business at all. It's not certain if they even had contracts. They were just thrilled to be performing in the West End, until, as Annabel says, 'We found out how utterly shite the place was!'

Annabel was in the show for eight weeks: 'it just took them that long to find a replacement!' Terry would always maintain that they couldn't find anybody else who could perform the toad song as well, but Annabel, although flattered, succinctly explains that lots of people have performed it very well since. Terry was adamant though that without Annabel 'it just wasn't working!' Besides, it was only Terry and Doug Fisher left from the original line-up. It was the perfect excuse to wipe the dust of other people's gambling debts off his shoes.

However, Annabel Leventon would still find time, during her studies at LAMDA, to rejoin Terry and Doug for the occasional, quite lucrative cabaret spot. There was one they were doing somewhere down in Barnes. It was the Harrods Works Dinner cabaret! The three of them were in the taxi travelling there, and they were working out the running order for the show. It was all a bit rushed and, once they had agreed on the sketches and songs, Terry spotted a nasty little gap where somebody had to go off stage and couldn't get back in time to do the next number. Terry decided that Annabel would have to do . . . something, to smooth over the awkward break. Of course, it had to be Annabel to fill the gap! She enquired what she was going to do. Rather brilliantly, Terry wrote something for her, on the spot, in the taxi. Even without a pause, Terry just said the lines. And all these years later, Annabel can still remember that moment. Terry was so clever. Almost without thinking about it, he told her to go on stage and say:

*'The bus conductor with his cap. The dustman with his dustbin. They're naked underneath all that, Isn't it disgusting!'*

Being rather churlish at the time, Annabel retorted: 'Well, that's not very funny!' OK, so he had just made it up. On the spot. But Terry wasn't hurt. He wasn't bothered. Terry said: 'Just do it fast!' And that was it. She went out and did it – fast – and it got a huge laugh! It brought the house down, in fact! Hardly surprisingly then that Willie Donaldson still had Terry in his sights. Having missed out on the Establishment debacle, Michael Palin remembers Donaldson as: 'a very funny man. Very dry.' He was a witty Kensington and Chelsea sort of type. A posh chancer. He was the one who got *Beyond the Fringe* together – two from Oxford and two from Cambridge – and promptly, and foolishly, sold his share in the show just before the team became popular. As a result, he had this spurious reputation as the man who put *Beyond the Fringe* together and then lost it! For Donaldson, Terry was his next big opportunity to make a theatrical success, and he gave him some money to do a thing called *The Love Show*.

Willie Donaldson sold the piece to potential backers by explaining it would be a trendy satire on the sexual revolution, but, according to Michael Palin, Terry was writing it in such a way as to take it down a very different path indeed. Whereas *Hang Down* had been a topical theatrical piece about capital punishment, *The Love Show* was to be a modish comedy about sex through the ages, something that Terry was quite interested in. That's an understatement. Anyway, despite his huge interest in the subject matter, Terry called Michael, who had by that point just left Oxford, and said: 'Look, I'm finding it a bit difficult to write this on my own, could you help?' Michael wasn't sure what he wanted to do next and so he agreed to help Terry. Michael admits that helping Terry was 'not quite as simple as it sounds, because Terry always knew what he wanted'. Terry always really wanted Michael to be there to discuss it, rather than lead in what was actually being written. Terry was the driving force, without doubt. It wasn't that he was stumped and couldn't write, it was that he needed some more ideas for sketches, which he would then flesh out in his own style. The basic idea for *The Love Show* was Terry's. Although Michael was really a sounding board for his ideas, they did actually write some of the sketches together. During the writing process, in December 1964, Terry had joined the comedy repertory company performing at The Poor Millionaire, a theatre club in the West End. He had a part in *The Carrierbaggers*, a parody of *The Carpetbaggers*, the Harold Robbins Hollywood exposure novel, which had been turned into a film released that spring. Terry stuck with it for less than a month. He gratefully relinquished his place in the team in early January 1965, with Nigel Pegram taking over, and returned to writing *The Love Show*. However, *The Love Show* didn't set the West End alight as Willie Donaldson had hoped. In the end, after being performed in a West End pub, it came to a halt, though it earned Terry fifty quid. At least, one hopes the cheque for fifty pounds that Willie Donaldson wrote out during a boozy meeting in a Sloane Square public house didn't bounce from there to Notting Hill Gate.

Donaldson still believed that there was money to be made from these young Oxford graduates, however. Perhaps sending them to America would be the answer. On 23 January 1965, Terry, Michael Palin and Nigel Pegram were rounded up by Donaldson for an intense and liquid interview with Bernie Sahlins, who ran the Second City venue in Chicago. In the end, Donaldson's attempt to showcase a more polished presentation of those ramshackle but really rather liberating 'Reject Nights' from the Edinburgh Fringe featured just Nigel Pegram from *The Oxford Revue*. Billy Wallace was the only one from Cambridge. The show was called, a little glibly, *The Oxford and Cambridge Revue*.

The group did perform 'The Custard Pie Sketch', the deadpan dissection of slapstick originally written for *Loitering with Intent*, so Terry's work at least made it to the Windy City, even if he didn't. That summer it was performed in Nottingham too, in the revue *Changing Gear*, while in September Doug Fisher and Ian Davidson would reunite with some of Terry's work for *Anyone for England?* The sketch's originator, however, found himself back at his parents' house in Claygate, and in very desperate need of employment. He had no desire to stay in Surrey longer than he absolutely had to. With the brief but heartfelt endorsement from David Frost and safe in the knowledge that he could turn out a good joke at the drop of the proverbial hat, Terry applied to work for an organisation that was frantically hoovering up Oxford and Cambridge graduates with experience of the Fringe. The organisation would be the beacon and the bane of Terry's professional life: the British Broadcasting Corporation.

# CHAPTER FOUR

## INSIDE THE BRITISH BROADCASTING CORPORATION

*As soon as I got to the BBC I discovered it was very much an anarchic organisation with very little bureaucracy. That suited me down to the ground!*

TERRY, although gleeful and often rambunctious in his criticism of the corporation, was a BBC man through and through. I remember vividly, one March evening in 2012 – Friday the 16th, to be precise – walking in Highgate with Terry and his dog Nancy between the house and the pub, avoiding the huge, ancient trees that grow out of the pavement. As usual, Terry and I started by chatting about what we had been doing that day. Naturally, Terry had been writing. A few pints before dinner was his treat for a good day, and his balm for a bad day. I had attended the memorial service for David Croft: 'Oh, I hadn't heard about that,' lamented Terry, 'I would have come.' For, you see, Croft was a BBC man through and through too. Indeed, the corporation had footed the bill for the party. Terry had been in the shallow end of the BBC's pool of talent when Croft was directing Hugh Lloyd and Terry Scott in the comedy series *Hugh and I*, while Michael Mills had commissioned *Dad's Army* a mere year or so before giving Monty Python the green light. While being very different comedy crafts-men, from very different backgrounds, Terry and Croft were cut from the same, old-school BBC cloth. Those two old comrades had never really served together but were working towards the common goal, of cheering up themselves and, in turn, cheering up the nation. So, it was fitting that we raised a pint or two to the legacy of David Croft that evening.

And, unsurprisingly, our conversation drifted back to the BBC and Terry's rather incongruous, but exciting, early days there. Even in that short but nerve-wracking hinterland between Oxford and Wood Green, Terry had been commissioned to write a television play called *The Present*. Terry wrote it and was paid for it – the princely sum of £200 – but it was never made and never heard of again. Mind you, those 200 notes kept the wolf from the door while Terry weighed up his options. Those options all seemed to point to a career in television. Akin to that educational crossroads when Oxford had offered Terry a place, only for him to be tempted by a later, more desired place at Cambridge, Terry's entrance into the world of television was a further embarrassment of riches. This time, though, there was no authority figure pressuring him to do the right thing. With the experience, if not the exposure, of writing for Willie Donaldson, Terry now saw his future in show business. To that end he applied to various television companies. Lots of television companies. He was offered, and accepted, a job as a copywriter for Anglia Television. As soon as he had accepted that position, the BBC came knocking. And that offer from the BBC trumped all others. Typically, Terry was rather bemused by, not to say dismissive of, this break. He accepted the role of script editor, although he never fully understood why it had been offered to him. Most importantly, however, this offer had come from Frank Muir.

Long before becoming the bow-tie-wearing panellist and presenter, and the fruity singing voice of the classic Cadbury's chocolate advert, '*Everyone's a fruit and nut case*', Muir was a powerful mover and shaker within the portals of BBC Light Entertainment. With his writing partner Denis Norden, he had created the popular post-war Jimmy Edwards radio sketch show

*Take It From Here*, and had nurtured Alan Simpson and Ray Galton through the corporation. A nod from Frank Muir was weighty indeed. Moreover, Muir nurtured and championed Terry, who was plonked down in his own, tiny office. Well, a shared office. With two very small desks and two even smaller typewriters. The script editor position also came with the opportunity of graduating to a trainee writer and, as such, Terry was given full permission to wander round Television Centre, just observing shows in production, receiving training in camera equipment, and general encouragement to sit around and chat with other writers and write jokes. Muir told Terry this was all part of the job, all part of being employed by the BBC. The Corporation was the gold standard. Worldwide. If Terry just kept his mouth shut and his eyes and ears open, he would never be out of work again.

Michael Palin remembers being impressed by Terry's enrolment, even if his old Oxford chum was swift to downplay his position: 'It was rather thrilling really. Terry working at the BBC, in the script department, this thriving hub of comedy.' But Terry told Michael that he was doing very little except sitting in an office. He would write a few little jokes that were used, but to all intents and purposes the job involved looking at scripts that were sent in. Basically, he would sit at his desk and say: 'This is good!' and 'This is not good!' That was it, really.

The earliest surviving BBC contract for Terry comes from his representation at the time, Tom Parkinson, of Players & Writers Limited, at 71 Great Portland Street. In a correspondence dated 8 April 1965, Heather Dean, of the BBC Copyright Department, records that:

*I hear from Ned Sherrin that he asked Terry Jones to write a sketch entitled 'Gibraltar' at an approximate length of three minutes for inclusion in* Not So Much a Programme, More a Way of Life. *I suggest a fee of 20 guineas for this sketch.*

That was £21 in real money, and *Not So Much a Programme, More a Way of Life* was a thrice-weekly, late-night cutting-edge commentary on modern life in Britain. It was a little more controlled by the BBC in the immediate wake of David Frost's *That Was the Week That Was* being cancelled ahead of the 1964 general election, but, with satirists John Bird and John Fortune and variety comedian Roy Hudd in the cast, the show was still sardonic and relevant. Sometimes too sardonic and relevant for comfort at the BBC. Not that any discomfort would worry Terry overly. Despite writing again for Bird and Fortune and Hudd soon after, his association with *Not So Much a Programme . . .* would be short-lived. The edition including Terry's very first sketch for television was transmitted on BBC1 on Sunday 11 April 1965. It was the last *Not So Much a Programme . . .* of all.

Still, Terry was on the sainted system at the Beeb and working with a group of people who were really very good comedy writers. Long established. Not only people like Frank Muir and Denis Norden, but also John Law, who would co-write the classic 'Class' sketch, descending from upper class down to working class across John Cleese and the Two Ronnies. It was a good little group of writers, and Terry was very charming. Terry liked a drink and all that. That was very good too, because he fitted in. The BBC was still something like a gentlemen's club in those days. The officer classes and the foot soldiers. All lads together. Being paid in guineas not pounds. A guinea was a pound and five shillings . . . so a little more buck for your joke!

Professor Alan Ereira, a contemporary from Queens' College, Cambridge, and fellow BBC staff member, who would, much later, produce and direct Terry's history documentaries, goes even further: 'The BBC was absolutely a gentlemen's club, basically run by MI6!' It was all quite peculiar. Ereira felt he was always a little bit of an outsider, and believes Terry was too. They had this business of staff files that were regarded as 'suspect, shall we say'. The files of employees they were keeping an eye on had a little Christmas tree drawn on them. Someone once told Ereira that his file had a Christmas tree on it – 'That explained a lot!' Although Terry's files are free from seasonal firs, his loyalty to the corporation was often counterbalanced by the boredom of his position. He was content rather than happy at the BBC. He yearned for a good friend. And then, as always one year behind, following his graduation from Oxford, Michael Palin applied to join the corporation too. He was less successful. The BBC took an awful lot of graduates at that time, but Michael was turned down for a formal traineeship. At least Terry's earliest comedy champion, Ian Davidson, was there, having also secured a role.

Undeterred, Terry used his growing influence to get his Oxford chum in. Michael recalled how, at the time, he didn't have a job that he could tell his father about: 'My father didn't approve of my plan to go into show business, not thinking there was any money in it.' Michael admits now his father was right. At first. It was a pittance. Three guineas – a joke. But it was work. People liked Terry. They were charmed by him and trusted his judgement. So Terry asked Michael if he could come in to the BBC every now and then. Of course, it was an opportunity Michael grabbed. Together, Terry and Michael would write some amusing links for performers like Winifred Atwell, the pianist. Russ Conway and *his* piano. Kathy Kirby, the singer . . . All these variety turns. There was the Light Entertainment Department and within that was Variety, and that was where Terry and Michael were beavering away. The entertainment shows fronted by a singer, Des O'Connor and that ilk, were filmed in front of an audience and the hosts all had to have a bit of material, some witty banter, that they could do at the piano. A bit of patter to the camera like:

'*Oh . . . I'm off to Spain.*'
'*Costa Brava?*'
'*No, costa fiver!*'

And then go in to the song 'Granada' . . . To Michael, this was 'Terrible, really, but we thought of the guineas and wrote those links. I was a bit shame-faced about that one!'

Terry was equally shame-faced about a link they had to put into one of Russ Conway's many appearances on *Billy Cotton's Music Hall*. Russ Conway's big hit was called 'Side Saddle'. It was pretty much insisted upon that he play 'Side Saddle' every time he appeared, and it was insisted upon that they give Billy Cotton the joke along the lines of:

*'I don't care what position you play it in, what's the number called?'*

Russ would then, usually, make a joke of that old joke, saying:

*'That's not funny, and it wasn't funny last week either!'*

After spending a morning thinking up dialogue like that, Terry had come to the conclusion that he was getting pretty good at writing silly jokes.

Having gone from freelancer to staff writer, Terry was already happily recycling previous material. In the spring of 1966, he had submitted a two-minute sketch entitled 'Radio Rave' to producer Kenneth Carter, for *The Lance Percival Show*. The toothy satirist, brilliant at topical calypsos, was another refugee from *That Was the Week That Was*. Now in its second run, despite being referred to in official BBC correspondence as the 'Lance Percival Series', its chief writers were Lew Schwarz and ex-*Goon Show* scribe Maurice Wiltshire, with John Law overseeing all the allotted material.

In a memo suitably dated 1 April 1966, Heather Dean, in the BBC copyright department, confirmed with both Carter and Law that they should:

*Please buy a sketch Radio Rave written by Terry Jones which was included in the first programme of the series. Also Terry Jones has done a complete rewrite of the sketch Human Flight by Bryan Wright. The original sketch has already been paid for in full, but Terry Jones did an extensive rewrite leaving only about two lines of the original dialogue. Would you please negotiate a rewrite fee.*

*Please note that Radio Rave was written by Terry Jones before he became a staff member.*

Still, it was another toothy comic genius, Liverpudlian purveyor of Happiness Ken Dodd, for whom Terry wrote his first major television sketch. The previous year, 1965, had seen Doddy's nationwide breakthrough, with his hit single 'Tears' being the top-selling record and his residency at the London Palladium selling out for a record-breaking and eye-watering forty-two-week season. During this mammoth mirth-fest, Terry was even invited to meet with the great man at the London Palladium. The citadel of variety. The Palace of music hall. Terry was not of that world, of course. He was of Oxford and the BBC. Upon walking into the dressing room of the great Ken Dodd, Terry whistled merrily to himself. Dodd, with the traditions of the clown in his very blood, had a fit. And not a funny one either. Whistling in a theatre is extreme bad luck. It basically goes back to the days when most stagehands were veteran sailors, used to giving signals in whistle form because those could be heard during bad storms at sea. A whistle out of place in a theatre could result in a tonne-weight piece of stage scenery being hoisted or lowered right on top of an unsuspecting person. Even on top of Terry Jones! Ken Dodd insisted Terry leave the room, turn round three times to restore good luck, and then come back in again!

Despite this outrageous theatrical faux pas, Terry still got to write some television material for Doddy. Based upon an idea by Oxford contemporary and oft-times writing partner Miles Kington, it was the first of Terry's recognisable, great visual slap-stick scenes for the small screen. The skit was a kind of Sports Day for Policemen, with all the coppers, notably Dodd himself, in full uniform walking the running track in that clichéd, knee-bending *Dixon of Dock Green* manner. Evening All! When the BBC news round-up of 1965 related that it had indeed been the year Ken Dodd was crowned the King of Comedy, it was Terry's gloriously silly policeman sketch that illustrated the story. It was a good gag. A lasting gag. It could also have been Terry's last gag.

Terry's comedy idol Buster Keaton died of lung cancer, in Los Angeles, aged seventy, on Terry's twenty-fourth birthday, 1 February 1966. Terry wasn't fighting fit either in the spring of 1966, and his housemates at 138 Black Prince Road had become increasingly worried. (It's long gone now, comedy location spotters, so knock yourselves out trying to find the original site.)

Terry's BBC champion Frank Muir had continued to encourage him, urging him to accept a place on the well-respected directors' course within the corporation. Terry had had an interest in film-making since his stop-motion days at home in Claygate. As part of his BBC course he wrote and directed a five-minute short entitled *The Body*, centred around the misadventures of a dull and uninteresting chap. The film, also known as *The World of Charlie Legs*, was to have featured Michael Palin as the central, annoying character, trying to win the affections of the girl next door. It was an embryonic Reg Pither-type, who would eventually resurface in Monty Python's 'Cycling Tour' episode. However, Terry didn't finish the course, as he became seriously ill. The diagnosis was peritonitis. For those of you of a squeamish nature do look away now, for, in layman's terms, peritonitis is an abdominal swelling, usually caused by an infection, which can be very painful. Without treatment, the condition can prove fatal within days. This was serious stuff.

Laid up in St Thomas' Hospital on Westminster Bridge Road, on a Saturday morning, Terry waited and waited and waited. No medical attention was forthcoming. And then his appendix – the cause of all the trouble – burst. Although Terry's memory of what happened over the next few days was, understandably, a complete blank, he had undergone a life-saving operation. His next recollection was finding himself lying in bed and seeing a few of his housemates walking down the ward. He was a little surprised because he could see them but they didn't seem to be able to see him. When they finally spotted him, the look of shock and worry on all their faces was a source of shock and worry for Terry. He had lost so much weight in those few days that his friends hadn't recognised him. He was seriously ill, sewn back up, gaunt and hooked up to various tubes and wires to keep him going and siphon out the horrible stuff from his stomach. One of the most common side effects of peritonitis is weight loss and, indeed, Terry did lose that Welsh chubbiness of his youth. His weight would fluctuate throughout his life though. That Welsh chubbiness would come back and go again.

Concerned for his welfare, and dubious about the care he was receiving, his friends got him out of St Thomas' Hospital and safely home as soon as possible. Terry would have a lifelong reminder of his near-death experience in the form of a big, angry white line of a scar. Unsurprisingly for him, this weak spot could also make him laugh, as his daughter, Sally, recalls: 'Where the appendix had been removed was always very ticklish for Dad. If you wanted him to literally just drop to the floor in hysterics, you could do it just by tickling him there!'

Once fit enough, Terry resumed his BBC duties, hoping to continue his comedy writing output and tickle the funny bone of the viewing public. Still, he never did resume his aborted directors' course. Instead, the BBC seemed to forget all about that and instead gave him an elevated position as a production assistant, fundamentally a gofer to the producer. Terry had had absolutely no training in this field. He wasn't even entirely sure what the job entailed. He was completely unqualified for it – 'whatever it was!', he would chuckle, years later. All he remembered about it was that he was so bad, so utterly hopeless, that the director once bellowed at him. On location, in the street. Notwithstanding his inability to do the job, the BBC, as per usual, happily kept him in it for a few months. Terry was still writing though, having established himself as a solo writer within a core unit of solo writers.

Meanwhile, Michael Palin was subsidising the BBC guineas by dipping his toe into presenting the Bristol-based commercial television pop music show *NOW!* By a very strange connection, he got the opportunity via one of Terry's ex-girlfriends at Oxford. Michael was paid £35 a day for basically donning silly costumes, larking about in front of the camera and doing such cutting-edge things as impersonating Harold Wilson and then saying: 'And now . . . the Kinks!' But that extra income enabled him to stick with Terry, writing their 'bits and pieces at the BBC'. It was at this time that Terry and Michael met a man who was to be a very important influence: Barry Cryer.

Cryer, seven years Terry's senior, had come from the variety world of Leeds music hall and speciality acts. The kind of acts that Terry had been writing jokes for during the previous twelve months. Cryer was just what Terry needed: a razor-sharp joke-writer of the old school who was still young enough and cool enough to coax and encourage the Oxbridge invasion at the BBC. The television programme that fully and forcefully utilised most, if not all, of the celebrated comedy graduates was *The Frost Report*. And here, at this point in our story, is the second appearance of a certain David Frost. A presenter who became, as Baz Cryer would dub him, 'a practising catalyst' at the head of a writing room that would see the five British Pythons together for the first time.

David Frost hadn't forgotten meeting Terry and Michael in Edinburgh in 1964. And he was as good as his word. He said, 'I remember you guys, I know you can be very funny, will you come and be writers for my show?' Terry and Michael were excited – this was a big deal. What they didn't realise at the time was that David had signed up 384 other writers as well as them! As Michael says, 'Basically, anybody who could write, who was over the age of seven, was in!'

Indeed, Barry Cryer would refer to that long, seemingly never-ending roll-call of writers in the show's credits, in very, very small print compared to the name of David Frost, as 'the Dead of World War Two'. Terry was on that roll-call from the very beginning; he had his first 'quickie' joke accepted for broadcast on 10 March 1966, in the very first episode of *The Frost Report*: 'On Authority'. In fact, Terry had two 'quickies' included. Both were policemen-based – in light of the Ken Dodd success, this was fertile comic terrain for him at the time. The other was the joke now simply referred to as 'PC Super'. That's the: *'Morning Super.' 'Morning Wonderful!'* gag from *The Oxford Revue*. There: it really was a quickie.

A *Frost Report* writer who was clearly on Terry's comedy wavelength was Marty Feldman. Even though Terry had always preferred a good book over the idiot's lantern in the corner, Marty was 'a television name to conjure with'. On the rare occasions when Terry would sit in front of the television set at his parents' house and watch, it would be a comedy. *The Army Game* or *Bootsie and Snudge*, even ventriloquist Peter Brough's television show with his dummy Archie Andrews. Marty's name would regularly pop up as the writer. So, when Terry was introduced to him, it was something of a thrill. Marty's influence was all over *The Frost Report*. Although only in his early thirties himself, he made a point of introducing the young Oxbridge blood to the established writers in the room. And it was an impressive bunch.

The way the show's writers usually worked was they would go to a meeting at the start of the week and be given a 'thesis' written by Antony Jay, who had been part of current affairs at the BBC since 1955, before going freelance almost exactly a year before Terry joined, in April 1964. Jay's 'thesis' was a sort of themed document about the particular topic for that week's show – traffic or money, for example. That was what everything was based on. They would write their sketches by spinning ideas off from that document. Then, at the end of the week, there would be another meeting where the writers would read out their stuff and see what Feldman and Jay picked up. These meetings would invariably take place on a Saturday, in a room above a Methodist church on Crawford Street, just behind Marylebone station, and Marty Feldman was particularly encouraging about the sketches Jones and Palin were producing. He told them: 'I've read your sketches and I'm sure you can make it as a writing team.' What an endorsement. For Terry: 'this meant a great deal to us'.

The abiding memory of everybody present at those writers' room read-throughs was that Terry would laugh and laugh and laugh . . . and he would laugh loudest when Michael read out the jokes they had written. It was undoubtedly nervous laughter. At least some of the time. Because Terry got the impression that John Cleese would accept it more readily if he thought Mike had written it and not Terry, it was Mike who read their material!

Certainly John, and his writing partner Graham Chapman, were far more stoic and certainly less inclined to laugh out loud during these sessions. John too, with the much, much more extra money he was earning for his regular, lead appearances on *The Frost Report* as well as writing it, could clearly afford to splash out a little. Terry recalled John once asking him to join him for a comedy conflab at the Angus Steakhouse. He couldn't remember a thing of what they talked about, just how impressed he was that John could actually afford an Angus Steakhouse! As for John himself, he remembers a lunch in the far more reasonably priced canteen at the Aeolian Hall in New Bond Street. His memory of this conversation is equally shaky, although he seems to remember disagreeing with whatever Terry said. This would be the blueprint for their relationship within Python, for they were both too alike, each convinced their opinion on comedy was correct.

Terry swiftly rose to the top of the heap of that elephantine and enthusiastic writers' room; his jokes were clearly met with great approval, as demonstrated by Heather Dean's continuing her correspondence with Players & Writers:

*Would you also confirm that Terry Jones would be agreeable to accepting payment at the rate of 7 guineas per minute for sketch and 'quickie' material which James Gilbert may accept for future programmes in* The Frost Report *series.*

Terry was more than agreeable to this. And even more so when he made the leap from 'quickies' to sketch-writer, beginning with *The Frost Report* episode 'On News', for which he picked up a higher than usual fee. His contribution, 'Non-News', starred Ronnie Barker as a desperate newsreader trying to make news out of nothing: 'The oldest man in Britain, Mr Amos Parkinson, who was 127 last birthday . . . is still alive.' The sketch weighed in at one minute thirty and earned Terry a princely fourteen guineas.

Terry was certainly still encouraging Michael Palin, not only in gag-writing but also by inviting his Oxford pal to perform spots in London cabaret clubs. Terry, Mike and Robert Hewison were enjoying a two-week stint at the Rehearsal Club, above the Royal Court Theatre. With the fading pull of the Establishment, this club swiftly became the new place to be seen. As Michael recalls: 'Paul McCartney turned up one night. And the following night David Frost was in.' Having loved them in Edinburgh, this was simply and rather endearingly to see his writers Terry and Michael in performance again.

*The Frost Report* had certainly given Michael Palin a sense of job security for, two days after the broadcast of that edition dedicated to 'News', on Saturday 16 April 1966 he married Helen Gibbins. Terry's date for the occasion was Astra Meesok, a young lady from

Thailand who had been on the scene, on and off, since Oxford. She was living at the same Black Prince Road address as Terry. Astra had done some work, backstage, for the Oxford revues, and had met Terry there. Assignations between the men's and the women's colleges were not easy, and with a 10.30 p.m. curfew – with fines, disciplinary action and shame tinged with triumph – you had to be clever. Terry had been very, very clever. Teddy Hall was one of the trickiest to get back into once the gates were shut and locked. The junior dean would be on duty to dispense punishment, along with the night porter recording disobedient names in his ledger. As a result, a late-night dalliance outside college would see Terry faced with two points of entry into the college to get back to his own bed. Either he would have to face the public gaze of passers-by on the high street, or gain entrance by climbing in through a chum's window. Alternatively, he could risk waking the dead by clambering over the ancient stone wall of the churchyard and hoping an obliging pal in the rooms facing would pull him through.

Although Terry and Alison Telfer never quite managed to meet at Oxford, Alison did know Astra, although she says she didn't find her particularly friendly. Like Terry, and most of the under-graduates presumably, Alison found the time restrictions imposed by the colleges at Oxford infuriating. Astra had a room near a door, with steps coming up, so you could just step into Astra's room; whereas Alison's room had a high window and you would have to climb up the roses on the wall to get in. One evening, Alison came back a little after midnight and saw Astra's light was on, so she knocked on her window and asked if she could get in. While Astra did let her in, she seemed to Alison to be less than thrilled about it.

After the Palins' church service, the wedding guests all went to a hall for the wedding reception, where there was a toastmaster who was calling out everybody's names as they arrived at the door.

Terry had discreetly whispered their names in the ear of this toast-master but, Oxford chum David Wood remembers, instead of saying Mr Terry Jones and Miss Astra Meesok, with great confidence the toastmaster announced: 'Miss Terry Jones and Mr Aston Martin!' Of course, Terry couldn't resist the silliness of this, but Astra was less amused. In the fairly monochrome world of 1960s England, having your 'foreign' name mangled or remarked on was presumably a regular occurrence that must have been annoying, at best. Astra and Terry's on–off relationship didn't last long after the Palin wedding day, with Astra leaving for New York and Terry moving out of his upstairs room at Black Prince Road soon after.

While Astra and Terry's relationship was fizzling out completely, the Jones and Palin collaboration was blossoming into full flower. A first joint BBC agreement had made the partnership official, with Heather Dean having signed off on behalf of the BBC. Michael Palin added his mark on 15 September 1966, and Terry, still signing T. Parry Jones, exactly a leisurely fortnight later, on 29 September 1966.

Terry could afford to take his time for it was TERRY JONES, alone, who had been cited throughout a lengthy and binding agreement that tied him to not one but two, associated, new comedy revue shows for BBC Light Entertainment, *Late Night Line-Up* and *Late Night Review*. Clause 3 of the contract specified that his talents as both researcher and scriptwriter would be employed, coming up with sketches and linking material for the programmes. Furthermore, it was agreed that the BBC '*shall have first call on Terry Jones for the services to be rendered under this Agreement*'.

Terry was also granted a modicum of freedom – writing from home, which at this stage was temporary accommodation and the sofa of willing, obliging friends until he moved in, once again with a bunch of chums, to a home in Wellclose Square, East London, just behind the Royal Mint – although the BBC was often a more restrictive and fixed place to work, within the corporation itself. Indeed, the contract confirmed that Terry was expected to show his face at the office and the studio when required. As a maverick, Terry would have baulked slightly at the BBC's strict rules and regulations, and the insistence that these were to be followed at all times. There would have been a modicum of relief at the contract's rather ominous – to everybody else – wording that this was to be 'for the time being in force for the conduct of broadcasting'. No doubt that 'for the time being' would have amused Terry, for, although the payments were not huge and life-changing, they were regular and accommodating of a comfortable existence. He was picking up £35 a week for scripting and editing duties on *Late Night Line-Up*, alongside the other subsidiaries for quickies and witticisms on other people's shows.

Perhaps most joyously of all, those of Roy Hudd, that youthful purveyor of music hall and briefest of pals from *Not So Much a Programme, More a Way of Life*, who was also adept at more contemporary comic commentary. A decade before the start of his long-running *The News Huddlines*, Roy starred in the television sketch series *The Illustrated Weekly Hudd*. Something of a forerunner to his radio success, this too was satire and silliness in equal measure. It was produced by Jimmy Gilbert, also at the time producing *The Frost Report* – a show that Terry was still heavily involved in. In the May 1966 report 'on Law', he wrote a blistering comic rant for High Court Judge John Cleese. Defendant Ronnie Barker is accused of arson, manslaughter, robbery with violence, rape, treason and three separate cases of murder. 'What have you to say for yourself?' demands Cleese. Barker sheepishly replies, 'I'm terribly sorry ...' It was so funny, no wonder Terry was commissioned as a writer for the Roy Hudd series too, with contracts issued on 14 September 1966 that required him to submit two minutes' worth of material for each of the seven episodes in the series, with weekly recording dates starting on

3 November. He was to be paid the princely sum of seven guineas a minute for his transmitted work, and now his fees would be filtered through a new agent, Kenneth Ewing of Fraser & Dunlop (Scripts) Limited, at 91 Regent Street.

*The Illustrated Weekly Hudd* was a crazy universe of comic coppers and cheeky convicts, prison breaks and seaside romps, naughty nuns and venerable vicars. With sketches entitled 'Beach Photo', 'Dirty Postcard' and 'Nasty Habit', these were Donald McGill saucy snaps made flesh – with a university education. They had one foot in the nostalgia of music hall and the other in high-brow deconstruction. A little Max Miller and a pinch of Arthur Miller, if you will.

And at last, around this time, fate decreed that Terry's path would finally and properly cross with that of Alison Telfer's. As soon as Alison left Oxford, she went to London to do a PhD in botany at King's College. She had assumed ('stupidly', she says) that she would be studying in the centre of town, but soon discovered that the laboratory was in Herne Hill, SE24. As far as Alison, who had grown up in Hampstead, was concerned, over the river was Dover and France. So she had to find somewhere convenient to live. At that time, she didn't have many friends in London, so there was no one to turn to for a flatshare. Thus began the arduous task of looking for a room. Eventually, she stumbled across an advertisement in the *Evening Standard*: '*Graduate!*' Fantastic. She went along to look at this room, in a very scruffy terraced house by Lambeth Walk. She got into conversation with the chap who had placed the advertisement, and it transpired that he had also gone to Oxford. They had so many connections that he naturally 'had to give me the room'. The room, being vacated by Mike Wyn Jones, was on the ground floor, with a little bit of garden at the back.

With her work placement beginning the following Monday, on Saturday 1 October 1966 Alison swiftly moved her belongings into

Black Prince Road. She had just finished when, suddenly, there was a knock at the front door. She opened it and there was Terry! Along with a friend. Surprised, Alison said: 'Hello! I know you. You were in *Hang Down Your Head and Die* in Oxford, weren't you?'

To which Terry replied, '*Yes!*'

Alison didn't even know his name. No doubt chuffed and flattered at the recognition, and probably immediately attracted to this pretty young woman, Terry explained that he had been living at the property until quite recently and had decided to pop back to say hello to the new housemate.

Once the formalities were complete Alison invited them in and made them a coffee. They sat around chatting until Alison remembered she had to go because she had arranged for a friend with a car to meet her at her parents' house in Hampstead to collect a table. She only had an hour to get all the way to north London, she suddenly realised. Clearly not wanting the conversation to end, Terry piped up: 'Oh, I'll give you a lift!' As it transpired, it wasn't Terry who had the car but his friend. A tiny little Mini, to boot. So, Alison had to sit on Terry's knee. All planned? Perhaps. Although this 'meet-cute' was a little painful for Alison – as she was getting into the car to sit on Terry's knee, she placed her hand on the edge of the roof, and he shut the door on it. Ouch!

Back at the flat later on, there was another knock at the door – it was Terry and his friend, back again. 'Then it turned into a party!' recalls Alison. They went to a chemist and bought little shiny stars, which they stuck round their eyes, for some reason – though the reason wasn't tipsiness. Despite the fact that it was the Swinging Sixties, Alison says that 'It wasn't booze in those days. It was cups of tea.'

After a couple of hours, Terry said: 'Ooh, I'm meant to be taking this girl out!' She was coming up from Claygate. So he whizzed off to Victoria station to pick her up, and brought her back to the house. Terry's mother had been wanting him to get to know people, and this lady was someone who he knew vaguely, and probably had esteemed parents or something. This poor girl was shoehorned into the party, though Alison remembers she seemed vaguely horrified. The party went on and Terry said: 'We should get some dinner. Shall we go to the Soup Kitchen in Knightsbridge?' – a very basic but very good restaurant. So they all went and had a meal before heading back to the flat. Again. Then, eventually, Terry said: 'Oh, last train!' So he took the woman back to Victoria and waved her off, not unlike that clichéd railway station sketch. And then Terry came back and the party went on into the wee small hours. Alison believes that Terry never saw the poor woman again!

That's how Alison met Terry. At last. Third time lucky.

# CHAPTER FIVE

## THE TWO OF US

*When you are so close to someone you don't*
*have to make jokes, you simply have jokes!*

TERRY was lucky all round. Getting paid to be silly is double the fun if your best friend is right there by your side. And since Oxford, Terry's best friend, Michael Palin, had been by his side. Terry and Mike laughed at the same jokes. Terry and Mike supped the same ales. Terry and Mike tapped their feet to the same tunes. In July 1964, on the verge of taking *The Oxford Revue* to Edinburgh, Terry and Mike had eagerly queued up together to each buy the latest long-playing album from the Beatles, *A Hard Day's Night*. In the wake of the first series of *The Frost Report*, in the summer of 1966, they had turned up, tuned in and tripped out to *Revolver*. While the Beatles were recording and audio-bending and fine-tweaking a little concept album by the name of *Sgt. Pepper's Lonely Hearts Club Band*, for what would become the defining event of the Summer of Love of 1967, Terry was slaving away on sketches for *The Frost Report* that were still not always cutting the mustard. Never discouraged, in the wake of *Sgt. Pepper* Terry turned his hand to psychedelia, writing lyrics for Barry Booth's groovy baroque comedy album *Diversions!* It was released on the Pye label, in April 1968, with titles like 'Henry Smith Addresses a Butterfly', 'A Concise History of Harry Shoes' and 'He's Very Good With His Hands'. Music and comedy were changing. Quickly. And Terry was at the centre of it. And now, with Michael Palin officially contracted as a writer for the BBC, the two friends were taking home a joint £60 a week. A momentary loss of a fiver in Terry's pocket from his solo contract notwithstanding, it was worth a crisp blue note to have a friend in the mix, a sounding board for silly, a chum with whom to discuss and dissect over a few pints.

During the closing months of 1966, Terry had also followed up on that wild and wonderful first day with Alison. Having lived at the house that she had moved into, Terry knew the phone number without having to ask. One day in November 1966, soon after that first day, he called her and asked her out to dinner. The rendez-vous was a rather smart restaurant. And it all went very well. Before long, Alison was invited back to Terry's house in west London. Just six weeks after that first meeting, Terry moved in with her. Alison was a good cook, with skills learned from her mother, and, alongside visits to good restaurants and good eating in general, Terry swiftly put the weight back on that he had lost during that bout of peritonitis. It would go on to his neck and then on to the belly. It was something he was self-conscious about, but he liked good food even more than he disliked gouging fresh holes in his belt. So, Terry was back in the house in which he used to live, but down in the basement this time. He gently persuaded friend John, who had a double bed in another room, to allow the fledgling couple in the lower room to have it. As Alison remembers: 'the deal being that, if John got a girlfriend in the meantime, he could have the double bed back!'

Although Terry was employed as a writer on *The Frost Report*, first and foremost that juvenile hope to be an actor still kind of lingered, and, if it meant delving into the dressing-up box to trans-form himself into an aged High Court judge or a potty policeman in an incongruous situation, be it a kiddies' playground or an Olympic running track, then so be it. Besides, Terry wanted the money – this glorified-extra work as part of David Frost's reper-tory company not only drip-fed his love for performing but also added an additional twenty quid a pop to his writers' salary. More than a help to his weekly grocery bill, these opportunities were fundamentally lifting him as a writer and wannabe film-maker.

Despite the prerogative of television seeping into his subconscious, whether he wanted it to or not, and his reluctance to ever finish that directors' course, vivid memories of silent slapstick Hollywood permeated his work. But while the ghostly shadow of the stone-faced, fearless mime of Buster Keaton was, and always remained, Terry's great comedy favourite, it was a contemporary clown on the Continent who proved the revelation. Keaton was the person Terry wanted to emulate, but the work of Jacques Tati convinced him that he should be able to do silent comedy in the sound world of television and film.

With that key to the comedy kingdom, Terry started a personal revolution from the best vantage point. From within. It was the pratfall rather than the brickbat that was Terry's bread and butter throughout 1967, but he willingly did both. A two-minute vignette of visual fun, 'String Quartet', was commissioned for an episode of *The Late Show* on 3 February 1967, while precisely a week later another three minutes of silly slapstick was requested for *The Frost Report*. Terry was allowed even more freedom of comic expression on *Late Night Line-Up*, broadcast much later in the schedule. Joan Bakewell, in the host's chair, was encouraging of little flights of mad fancy, as witness one surreal moment, with Terry sat at the piano, tinkling the ivories and discussing the most banal of matters. Where he was thinking of going on holiday that year. What he was going to prepare for dinner that night. Anything, in fact, except the wonderful classical music that was coming from his fingertips – courtesy of old Oxford revue composer and pianist John Gould. This sort of twisting of television convention was, or, more to the point, would become, Terry's signature style. This trope of casual pianist chatting to the unseen viewers was ripe for mockery and second nature to Terry, who had previously put all those corny comic introductions into the mouths of pianists Winifred Atwell and Russ Conway.

In April 1967, *The Late Show* indulged Terry's love of Chaucer with some jester slapstick for the 'Medieval Revue', a three-minute sketch that was also referred to as 'Before the Fringe', which basked in comic cachet by twisting the title of the genre-defining show *Beyond the Fringe* and revelled in the fact that satire and silliness were certainly at play long before the Edinburgh alternative arts festival! It gently baited the spectre of satire that was still nipping at light entertainment five years after its glory days. With a finger on the pulse of the future, there was 'The British Space Race' sketch too, which targeted the lacklustre and make-do-and-mend mentality of the nation's involvement in the exploration of the solar system.

It wasn't the first time that Terry had mined a certain sense of British mediocrity for laughs. The previous month, he had submitted a gaggle of like-minded film inserts and studio sketches, including a send-up of the supersonic airliner Concorde, still in prototype stage; a frolic with the lions of the recently opened Longleat safari park; and a pastiche of gangster cinema, just ahead of the release of the film *Bonnie and Clyde*. All 'ripped from the headlights' comedy there, alongside the much more prosaic humour of the humble 'Helpful Postman'. Of course, in Terry's hands even the most dull could be hilarious, the most pedestrian engaging.

That same month of April 1967, Terry's contributions to *The Frost Report* had been upped from three minutes a programme to five minutes per week, commencing with programme three, a report on the armed forces. In the end, the three 'quickies' were initially accepted but then discarded and not used. Although Terry did secure a script consultant fee for the 'Army Recruiting' film and spent a day on location during the making of the skit. The 'Haunted Wood', a sketch for *The Frost Report* on 'The Countryside', with a planned location shoot, and set for broadcast on 11 May 1967, was also accepted but not used. It was like a weekly comic newspaper. Some editions, your hard-grafted copy just wouldn't make the edit. Terry was very much on the staff though, and *The Frost Report* had proved so instantly a comedy talking point that the BBC cobbled together a compilation edition, *Frost Over England*. It had been transmitted on 26 March 1967, and a Terry Jones and Michael Palin-scripted sketch had been included. It was one of three wedding cake quickies (the other two were written by Eric Idle, and Jim Franklin). Terry and Mike's 'Karate' variant had the groom cutting the cake with a martial arts chop. It did its own little, very tiny bit in winning *The Frost Report* and the BBC the Golden Rose of Montreux, the international seal of excellence in television since the first ceremony in Switzerland in 1961. In May 1967, David Frost celebrated the victory with a lavish garden party at his home in Kensington. Typically of Terry, that award-winning vindication of his work on *The Frost Report* seemed to draw a definite line under the show. He had achieved all he could within its boundaries. It was done. Time to move on. Certainly, he felt the less restricted mentality of *The Late Show* was far more him. Despite the fact that he had a bit of a battle on his hands. Maybe because he had a battle on his hands. A new avenue.

The initial premise was to bring back satire to television comedy, though Terry thought this move was a little late in the day. His mind was set to silliness rather than satirical, but they were paying him to write jokes and, as he later sighed with relief, 'there weren't many so it wasn't arduous'. Added to the writing team for *The Late Show* were Barry Cryer and old Oxford cohort Robert Hewison. Terry had also brought in Michael Palin, which proved revolutionary. Together they did touch upon satire but in a more general, countercultural pastiche kind of way.

*The Late Show* now included 'Hibachi', a spoof of the Japanese samurai craze started by Akira Kurosawa's films and galvanised by the 1962 release of *Harakiri*; and a sketch about fantasy commuters fighting their way to work through a jungle. There was even a send-up of Michelangelo Antonioni's commercially successful art-house film *Blow-Up*. Indeed, Jones and Palin were having so much fun just larking about that they got into trouble with the BBC bigwigs. One night, they did a sketch for *Late Night Line-Up* in which they were jumping off chairs, dressed up in Batman suits. They recorded their segment and then went home and sat by the television set to watch the show go out. This was such a big deal for them that they had invited family and friends to watch it with them. Anyway, their sketch came on and then, immediately after it had finished playing, there was a ponderous panel discussion, a familiar element of the *Line-Up* programme. As Terry remembered: 'it was about the future of the arts or something'. Sitting on the panel was TV playwright Dennis Potter, whose pivotal political plays *Stand Up, Nigel Barton* and *Vote, Vote, Vote for Nigel Barton* had been broadcast in December 1965. Forthright and opinionated as ever, Potter said he hadn't come all the way from Gloucestershire to take part in a programme that could include such idiots dressed as superheroes. As a result, Terry was suspended from the show. But not dismissed from the BBC. Still, as a mild punishment, his next assignment saw him moved to an office where he sat next to the man who wrote *Pinky and Perky* – those cute puppet pigs who performed pop songs in their own unique, high-pitched style, until the BBC put them out to grass in 1968. Terry sat trying to think up jokes while all the while he could hear a typewriter banging away as another completed *Pinky and Perky* sketch hit the paper. It would have been all oinks and snorts and haphazard jamming of contemporary smash hits, but the relentless pounding of the typewriter keys was frustrating and oppressive for Terry. In his mind, despite the porcine nature of the material, someone in the building was being productive and hilarious while he struggled to come up with Corporation-friendly funnies.

A happier writing space was Terry and Alison's new basement flat in Black Prince Road, Lambeth, where Michael Palin and Terry would work together, side by side, writing their stuff for *The Frost Report* and everything else. Both Terry and Alison were amazingly tolerant because Michael was a smoker at the time and they weren't. As Michael recalls: 'Nowadays, you can't conceive that one person would be filling a basement with second-hand smoke all day long, while the two who were the couple who rented it, and who had to live there, were non-smokers! Nobody complained, though, because the world was full of cigarette smoke at the time.'

Michael, having secured a flat in Belsize Park with young bride Helen, would also host Terry for writing days. They would sit together and take half an hour to each scribble down some ideas, and then say: 'Well, what have you got?' If Terry had a great idea – which was often – they would develop that. If Terry loved one of Michael's ideas, they would develop that. The flat was right next door to the pub and, as Michael recalls, 'That was great. I have to say that having a drink was quite an important part of it!' That was their reward for doing a good day's work.

The Batman sketch that proved such a debacle on *Late Night Line-Up* had been Terry's idea. Hands up. And childish or not, it got them talked about in the press. These wonderfully silly television appearances had also won them a little fame. Such recognition, indeed, that Terry and Mike were invited to officially open the public toilets in Lambeth Walk. 'Fame at last,' as Michael remembers it. 'We had to go in and christen this place with a pee, and then just leave. All while the mayor was standing outside.' The pressure, not to mention the glamour, of show business! It was all about to get a little more glamorous, though, and certainly a lot more silly. Now, larking about in superhero outfits would be almost expected rather than frowned upon.

In the spring of 1967, director Tony Palmer was desperately trying to pull together a show that was definitely up Terry's street. Not satirical at all, just Oxbridge graduates being silly in a very clever way. By 28 March, Palmer had been actively courting Australian critic and wit Clive James to join the team. James was keen to prove himself an actor but Palmer wanted him in the writing room, and urged him to reconsider turning down the assignment as 'the performers are ten a penny but scriptwriters of your calibre are few and far between.' In the event, Clive James did not appear, although Germaine Greer did.

The show was *Twice a Fortnight* and, as Graeme Garden explains, it was: 'a showcase for me and Bill Oddie, really. [Studio G, at Lime Grove] was a madhouse. The audience had been liberally supplied with alcohol before recording so they would laugh loudly. At everything. I remember asking friends at the time whether they had seen the show and when they said "No!" I would reply: "Good!"'

Graeme's overriding glee with regards to *Twice a Fortnight* is that very little of it survives in the archives. What does survive are the filmed inserts. 'I knew Terry was very keen on making these little comedy films,' remembers Graeme, 'so I suggested that Tony Palmer invite Terry and Mike to contribute one or two per show. Although Tony was ostensibly the director, those films were very much Terry's babies. He had his hand on the tiller throughout.'

Graeme Garden and Bill Oddie would appear in these little films, but only as supporting players. On Monday 10 April 1967, the team was filming at Stonehenge. The pilot show for *Twice a Fortnight* would include this four-minute filmed insert, 'The Butler Trials', written by Terry and Michael. As if to embrace Palmer's dismissal of performers, Terry and Mike took part as well. Terry's skill for physical comedy was to the fore, in the role of the aged butler to an even more aged master, Lord Churton-le-Willow, who was played by Jonathan Lynn and described in the script as being an 'Old Queen, aged 304'. Germaine Greer was a country type, and quite youthful at a playing age of eighty-four! Palin was cast as her butler. And, as if to fully capitalise on the Stonehenge setting, Bill Oddie wandered in as a Druid. Still, it was

Terry who was on decidedly scene-stealing form, eagerly playing with the conventions of filmed comedy by walking away from the camera towards the distant horizon, falling over with silent slap-stick elegance, getting up again, desperately trying to regain his authority, and staggering away once more, deflated.

In a note to Tony Palmer penned after the show was broadcast, Bill Oddie gushed:

I can't say what a great job you did flaunting the 'rules' of TV direction, & showing them just what can be done.

Indeed, the show did point, inevitably, towards not only *The Goodies* but Python too. However, Palmer was under no illusions. Terry had been the stand-out comedy turn, not to mention the director, and, although it is certain he would have filed away Palmer's techniques and freedom of expression for later use, he clearly got the core sense of fun at the heart of *Twice a Fortnight*. So much so that, on 17 April 1967, Palmer wrote:

Dear Terry, I think you are the oldest and most senile butler in the business. Why don't we make a [feature] film about the butler trials? I think Stonehenge would be a great place to do it.

Stephen Hearst, who had directed much of the studio material and was executive producer of music and arts programming at the BBC, noted to Terry on 25 April 1967: 'the fact that we've got over the worst hurdle, namely to get the series accepted, is proof that we weren't blowing South Seas bubbles. It will be great having you as part of the team.' The show was up and running, and Terry and Mike were in – doing comedy the way they wanted to do comedy. In a very silly way.

Right off the bat, they were down in East Sussex, at Old Roar Gill to be precise, on Thursday 3 August 1967. That Spring of Love had given way to the Summer of Love, although the Terry and Michael-scripted film 'A Game of Croquet' for *Twice a Fortnight* was not of the zeitgeist at all. It was just all very silly. Again. Terry and Mike were cast as choirboys, peasants and gangsters. In a scenario that heralds Python's conjoining of Sam Peckinpah and Julian Slade, with the squire (Jonathan Lynn) and the vicar (distinguished radio announcer Ronald Fletcher, who would lend his weighty BBC newscaster tones to the narration of *Ripping Yarns*: 'Escape from Stalag Luft 112B') caught up in the furore. The script sets the scene of some of Terry's, admittedly minor, action in the adventure in support of the squire: 'immediately his peasants, armed with pitch-forks, crossbows and large size mallets and balls appear from the undergrowth . . . the vicar's wife [Julie Covington] strips off to reveal she is a Red Cross nurse . . . [and] the battle of the croquet lawn rages. Up the garden path comes a Chicago-gangster unit, driven by the curate in a hearse. Eventually the croquet lawn is strewn with the dead of battle. Only the vicar is left . . . he staggers to his feet with his last efforts and plays his last shot. He hits the winning post and gives a grateful glance to heaven before he expires . . .'

Terry was in slapstick paradise. It was perhaps those films where, for the first time, he realised how much good filming could add to comedy. Palmer wasn't very sensitive in a way to what they were doing, but he had a tremendous visual sense – he knew how to get a good picture and it looked terrific. He paid attention to detail as, for him, the aesthetic was much more than a mere backdrop for the joke – it could and should add gravitas to the comedy. Terry became aware then that you could marry beautiful pictures to comedy and get something really amazing. Plus, if a scene looked right, the brain wouldn't have to worry about thinking about how it didn't look right. Thus, historical accuracy – in, say, *Monty Python and the Holy Grail* – frees the brain to simply laugh at the comedy. In that respect, *Twice a Fortnight* was an education.

And far more use than any BBC directors' course, for, here, Terry had the freedom and the encouragement to pitch in with a filmic pastiche sending up Ingmar Bergman here, and a historical romp like a Battle of Hastings sketch there.

To go full circle, early, Terry threw in a favourite bit of material that had already been trotted out multiple times, his beloved 'Slapstick' sketch – the joke about joke-making, now called 'Humour Lecture', which for the *Twice a Fortnight* of 22 December 1967 earned him forty quid in a four-minute reappraisal. It was the sixth show of the series and a riot.

Despite the *Late Night Line-Up* embarrassment, Terry was still very much in with *The Frost Report* people. And every guinea helped. Even those that were earned off sketches written but relegated to the bottom drawer. On 21 June 1967 it was noted that *The Frost Report* 'On Woman', which had transmitted on 13 April that year, had commissioned additional material from Terry and Michael that had been accepted at the read-through stage but subsequently not used. These were 'quickie' sketches: 'Sometimes I Don't Understand You', 'Supper's in the Oven', 'Unbuttoning Blouse' and 'From Here to Eternity'. So far, so self-explanatory. Obvious humour was to be gleaned too from a 'Film Idea' of Terry's, entitled 'Driving School', although that didn't make the programme either. But still Terry was a BBC man. Through and Through. By October 1967 Terry was back with *Late Night Line-Up*, although his presence was less revered and certainly less acknowledged. For the edition broadcast on 5 October 1967 – two years to the day before a certain *Monty Python's Flying Circus* first took flight – the sketch 'Outer Space' was credited in internal BBC correspondence just to Michael Palin. The gag relied upon a clever Dream Screen box, designed by Michael Sutin, which projected shapes from outer space over which a narration dealt with the problems radio programmes have when covering visual events of this nature. The joke was made a lot easier by being on television!

On 23 October 1967 it was noted on the remittance order that: 'both boys wrote this one, so I have added Terry's name.'

There had also been a satirical and surreal sketch show *A Series of Bird's*, for the autumn of 1967. It was produced by Dennis Main Wilson, who had been part of that immediate post-war influx of ex-military types who steered BBC's comedy output through the insanity of *The Goon Show* and the pioneering domesticity of *Hancock's Half Hour*. The producers, directors and writers of this breed who had shaped and sometimes stagnated the corporation were very in control when the bright young things of Oxbridge joined the Beeb in the freewheeling Sixties. All of these establishment authority figures were characters in Terry's collective memory of the BBC, a place where old-school military clout indulged and embraced the new kids on the block. The new kids from old education.

Indeed, *A Series of Bird's*, with a slot just after 9 p.m., had shades of both, and pushed diminutive Cambridge wit John Bird to the fore. Bird described the show as 'satire by the back door'. Indeed, its working title had been simply 'The John Bird Series'. That wasn't to deny satirical activism from Bird's fellow student wag and long-time collaborator John Fortune, who was recruited for the series too. Terry's contribution was to deconstruct the very production of television, once again standing on the shoulders of giants Michael Bentine and Spike Milligan.

Peter Cook and Dudley Moore had their feet well and truly under the BBC table too. Terry would cross paths with Pete and Dud for the 1,000th episode of *Late Night Line-Up*, on 30 June 1967. They were dining at the Villa dei Cesari Italian restaurant in Pimlico. Terry played the waiter. With Cook and Moore safely gathered in, noises from within the BBC were already being made to poach Marty Feldman from commercial television. Thus the surrealism of the Goon generation was now less than pioneering and more pretty much the house style of BBC sketch show comedy. Crucially for Terry's sketches, *A Series of Bird's* allowed him to indulge in longer bursts of sustained comedy for the first time. These were not the 'quickies' of *The Frost Report* but rather more intricate, sophisticated commentary on the Britain of 1967 and, most interestingly of all, the television of the Britain of 1967. The sketches would take peeks behind the scenes, and playfully expose the making of documentary films, noises off, 'see-through' scenery, and a daring, although again not revolutionary, lifting of the lid of the box in the corner of the living room. Figuratively speaking.

*A Series of Bird's* lasted just one series, broadcast on BBC1 from 3 October to 21 November 1967, but had galvanised Terry's repu- tation. And while Marty Feldman was on the verge of skipping over to the BBC from the commercial environs of Rediffusion London, Eric Idle had been approached to write and star in a show for that very same television network. As Eric remembers: 'this was a huge deal. My own show. And I knew I wanted Terry and Mike to be in it too. So I told the producer I would do it, but only if Terry and Mike joined the team.'

The resulting television programme would be a sketch show sensation. With real adverts. A show absolutely planned and created for children, which soon, through no fault or forethought of anybody involved, became the comedy that grown-ups adored too. The comedy beat combo the Bonzo Dog Doo-Dah Band would be along for the ride as well, performing the latest pop songs week in and week out much as Pinky and Perky were doing over at the BBC. As Terry well remembered. But the Bonzos, under the insane leadership of Vivian Stanshall and with Neil Innes on the more wistful lead vocals, were the real deal of madcap rock 'n' roll. This was hip stuff for hip kids. And hip adults. Even the title of this new television show was a knowing reference to technical hitches within broadcasting. When this ragbag collec- tion of no-longer-fledgling but just-about-ready-to-fly-the-nest comedy movers and shakers hit the small screen, the announcer would mutter, 'Do Not Adjust Your Set!'

For Michael Palin, it was wonderful to be able to write and perform material that could not be found anywhere else on television at that time. Children knew all about silliness and anarchy and he and Terry wanted to reassure them that some adults did too. *Do Not Adjust Your Set* was transmitted in the renowned 'children's slot', between 5.25 and 5.55 p.m., and, as Michael recalls, a rather niche audience – London's Italian waiters – were the first vocal grown-up fans of the show! 'These waiters were just getting up and getting themselves ready for a long night's shift at work. As they tucked in their dress shirts and secured their bow-ties, they tuned in to our show with ever-increasing enthusiasm.' This was the first time that Michael was recognised from a TV appearance – by the head waiter at La Terrazza, in Soho, Mario Cassandro and Franco Lagattolla's go-to Italian restaurant.

Terry found out that they were also a hit with London's Chinese hospitality community. Alison recalls that after a recording of the show they would all go for a meal. One particular evening they went to a lovely Chinese restaurant that turned out to be run by fans of the show. It was a restaurant they often frequented, so it would stay open especially for them! One evening the waiters alerted Terry to the fact that the following week was Chinese New Year. At the time, the gang didn't really know anything about Chinese New Year and its tradition of eating copious amounts of great food in symbolism of the hoped-for abundance for the next twelve months. The celebrations can last up to sixteen days. Naive to the glorious excess, the *Do Not Adjust Your Set* team and their guests agreed to dine again after the recording the following week. The waiters brought out the first course and the team ate everything. Then they brought out the second course and they ate everything. By the time they got to course fifteen – which was the whole fish and followed by the whole duck – they couldn't eat anything at all.

Jeremy Isaacs, at Rediffusion, had had his sights set on the

BBC's stash of comedy talent for a while. Humphrey Barclay, producing the Cambridge Footlights boys in *I'm Sorry, I'll Read That Again* – radio's 'wonder show', itself bearing a title derived from a broadcasting hitch – was Isaacs' first and only choice to produce the new commercial comedy sketch package he had in mind. He invited Barclay for a meeting, though Barclay thought that the summons was merely because Isaacs wanted to buy some old radio material for the television. When he heard what Isaacs was planning, he jumped at the chance to assemble and cast this silly show for kids. Isaacs already had the title. *Do Not Adjust Your Set* was set in stone. Isaacs just needed Barclay to conjure up an off-the-wall series that fitted that title.

Barclay selected a team, pick 'n' mix, boy- and girl-band style. Cambridge wunderkind Eric Idle, who he already knew, was the first to be signed up. Barclay had seen Terry in ****, back in the Oxford days, and he knew of his sketches for David Frost and John Bird and, moreover, trusted Eric's judgement – but really only where Terry was concerned. Despite Eric suggesting Michael Palin too, it was Terry that Humphrey Barclay wanted. Barclay phoned Terry and asked him if he would be interested in doing a television series with Eric Idle. Terry only knew Eric from Edinburgh, but that Oxbridge meeting of minds – particularly in playful improvisation – had clicked. Terry was in, for sure, but insisted to Barclay that he would only do the show if he took on Michael Palin too. Michael explains that this was typical of Terry. 'Terry had his own sense of integrity within his own little world,' he says. And when Terry was determined, he invariably got his way. So Mike was in too. Those consciously non-uni talents Denise Coffey and David Jason came from legitimate theatre and end-of-the pier farce respectively, and had respected acting chops. Having trained at the Glasgow College of Dramatic Art, Denise had joined the repertory company at the Gateway Theatre in Edinburgh. Having juggled working as a reporter for the BBC and distinguished stage work in *A Midsummer Night's Dream*, by the time of *Do Not Adjust Your Set* she had left Scotland in favour of the West End stage. While David had been doing a Ray Cooney farce in Bournemouth and playing Bert Bradshaw in the television soap opera *Crossroads*.

Terry was keen to get started, but he received less-than positive vibes from his agent, Brian Codd, who was very reticent about children's programmes. His advice always tickled Terry. Brian told Terry to write a stage revue for BAFTA-winning screen and stage actress Dora Bryan, who, in October 1967, was just about to close at the Theatre Royal Drury Lane as the star of *Hello, Dolly!* Codd said that a comic capitalisation of Dora's West End popularity would be much more productive and profitable for Terry in the long term. Nothing against Dora Bryan but Terry didn't want to do that, though he had written for her before, when she had appeared in *Before the Fringe* earlier in 1967. It had been fun but not at all what he had his sights on. Whereas *Do Not Adjust Your Set* was exactly what he always wanted to do – write silly sketches for him and his mates to act out.

Terry was, however, very aware that none of the writing team – himself, Mike and Eric – had children at that time. So he simply turned his 25-year-old head back a decade and accessed the comic strips and wireless shows that had made him laugh as an adolescent: 'It was pretty much what made me laugh at the time and still makes me laugh now, which helped us get that audience across the age groups, I suppose.' So the jokes revolved around school – history sketches and playground games – as well as his old favourite, television itself. Terry's attitude was never to write down to his audience, and certainly not if that audience was children. He would tone down the saucy stuff. Just a little. But, fundamentally, he decided to write the sort of sketches he had always written. Although now, having been taken out of the BBC and thrust into commercial television, for the kind of money that he had only ever dreamed of.

Michael Palin recalls: 'My God, we were paid! Really well paid!'

It was big money, yes, but also a lot of work to write and perform the material. Twenty-nine episodes of *Do Not Adjust Your Set* were made in total. Although Michael jokes now, 'At the time I would have happily signed up to do it for twenty-nine years!' The fee, for writing and performing each episode, was £100. Split three ways. A lot tastier than the fourteen guineas over at the BBC.

The very first *Do Not Adjust Your Set* was recorded on Monday 6 November and scheduled for broadcast on Boxing Day 1967. Terry and Alison spent that Christmas – their second as a couple – separately, with their own families. Alison had a toddler sister, while Terry had an ailing mother. So, with duty and dread pretty much in equal measure, Terry made the journey to spend the festive season with his parents in Surrey. At least he had the thrill of being on telly not once but twice over the Christmas period: 'it's something every writer, every actor gets an extra buzz out of. I know it can't just be me. To be on television over Christmas. I didn't get my name in the *Radio Times*, but still . . .' A forty-minute *Frost Over Christmas* – the last of *The Frost Report* – was screened on BBC1 at 7.30 p.m. that Boxing Day Tuesday, just ahead of the Beatles film *Magical Mystery Tour*, featuring the Bonzos. Not that Terry would have been in the mood to tune in at that time, for his pet project, *Do Not Adjust Your Set*, which he had written and starred in, had not had a smooth broadcast. Still, as one pivotal television success, *The Frost Report*, was about to come to an end, another pivotal television success was about to start.

*Do Not Adjust Your Set* was much publicised and eagerly awaited. However, as if jinxed by its own title, the wrong episode had been loaded up for transmission. In actual fact, it was the first episode of the series, scheduled for broadcast on 4 January 1968, that viewers gazed at over their left-over-turkey sandwiches and fifth glass of sherry. Terry would have turned to his mum and dad in horror and reached for the nearest bottle as he watched helplessly. The tape they were broadcasting hadn't had the adverts spliced onto it, so there was a blank patch for about three minutes in the middle where the ads were supposed to be. It was terribly embarrassing.

Even more embarrassing was that this episode was too long for that 6.35 p.m. Boxing Day slot of twenty-five minutes. Two established comedy greats were lined up in the schedule, with *The Benny Hill Show* from 7 p.m., followed by the Peter Sellers feature film *Waltz of the Toreadors* from 8 p.m., both shot in colour but screened in black and white by necessity of the broadcaster (colour commercial television would not come along until November 1969). So in a ham-fisted attempt to get the schedule back on track, *Do Not Adjust Your Set*, the introductory programme to a new thirteen-week revue for teenagers, as the *TV Times* had it, was phased out in the middle of the closing sketch and a muffled, apologetic announcement made before programmes continued. It was a foul-up that, rather wonderfully, set up the very anarchic, convention-twisting ethos of the series as a whole. Moreover, the mistake made the national press the following day. It was the kind of unexpected, extra publicity that the programme makers could only have hoped for. And for Terry too it proved a blessing.

The cringe-worthy error was soon forgotten, *Do Not Adjust Your Set* was billed as the grown-up comedy for children, and Terry and Michael were at the forefront of the sketches, performing as children in positions of high power and authority. The barbs were cheekily aimed, for the very first time for the juveniles, at such previously untouchable targets as the police, the military, politicians and pop stars. Even schoolteachers. Much to the joy of every young viewer watching.

That Christmas cock-up notwithstanding, *Do Not Adjust Your Set* provided the long-awaited opportunity for Terry and Michael to both write and act in leading parts – 'we were desperate to start performing our own material!', Terry remembered. He could play everything from a gurgling baby to an overzealous soldier asking:

'Friend or foe?' When the answer came back – 'Foe!' – and Terry fired his weapon, the wounded enemy congratulated the squaddie on his skilful marksmanship. That the foe in question was played by Michael Palin was a glorious encapsulation of Oxford comradeship, comedy shorthand and friendly banter, as well as a shadow of things to come. Indeed, from the very beginning, sketches were starting to fade and merge into each other, and the very dynamic and conventions of television were questioned and mercilessly sent up. It evoked the madness of Spike Milligan's Q, but without the malice or delight in awkwardness of the arch-Goon. *Do Not Adjust Your Set* was insanity that kept its mittens on.

And, apart from Terry's lovingly filmed inserts, the show was recorded as live, with absolutely no editing in post-production. In those days, to edit footage you had to physically cut the tape. The editor had to look at the tape through a magnifying glass and see where the magnetic pulses were, cut there and then join the pieces together. That was all too much like hard work for Humphrey Barclay and Rediffusion. And far too expensive, more to the point, as the tapes cost forty quid each. So, all the studio sketches were performed with the angst and energy of a live show. Recorded and broadcast, warts and all. There weren't that many warts, thankfully, but any mistake was gladly embraced as part of the free-for-all fun of the thing. It was a student rag week, essentially, only better written. Indeed, *The Sunday Times* went rather round the houses but still planted a lovely compliment within its review, stating that *Do Not Adjust Your Set* was: 'Not only quite the funniest of all the children's programmes but also in its way as funny as anything on television at any time of day or night.' The series went on to win the Best Children's Entertainment Programme Award at the International Prix Jeunesse festival, in Munich in 1968.

The one negative, for Terry at least, was that he couldn't play every character he wanted to. That ambition of writing and acting all your own work simply cannot be completely achieved within a talented group, and certainly not a group that includes brilliant slapstick clown David Jason. The character of Captain Fantastic had always been intended for David. Michael and Terry thought it would be a good idea to have a running gag throughout the series, and they could do these on film, as inserts, which would give them a bit of a breather in the studio. Terry was later sure Captain Fantastic – a greengrocer who didn't do anything fantastic at all – was his idea, developed with the help of Michael. All of these segments were directed by studio director Daphne Shadwell and comprised various scenarios that were rather ambitious, with lots of wonderful visual ideas. One was Captain Fantastic and the World Eaters, fiendish foes who were, indeed, going to eat the world. This short film involved very elaborate gags with alien people eating huge things and those huge things disappearing. Unfortunately, it was sometimes a little too ambitious. Michael and Terry couldn't be in them because they were busy writing the next show. More frustratingly for Terry, this meant he couldn't be on location to oversee the shooting of the scripts. David and Denise would go off to film the segments, and use the basic ideas that Terry had come up with, without filming much of the actual script. It was really just David doing a lot of brilliant slapstick in something of an improvisation on the vague themes that Terry and Michael had plotted. Terry found this quite annoying, to say the least, and at one point insisted to Humphrey Barclay that, as he was pretty good at the silent slapstick stuff himself, he could play Captain Fantastic. He could have done, certainly, but not halfway through an established series with the original actor still in the team!

The frustration over not playing Captain Fantastic could, on occasion, blunt the sheer joy of all those other hilarious and freewheeling characters of *Do Not Adjust Your Set*. To such an extent that, on occasion, Terry even had a mild grumble about a beloved old colleague. That beloved old colleague was Marty Feldman, Terry's champion on *The Frost Report*, and the mild grumble was very mild indeed. Terry would certainly pooh-pooh any notion that, with the commitment to their own, very lucrative show in *Do Not Adjust Your Set*, he would consider turning down writing exclusive material for goggle-eyed comic genius headliner Feldman as well: 'Not at all, no,' he would chuckle. 'We were raring to go.' After Feldman had been the stand-out star of *At Last the 1948 Show*, the BBC had headhunted him for his own sketch show. In full colour. *It's Marty* or just *Marty* – it answered to both – secured the Jones and Palin partnership a well-paid writing deal.

Besides, as Terry often said, 'we owed Marty an awful lot'. It was only a year or so since *The Frost Report* and both Mike and Terry were chuffed to bits for him for making it big as a performer, having been such a brilliant and well-established writer. They went to see Marty at his amazing home in Highgate, a huge Gothic mansion with a double staircase, like something out of an old Hollywood musical. At the stroke of one o'clock in the afternoon, Marty appeared at the top of the stairs, dressed in a silk kimono and smoking a cigarette. Terry thought: 'God! Is this what happens when you become a star?' Marty was as lovely as he had always been. Terry remembered that he was very kind and encouraging, very fulsome in his praise of their writing. They were chuffed to be working with him once more.

However, the old frustrations about writing for other people were soon coming to the fore again, in particular with what was known as 'The Gnome Sketch'. I shall allow Terry to set up the premise: 'It was all about this gnome going to see a mortgage advisor. The guy behind the desk [played by the ever-incredulous John Junkin] is a bit surprised but the gnome speaks very sensibly about collateral and everything else. Eventually, the mortgage guy relaxes and asks: "What's the property?" and the gnome matter-of-factly replies, "It's the magic oak tree in Dingly Dell!" Mike read it out at the script meeting and everybody laughed and said, "That's great!"'

The star comedian liked it a lot and Terry and Mike were pleased to have got a sketch into their old friend Marty's very successful show. However, when the show was being recorded Marty came out dressed as a gnome, which was all well and good, and he sat cross-legged on the desk of the mortgage guy. But instead of doing the first line, he started cracking a lot of gnome jokes. Marty loved to get reactions from the studio audience, sure, but it seemed to Terry that he didn't have faith in the scripted material to get him the laughs. But there were no huge laughs forthcoming. Marty insisted on doing it again and started putting more obvious jokes in to try to get the response he wanted. As Terry later said, 'He just destroyed the sketch!'

Forty years after the event, this still seemed to grate on Terry. I said that I had seen the sketch and explained that it had ultimately been broadcast pretty much exactly how he and Michael had written it. This seemed to please him and he pondered why they hadn't used it on *Do Not Adjust Your Set*, as he felt it was a perfect sketch for the children's show that adults loved. He thought Mike or Eric Idle would have been great as the gnome. Or, even better, he said, they should have kept it for Python and given the gnome to John Cleese. Which, to be fair, would have been very funny indeed. Either way, Terry insisted, 'It would have been better if one of us had done it. Too late now!' The way in which this one sketch still bothered him years later shows that it was a catalyst moment for him: Terry knew then that his days of writing for other people – other than himself and the little gang of like-minded writer-performers he admired – were over. Thanks, again, in a back-handed kind of way, to Marty Feldman.

Terry did however remain very grateful for the work, the exposure and the money. Moreover, Marty gave Terry the occasional opportunity to do a bit of acting on the show too. There's a particularly good World Cup sketch with Marty as a Dopey-like footballer, continually going round and round the group of players in order to get another kiss and yet another kiss from the Snow

White-like royal greeting the team. And right there in the football sketch is Terry, jogging and grinning and awkwardly trying to get on with the match. The Terry Jones frustration is writ large there – enjoying himself, despite himself.

In 1968 the BBC was still keen to keep using Terry's sketches, and he remained for the moment, eagerly delivering the funnies for other people and other people's shows. That was where the guaranteed work – and the guaranteed money – was, after all. Despite the sheer, unmitigated glee of *Do Not Adjust Your Set*, there was still a little bit of Terry that saw himself as a writer who performed, rather than a performer who wrote. On 14 June 1968, Terry was commissioned to write material for each programme in a series of six called *Broaden Your Mind*. Subtitled 'An Encyclopaedia of the Air', this was produced by Sydney Lotterby, whose name had been used for multiple idiotic characters in *At Last the 1948 Show*. Lotterby clearly had not been offended, or had not watched the programme, for *Broaden Your Mind* starred *1948 Show*'s Tim Brooke-Taylor. This material was very similar to what Terry was writing for *It's Marty* at the time, a show which Tim was also heavily involved in. Very much in the vein of *Twice a Fortnight*, with sketches written and, in the main, performed by Graeme Garden and Bill Oddie, in the end *Broaden Your Mind* also included filmed inserts, many written by and featuring Terry and Michael.

To Terry, though, these were really just bits and bobs, contributions to help out the production and, frankly, to earn him a little extra beer money. Increasingly, it was the long-form narrative rather than a silly sketch that was of interest to him. In February 1968, he and Mike had accepted a joint fee of £450 to write a thirty-minute script for *Comedy Playhouse*. The series had first launched in 1962 as a showcase for writers Ray Galton and Alan Simpson. That first batch had begotten the sitcom smash *Steptoe and Son*, and by 1968 *Comedy Playhouse* was an active playground for lots of writers, all trying out fresh and, hopefully, funny ideas from which, possibly, just possibly, a full-blown series would emerge. In the early Seventies, *Last of the Summer Wine* and *Are You Being Served?* started under its auspices.

In the end, although Terry and Michael adhered to the urgent nature of the contract, for the script to be delivered 'as soon as possible', the BBC turned down the effort. The aborted *Comedy Playhouse* script was 'The Dangerous Animal Policy', and John Cleese was set to star as Mr Burster, a zookeeper who hated cuddly animals and only wanted to keep cold-blooded killers. Ideally, lions and tigers and bears, oh my. Still, good ideas never die, they merely bide their time. And this one bided its time for a long, long time – twenty-five years, in actual fact.

Following the smash international hit of *A Fish Called Wanda* in 1988, John Cleese telephoned Terry with a notion. He explained that he had a brilliant idea of extending the half-hour script of 'The Dangerous Animal Policy', as long as they weren't thinking of doing anything with it. To be honest, Terry had pretty much forgotten about it, so he said, 'Fine'. When Terry told Michael, he was furious. The first thing he said was: 'Didn't you talk money?' But Terry was always sure John would see them right, as it were, and he had been fairly generous. John's film, *Fierce Creatures*, was eventually released in 1997. Mike was in the cast again, of course, along with fellow *A Fish Called Wanda* stars Kevin Kline and Jamie Lee Curtis. Ronnie Corbett and Robert Lindsay were cast too, but not Terry. Knowing Terry, he would have licked his wounds, shrugged his resigned shoulders and listened to *The Beatles Anthology*. The group that Terry and Mike had loved since the Sixties was breaking all kinds of records, once again, in the 1990s. Now in his comfortable comedy skin, Terry was as free as a bird too. Free to do what he damned well pleased. To be creative for the sheer fun of it.

# CHAPTER SIX

## 1969 AND ALL THAT

*My shirt was sitting next to me*
*One sweltering Summer's day*
*When suddenly it yawned, got up,*
*Then stretched, and walked away!*

IN that last year of the Swinging Sixties, when men walked on the moon for the very first time and Jimi Hendrix closed the over-running Woodstock Festival as the sun rose on a bleary Monday morning, the wheels were set in motion for a BBC comedy sketch show that would change, cement and secure Terry's life and work for the rest of his days. And beyond.

*Monty Python's Flying Circus*, which took flight in October 1969, really was a pivotal moment. A slow start, almost underground cult success, that would blossom into a surreal, internationally acclaimed universe of bizarre comedy. Not that Terry, or any of them, would have known that at the time. It was just another sketch show. Sacrilegious? Hardly. Even if it continually claimed to have a sketch that would be 'Something Completely Different', those something-completely-differents would go on to become such a familiar part of the society it aimed to debunk that it would be categorised, even pigeonholed, as Pythonesque.

Still, for Terry, 1969 started much like any other year. He was still feverishly writing for other, well-established, solidly well-respected figures in British entertainment. The previous August he had capitulated and signed up to write skits and sketches for

Dora Bryan's television series *According to Dora*, mainly to appease and reassure his agent, Brian Codd, who still wasn't sure about a comedy sketch show for kids. And yet, *Do Not Adjust Your Set* had been given another seasonal special, *Do Not Adjust Your Stocking*, this time on the Christmas Day of 1968 itself – and, on this occasion, the powers that be even managed to stick the correct tape on. Although the show was now beaming out from Thames Television and under new management.

Much more respectable in the eyes of some was the gloriously crusty, military bearing of Kenneth Horne. He had been broadcasting since the war and had been one of the comedians Terry had tuned in to. In the late Sixties, Horne was still the safe pair of hands for the comedic grotesques of the radio sketch show *Round the Horne* to gambol around. The show was written by Barry Took and Marty Feldman – two figures who loom large in Terry's legend – and Terry was one of the last to write for Horne, contributing one-liners to the Thames telly show *Horne A'Plenty*, which came to an end on New Year's Day 1969, just six weeks before Horne's untimely death at the age of sixty-one. Meanwhile, Marty Feldman's colourful flagship BBC2 sketch show *It's Marty* – for which Terry was still writing – had returned for a second and final run at the end of 1968 – the last episode aired on Monday 13 January 1969.

As for *Do Not Adjust Your Set*'s originating producer Humphrey Barclay, he was now working under the guidance of Frank Muir, at London Weekend Television. Frank Muir had, of course, been the wet nurse to Terry's career over at the BBC. Barclay recalls that Muir was still 'God to a lot of us, and one mad day Frank came along waving a script! He said it was written by my friends Terry Jones and Michael Palin . . . and was really very good, albeit with an unnecessarily long title!' This was *The Complete and Utter History of Britain*.

Barclay's immediate response was indeed that: 'the scripts were a joy . . . and very demanding!' He wasn't kidding. Within the first few sketches, the script called for a location shot within Stonehenge, which cast Terry as a rather awkward, jittery, child-like potential home-buyer – the home being Stonehenge, of course. Although Terry had filmed *Twice a Fortnight* at Stonehenge, *Complete and Utter* was denied access to the sacred site, which necessitated a duplicate Stonehenge to be constructed on the South Downs. Out of enormous polythene blocks: 'As one of these things was hauled into position, I remember thinking, "This must have been what it was actually like!"' Terry recalled.

*The Complete and Utter History of Britain* knew no bounds. If it wasn't rebuilding Stonehenge, it was King Canute holding back the waves. It was certainly all too much for David Bell, the director who Humphrey Barclay initially assigned to the project. More used to staging song and dance spectaculars, Bell panicked and put his hands up in defeat. In fact, he disappeared from a scheduled meeting at Barclay's flat twenty minutes before Terry and Michael arrived to meet their director. The call was out to get somebody else and Frank Muir suggested Maurice Murphy, a wonderful, eccentric, curly-haired Australian who had directed the ambitious variety show *I'm Alright Now*, for the Australian Broadcasting Commission, before becoming something of a Muir protégé since joining LWT in 1968. Murphy stayed with LWT until 1971, steering the first few episodes of *Doctor in the House* to popularity, as well as Ronnie Barker's influential sketch show *Hark at Barker*.

For *The Complete and Utter History of Britain*, Barclay's plan was to have Terry and Michael front and centre of the sketches, with a supporting cast of good, reliable comedy actors. There was even a wild, brief thought to include the rest of the *Do Not Adjust Your Set* team too, but Barclay decided this should be a star vehicle for Terry and Mike. And Terry and Mike agreed. The promise of more of the roles they had written to play, and more editorial control, was very attractive. Indeed, Barclay's maxim was always, but always to be truest to the sense of humour of the writer: 'you ignore the writer at your peril!'

This ambition wasn't helped, though, by the powers that be at LWT considering the seven scripts proposed for the series as a little underwhelming. It was swiftly suggested and decided that the material was only strong enough to sustain six episodes. This was frustrating to say the least, particularly as it was after the fact of all the material being filmed, but, rather than risk the cancellation of the entire series, Terry agreed that episodes one and two should be spliced together to make episode one. Even though the decision rankled; for years after, Terry would recall that they weren't particularly brilliant episodes, although certainly good enough. Two very funny shows, reduced to one extremely funny episode. Looking back on it, it was quite insulting, but Terry was used to seeing his sketches reworked and rejected, with Marty Feldman, and *The Frost Report*. And Terry would still be fighting for his sketches when they 'went back to the BBC for the wider group of Python, of course!', he would say with a wry grin. Not to mention, as the Stonehenge debacle would prove, the squishing together of two episodes still held more than enough ambitious material for a limited television unit to cope with.

In the end, *The Complete and Utter History of Britain* remained a mouthful of a title for a show reduced to six episodes. Namely 1. 'From the Dawn of History to the Norman Conquest'. 2. 'Richard the Lionheart to Robin the Hood'. 3. 'Edward the First to Richard the Last'. 4. 'Perkin Warbeck to Bloody Mary'. 5. 'The Great and Glorious Age of Elizabeth'. 6. 'James the McFirst to Oliver Cromwell'.

The basic premise at the core of Terry and Michael's comedy chords for *The Complete and Utter History of Britain* was what if television cameras had been around at major turning points in our collective heritage? It was modern technology recording and reflecting upon such epoch-making moments as the Battle of Hastings, which was related like a post-football match interview in the communal bath. The Roman invasion of Britain was shown as a home movie, with a dull, repetitive and unnecessary running commentary: 'That's me getting on the boat . . .' Samuel Pepys and Oliver Cromwell were pitted against each other, but in the environment of a television studio political chat show debate. Then there was the non-event of the 1065 scrapbook, with merchants moaning that nothing ever happened and that their souvenirs marking the year are pointless . . . and that they would not be bothering next year. Like, nothing's going to happen in 1066 either, right? In the fifth episode, William Shakespeare – actually four actors all playing the famous scribe – were found reciting their latest sonnet all at the same time. So far, so Python.

In the main, *The Complete and Utter History of Britain* was achieving what Terry wanted it to achieve. That being a somewhat daredevil, revue-like freedom of comic expression. Sketches that would look right, and felt funny. You can see the clear intention in Terry's performances from the very start of the series. In a celebration of prehistoric Britons, who stand to attention for 'Rule Britannia', Terry is cheeky, pulling faces and enjoying himself. This is comedy acting based on the pratfall and the slapstick. Grappling with a blond nymphet, Terry's prehistoric Briton quickly learns how to use his hands. So far, so Benny Hill. However, this mixture of sauce and serious history was what *The Complete and Utter History of Britain* was all about.

However, the show, although a Bayeux Tapestry of importance in the timeline of sketch comedy, received decidedly mixed reviews when it was transmitted, late on Sunday evenings – just before 11 p.m. – in the January and February of 1969. The *Sun*, commenting on that very first episode, considered it a 'self-indulgent, unfunny jumble', while Peter Black, writing for the *Daily Mail*, reasonably reasoned that it was: 'undergraduate if you don't like it and fresh and gay if you do.'

The comedy certainly was fresh. Thirty years later, its style of relating history with a contemporary twist was polished and reinvented by the *Horrible History* brigade. Indeed, so innovative had *The Complete and Utter History of Britain* been that, in the late 1990s, Columbia Television tentatively discussed re-filming all the sketches anew. They were not of an age, but for all time.

Humphrey Barclay had brought together a stellar cast of performers, some of whom fitted Terry's requirements perfectly. Diana Quick, who had been a contemporary of Michael Palin's at Oxford and, indeed, had been part of the troupe of the 1965 Edinburgh Festival Fringe show *The Oxford Line*, was very much in tune with the gang's mentality. Michael, as performer, writer, producer and director of *The Oxford Line*, was aided and abetted by Terry's beloved *Hang Down Your Head and Die* colleague David Wood. Terry had started working for the BBC by then, of course, but still had an old, unused sketch, 'Tinpally', included in the revue. So Diana Quick understood Terry's humour instinctively. Colin Gordon, however, seemed less in step with the style of *The Complete and Utter History of Britain*. A distinguished stage actor and director, and part of the backbone of officious authority figures in British film and television, Gordon was drafted in as the narrator-cum-host-cum-historical-pundit within the studio setting. Brilliant as pompous doctors and humourless men from the ministry, here he was a sort of ringmaster. Gordon's erudite delivery and newsreader demeanour was to act as a linking device between the silly sketches. But he appeared unable to get the intrinsic joke at the heart of the series – this was a send-up of earnest broadcasters. For Terry, Colin Gordon just delivered the dialogue as if hosting a serious history.

Having taken against Colin Gordon, Terry began to find fault in the supporting cast of the sketches too. Even thoroughly dependable character actors like Wallace Eaton, who had been part of Frank Muir's repertory company since the radio days of *Take It from Here*, and Johnny Vyvyan, diminutive stooge to Tony Hancock and Benny Hill, were deemed ill-matched to the style

Terry wanted. Still, Terry was most distressed by the wide-eyed overacting of Roddy Maude-Roxby as the manic Professor Weaver. Terry couldn't quite believe Roddy. In every sense. He was a lovely bloke, but he was an actor who thought comedy was only funny if it was shouted and performed in a very 'funny' way. But the scripts were funny. The laughs were in the writing, not in an exaggerated performance.

Some of the comedy supporting actors did fit Terry's vision though. Lanky and bald John Hughman would crop up in all six episodes. He would crop up in Python too, playing such diverse characters as a gasman and Alfred Lord Tennyson, as well as enjoying roles in *Jabberwocky* and *Time Bandits*. He was out of work for the last decade of his life, and, unbeknown to anyone but immediate family, Terry made sure Hughman was happily looked after in a residential home until the end of his days. He would even visit him often to check in on him. And, thirty-odd years after the series was made, Terry could admit that he may have been a bit harsh on some of the other *Complete and Utter* performers too.

In 2014, Terry and Mike were invited to re-record some material that had been lost in the archives for a special DVD release of the series – *The New (Incomplete) Complete and Utter History of Britain*. Terry rewatched the surviving footage from 1969 and he felt he may have been wrong in his initial judgement of Colin Gordon. 'He was really very, very good. Maybe I've got nicer with age or something, but what Colin did was brilliant. Very funny. Very dry. He was perfect, actually. Playing it straight, a bit like John [Cleese] would do, was the right balance with what me and Mike were doing. I must have been a hot-headed youth, anxious for exactly what I had written. To be honest, I'm rather sorry I never had the opportunity to say how good Colin was to him and I'm rather sorry more of Colin's performance isn't around.'

Sadly, Terry wouldn't be around for the final historical twist concerning *The Complete and Utter History of Britain*. The missing material wasn't actually missing . . . and never had been. For in 2023, all the episodes of the series were found to have been safely gathered in and stored in an incorrectly labelled set of film cans within the ITV vaults. This comedy milestone could now be made available to the nation, albeit unceremoniously dumped onto BritBox with absolutely no historical fanfare whatsoever. Did Terry and Michael waste their time re-filming material in 2014 that was actually already extant in the archives? Of course not. Now we have the lot. From both 1969 and 2014. It's Complete and Utter beyond complete and utter . . .

But, wait a minute. Is nobody interested in history? 1969 history, that is. *The Complete and Utter History of Britain* was broadcast to something of a splat rather than a clap in 1969, but the Wednesday after that last Sunday-night episode on 16 February saw the full-on return of Terry's flagship writing and performing pride and joy, *Do Not Adjust Your Set*, following on from the Thames Christmas special. Terry's faithful Oxford champion Ian Davidson had produced the show, with Adrian Cooper directing. And it was still marketed as a children's show, with a reassuringly child-friendly slot of 5.20 p.m. Throughout this run of thirteen episodes, culminating in the middle of May 1969, Terry enacted some weird and wonderful scenarios. He was particularly proud of another sketch about Concorde, the super-sonic jet plane that made its maiden flight and plenty of headlines while the show was airing. It was a pretty straightforward sketch about tea-drinking English boffins who get it wrong and think Concorde is an ocean-going ship. Terry and Michael are hard at work on HMS *Concorde*, much to David Jason's Frenchman's bewildered chagrin. Still, as Terry said: 'It made me laugh, anyway!' and that was always the point.

And, in echoes of Monty Python, so close now it hurts, each episode of *Do Not Adjust Your Set* was given a hilarious alternative title, ranging from *The Loose Denture Show* to *The Original*

*Broadway (Ealing) Cast*! Typically, Terry and Michael were writing as a team, with Eric Idle on his own. Then the three would come together, fashion the structure of the shows and shape the scripts. Graeme Garden, who was sharing a flat with his Cambridge contemporary at the time, recalls that: 'in a way our flat was the breeding ground for Python. Eric would invite Terry and Mike around a lot, and they would be writing sketches and chatting about the show. And, later on, a crazy American would start appearing there too!'

That crazy American was the crucial addition to the London Weekend Television editions of *Do Not Adjust Your Set*, for now this already extremely strong sketch-writing base was cemented, supported and made even stronger with the animations of Terry Gilliam.

Terry J. was, at first, a little suspicious of Terry G.: 'Here was this American guy, sat in the corner, in this strange, huge sheepskin coat. With all these psychedelic patterns actually painted on it!' Now, it's uncertain whether it was merely coat envy – Terry Jones having been known for his big fluffy coat at Oxford – or quite reasonable feelings that, with Terry's history of brilliant stop-motion film-making, this new Terry chap couldn't offer anything that our Terry couldn't have done himself, but something rankled. Moreover, there was within Terry Jones a sense of nervousness at some unknown quantity coming into the show. His show.

He had by this point slowly but surely eased himself into the spearhead position on *Do Not Adjust Your Set*, ingratiating himself more and more with the production side. Ian Davidson, of course, was more than keen to embrace Terry's input, as he had done in the earliest days of Oxford. For Terry, 'we had to get everything absolutely right'. He would later ruminate and conclude that he was trying to control everything on behalf of the group. He did get a little anxious if new people came in and tried to tear off in a different direction. And, a little like David Jason simply taking on the rudiments of Captain Fantastic, Terry felt he was the best person to interpret his own scripts.

Terry trusted and admired Eric Idle, though, and, for Eric, Terry Gilliam and that coat were of equal fascination. It had been bought in Turkey while Terry G. had been hitchhiking and it was a talking point, for sure. The animator angle was also of interest to Eric. Terry and Mike soon clicked with the fascination too. Ultimately, Terry Gilliam would bond and fall in with the Oxford boys over the Cambridge contingent within Python's tight-knit group. And it was Terry G.'s animations that struck Terry J. as the key to making his comedy truly stand out. The unique selling point, as marketing executives would have it today.

Although a lot less of this second series of *Do Not Adjust Your Set* survives in the archives, several of the groundbreaking Gilliam animations do. The one that Terry Jones talked about and analysed endlessly at the time, and for decades after, that students of television would point to as a breakthrough moment, was a little Gilliam cartoon called 'Beware of the Elephants' that starts with an unsuspecting man ignoring the sign and being jumped on by a pachyderm. It is this sort of thing that Terry Jones saw as the future. Following his initial hesitancy, in those dying days of *Do Not Adjust Your Set* he had quite quickly embraced Gilliam, and encouraged him to go further and further with the outrageousness of the animations: 'it was this stream of consciousness. No real theme to it, it just went from one very funny idea to the next. I thought, "This is it! The lightbulb moment. All comedy should be like that!"'

With Terry Gilliam now within Terry Jones's trusted inner sanctum, the four-man creative group of *Do Not Adjust Your Set* became very tight indeed. Our Terry admitted that his determination to do right by the show could be seen as stubborn, even aggressive at times, but his vision was clear. If he was very guarded about everything, it was because he was so aware of things getting diluted and ruined. There was always a fight to get anything onto the screen in the way that he had imagined it. Indeed, there were so many things that Michael and Terry had written that had been altered, so many things that had been screened in a form they disliked. Terry's defensiveness simply came from the barriers he always seemed to face in getting his own stuff together and the feeling that somebody else would then take them off in a totally different direction. Though not all alternative directions are bad, of course.

This second series of *Do Not Adjust Your Set* had been enjoying a repeat season, aired at 7 p.m. because the channel was getting complaints from company directors that their employees had been leaving work early on Wednesdays in order to get home in time to watch. Which made Terry very happy. There was now a very appealing offer on the table to make the core comedy of *Do Not Adjust Your Set* into an evening sketch show, aimed at the adult audience who had been, rather clandestinely, enjoying the original. Terry was particularly excited about a suggestion that he could be even more hands-on with regards to directing the shows. And LWT was eagerly outlining a plan to give them forty-five minutes per week.

In the event, as often happens in the business, nothing came of it. Michael Palin, for one, was reluctant to plough on with more *Do Not Adjust Your Set*, even if he and Terry were to be given a lot more freedom within the framework of a show for adults. Terry agreed that the fundamental joy of it had been subversive jokes for a junior audience. Not to mention that their silly sketch show for adults, *The Complete and Utter History of Britain*, had faced uncertainty from both the public and the production heads. An adult take on *Do Not Adjust Your Set* needed something else. Something just a little different. Something more from the Cambridge Footlights . . .

Although John Cleese, an avid follower of the Oxford boys, had phoned Michael Palin following the airing of the last episode of *Complete and Utter* and basically written it off by saying, 'Well, you won't be making any more of those, will you?' he and his writing partner Graham Chapman were admirers of *Do Not Adjust Your Set*. For Terry, the admiration was mutual.

Terry had loved what Graham and John had done in *At Last the 1948 Show*, from the autumn of 1967. Their sketches had an anxiety and a rage hilariously funnelled through John's pent-up performances and Graham's other-worldly vagueness. And of course Terry and Mike and Eric and John and Graham had rubbed shoulders at the Edinburgh Fringe and on *The Frost Report* and within the Marty Feldman writers' room. It's very fair to say that Mike and Terry were being influenced by John and Graham, in terms of how and what they were writing at that time. They were impressed by the surreal elements of what they were doing, when the sketches took off on real flights of fancy. And fantasy. At those sketch read-throughs, Terry would just sit back and wonder: 'How on earth did they think of that?' Graham and John had delivered, week in and week out, the cream of the crop for both David Frost and Marty Feldman, so it would certainly have been in Terry's mind to keep those special talents close within a writing and performing collective.

In May 1969, John and Graham attended the recording of an episode of *Do Not Adjust Your Set* – suitably enough for the final episode, broadcast on Wednesday 14 May 1969 – and, in a historic summit meeting, they hooked up with the two Terrys, Eric and Mike. Palin says that: 'we all got together at my house, got hungry, and went to the Light of Kashmir for a curry. All I can remember is that we argued about who would pay the bill, but we did talk about maybe doing some comedy together. As a team.'

Less than two months later, the first Python sketches were being shot. Fundamentally, it was *Do Not Adjust Your Set*, in colour, for adults. At that time, in the late 1960s, Huw Wheldon was in control of BBC1 and David Attenborough ran BBC2. Both were very enlightened men. Terry remembered them saying that the BBC was very much an anarchic organisation in a way, in that there was very little bureaucracy or personnel management. That anarchy appealed to Terry. Such personnel management as there was shared one tiny office, as opposed to occupying an entire building as they went on to do. The producer would be handpicked from the pool of BBC staff and would have a programme assigned to them by their head of department. The producers were the ones who decided what was going to go on the air and they took full responsibility for the programmes they made. As Terry wistfully recounted: 'If somebody objected to something that had gone out, then the producer would be asked to account for himself. But it was all after the fact; there was no censorship at all.' I'm sure you can see the appeal.

What Terry knew was that he wanted to keep his gang together and head back to the BBC. It was a corporation Terry knew, understood and, grudgingly, respected; and, perhaps foolishly, like the offer at LWT, he thought he could have complete control over the product at the BBC too. So Terry went to Barry Took in the hope of a brand new sketch show, for the BBC, with Mike and Eric and Terry G. in tow. Took, who until June 1968 had been head writer on radio comedy *Round the Horne*, had been something of a comedy patron. When offered *The Complete and Utter History of Britain*, he had liked it, although he'd promptly sold it on to Frank Muir at London Weekend Television. During that final flurry of *Do Not Adjust Your Set*, Took had been making noises about coaxing Terry and Michael back to the BBC. Certainly he thought it would be something of a feather in his cap getting them over from commercial television. In response to the tentative approaches, Terry was insistent that Eric and the other Terry be in it too, though.

While all this was going on, John Cleese had been really wooing Michael Palin. Indeed, Michael had worked with John, Graham and Tim Brooke-Taylor in the London Weekend Television one-off comedy special *How to Irritate People* in November 1968. Terry remembered that: 'John phoned Mike with the suggestion of doing a series together.' And, just as Terry had been loyal to Michael with regards to making sure he got to work on *Do Not Adjust Your Set*, Michael was, in turn, loyal to Terry: 'To be honest, I think John just wanted to work with Mike, but I came as part of the deal!'

Many millions of words have been written about Monty Python, some of them even by me. Suffice to say here were six young men, hungry for creativity – once their hunger had been sated by that curry – and eager to fully cross-fertilise their styles and strengths. Terry and Mike and Eric and John and Graham had been swimming in the same comedy ken for most of the 1960s, and Gilliam's animation was the added ingredient that would make the sketches flow. When cajoled to ponder the roots of Python a little deeper, Terry Jones would be characteristically perceptive and eager to reason on what exactly was the key to its success. On the one hand he would say: 'It was just another sketch show really, wasn't it?' And however a Python devotee could argue that, no, it was something much more than that, in its basic form, on paper, that's exactly what it was. For Terry, there was one element that made it stand out, which was simple but essential: 'We had colour! That's it really, it was John and Graham doing what they had done in black and white on *The '48 Show*, and the rest of us doing what we had done on *Do Not Adjust* in colour. I mean, that's putting it simply, but that's what it was. If we had made Python a year earlier, maybe even six months earlier, it would have been in black and white, and maybe forgotten about. Who knows?'

Who knows, indeed. An imponderable, but what is a cast-iron fact is that *It's Marty* – which made a star of *1948 Show*'s Marty Feldman, with Tim Brooke-Taylor willingly sticking with it as his chief support stooge – had broken the sketch show, in colour, on BBC2, in the spring of 1968. Benny Hill, and Peter Cook and

Dudley Moore had been tempted over to ATV. Still that Benny Hill special, which followed *Do Not Adjust Your Set*, and the Pete 'n' Dud series *Goodbye Again*, in April and May 1968, were shot in colour but screened in black and white. It was David Frost who launched commercial colour television, in November 1969. A year earlier, in the autumn of 1968, *The Morecambe & Wise Show*, recorded and broadcast in colour, made its debut on BBC2. Still, Marty Feldman was the corporation's flagship comedian in colour.

Less than a month after *It's Marty* had come to an end, the corporation couldn't leave Feldman be. And Terry was back in harness in the writers' room. On 2 March 1969 an internal BBC memo had recorded the fact that Terry was writing more and more slapstick antics for Feldman. Indeed, one extended, on-film and on-location sequence, cast Marty as a bowler-hatted business-man. The comedy camera would follow him as he left home for work in the morning: '*but is then broken by Marty Feldman crash-ing through the front door and leaping over the gate.*' This was the homage to Buster Keaton and Harold Lloyd that would become known as 'Stuntman Goes to Work', utilising the familiar iconog-raphy of a City gent within the incongruity of the dangerous and precisely timed career of a professional fall guy. This particular, unforgettable foray into physical, wordless slapstick was the centrepiece of the programme *Colour Me Marty*. A further colour-ful one-off show, *Marty Amok*, would follow early in 1970. And Terry was still happily in that writing room. The corporation was a hub of comedy. Ideas fizzing and developing like hilarious Catherine wheels.

Indeed, BBC2 was the place that was really something of an experimental playground. BBC1 didn't offer a full colour televi-sion service until Saturday 15 November 1969, a day before the first transmission of the fifth episode of that first series of *Monty Python's Flying Circus*. Thus, that opening month of Monty Python, in full colour, was something of a novelty, something, if not completely different, then a treat. A colourful treat. And it was a treat 200,000 homes were now enjoying. That BBC and ITV colour television service had doubled the viewing audience – in March 1969 there had been just 100,000 colour sets across the country.

For Terry, this liberating and encouraging time at the BBC was personified by Barry Took, the champion of his comedy, whose utter, blind faith in the team saw them dubbed *Von Took's Flying Circus* for a time. It was thanks to Took that this idea of a new sketch show, utilising comedy talent well established on commercial television, landed upon the desk of Michael Mills. Again, the anecdotes are so well told there are leather patches on their elbows, but it is true, as Michael Palin attests, that Michael Mills really did say to them that he wasn't completely sure about Monty Python but that he trusted them . . . and he said, 'you can only have thirteen half-hours. And that's it!' It's become almost apocryphal now, but it really did happen. As Michael says, they didn't argue! Of course. They took those six and a half hours with alacrity!

Mills, an extremely experienced producer, had been the head of comedy at the BBC since 1967; he had been attached to the BBC before the war, and had rejoined in 1947. That military expertise within comedy again. That BBC stamp of authority. The military veterans at work within the BBC and the military overtones of the *Flying Circus* title inspired overzealous copywriters at work on the official press release for the show to cast the main players within a fictional Second World War memoir. It was Mike 'Smudger' Palin and Terry 'Pud' Jones – which was a slightly kinder variation on what many of the inner sanctum of the team called Terry: 'the fat Welshman'! Terry was conscious of his fluctuating weight but far too excited to take any offence.

Terry relished at the BBC not only that freedom of creativity but that freedom from responsibility. The fact that, once a programme had been commissioned, the head of comedy would not interfere. Not at all. He would believe in the expertise and judgement of the show's producer who, for the first four shows, was John Howard Davies. The buck would stop with Davies, and it was Davies who took on any negative feedback from audience and the corporation alike. As a result, Terry would seize the opportunity to push the boundaries of good taste even further. To breaking point. Safe in the knowledge that their producer trusted them.

Subsequently, their director was Scottish madman Ian MacNaughton, who was also producing the show, and Terry would plead with him, even dare him to include a sketch that Michael and he had written. Or any of them, actually. The six of them were thinking as one. They agreed on what was good for Python. Against MacNaughton's better judgement he included some sketches that he really deemed far too controversial. With this freedom of expression, in full, glorious colour, Monty Python took flight. Not that it was instantly popular. Far from it.

Still, the BBC had faith in the team, and the team had faith in their comedy. Such confidence was laudable when you consider how extremely young they all were. Terry was just twenty-seven at the time he was writing the first series of Monty Python. The same age as Paul McCartney was when *Abbey Road* came out. The Beatles' end, as it happened, came almost in parallel with the Pythons' beginning. Like Paul, Terry would become the keeper of the flame for the group, the glue, the archivist and, as often as not, the one who would send out the rallying call when he felt it was time the group got back together and actually did something. Terry was, more than most, the one who drove Python forward. Even when he himself was unsure which direction it was going in.

It is undeniably pretty cool to have your own show, on BBC1, when you're still in your twenties. Michael Palin agrees: 'it is pretty cool, but that was the Sixties. Sorry to sound like an old man, but I am an old man! I'm unapologetic about that, and I'm unapologetic about the fact that the Sixties really were great.'

Quite a lot of things were able to take off in the Sixties. There was a much more relaxed attitude to experimentation, be it in music or fashion or art or comedy. If you had a good idea, you could do it. There was money around, there was confidence. The establishment was no longer the dead hand on comedy or culture. It was a good time to be able to try out new stuff. A very good time. The Pythons were sort of aware that, in comparison with the Fifties, there was a tangible freedom but, as Michael says: 'honestly, we didn't know how lucky we were. We had never had it so good, as old Harold Macmillan had said.' Having gone to London and found this whole atmosphere in the Sixties, they just thought that was the way the world was. They couldn't really compare it with what had gone before. There was no conscious judgement. That's just the way it was. Michael further reflects on that time: 'When you are young, you just carry on and do everything. Every opportunity that came along to write, and earn a bit of money, was very important to Terry and I.'

Even now, at the start of Python, it was a living. A job. A fun job, but a job nonetheless. Certainly, nobody in that initial meeting in the office of Michael Mills was aware or even dared to think that what they were about to do would rock the very foundations of comedy and establish a franchise that became so cataclysmic, so completely different.

The birth of Python, while revolutionary in terms of comedy, also coincided with Michael Palin's decision to give up smoking and take up keeping a diary. Terry had long kept a diary, although it could be a source of absolute panic for him. So busy would he be living his life and writing comedy that one, two, three, even four days would go by without him having written up his daily entry. Alison Telfer recalls that: 'by Friday Terry was frantic. He would say: "I've forgotten what I did on Monday!"' In the end, she advised him to keep notes of what a day had involved. Just bullet points on pads of white paper. Michael Palin was a little more strict on himself. The diary had been a way of helping him to give up cigarettes – it was either put pen to paper or give in and put a fag in his mouth. For Michael, it was pen to paper. He was dedicated to it, a little bit addicted to it. Sir Michael gracefully gave me permission to plunder and quote from his, at the time of publication, four-volume-strong collection of diaries: 'because Terry is all over them, obviously. Particularly in the first volume.' The discerning reader is advised, nay, urged, to acquire and devour the tomes. And, after such a fulsome recommendation, I will refrain from quoting them in great swathes here. Suffice to say, it is worth citing Michael's introduction to that first batch of diaries, in that: 'For the historians' sake I should probably have noted every detail of the birth of Monty Python, but it seemed far more important to me to record the emergence of my new family than the faltering steps of a comedy series that would probably last no more than two years. And that, I feel, is as it should be. Legends are not created by diaries, though they can be destroyed by them.'

Legends, indeed, although – thankfully – unknowing legends. That first snapshot of the group sees them relaxed and ever so slightly cocky. They look very much like a prog rock outfit. All apart from John Cleese, that is. In suit and tie and rather subversive sideburns, John looks like an area branch manager of a new town bank, about to refuse you an overdraft and smile as he does so. Perhaps the reason is that John knew he was on £300 a show from the BBC. The others were on £200. All, that is, apart from Terry Gilliam, whose animations and bits and bobs were earning him just £60 an episode.

In the photograph, Terry Jones is all tousled hair and crooked smile, a stunning 27-year-old, sporting a fairly tight pair of 'Kensington Gore'-coloured trousers and a pastel-pink shirt, haphazardly tucked in, and haphazardly unironed. The shirt sleeves are rolled up. He is ready for comedy action. It was taken on a blistering hot day in July. That first day of filming, Tuesday 8 July, to be precise, saw the team on location at Ham House, a seventeenth-century Jacobean pile on the bank of the River Thames, in Richmond.

In what could have been squeezed into or out of *The Complete and Utter History of Britain*, Terry's first filmed Python sketch saw him reassuringly in drag, a state in which he would find himself in many a Monty Python scene. In this pioneering Python moment, Terry is dressed as the Empress of India herself, Queen Victoria. Forever referred to as 'The Wacky Queen' sketch and a filmed insert included in the second episode of the series, this particular *Monty Python's Flying Circus* was given the alternative title of 'Sex and Violence'. In 'The Wacky Queen' sketch, it is Terry indulging in silent slapstick comedy again. The Queen Victoria footage starts off as a straight historical documentary though, with John Cleese intoning the serious commentary, before Michael Palin takes over and the narration morphs into that 'oh so crazy, oh so Sixties' compilation of 1920s comedy films. Terry was well aware of these compilations and would enjoy them, if only for the rare footage. Still, these cut-and-paste celebrations, which were thrown together by producer Robert Youngson, were ripe for parody. Indeed, Ronnie Barker and Ronnie Corbett had already sent them up on *The Frost Report*. These fast-paced salutes to the dawn of Hollywood were hugely popular throughout the Sixties, in an era when *It's a Mad, Mad, Mad, Mad World* and *The Great Race* and *Those Magnificent Men in Their Flying Machines* not only glorified slapstick humour but hoovered up several of the surviving exponents for one final custard pie in the kisser.

Terry displays real joy in giving the regal personage of Victoria some physical pratfalls to perform, stripping away that severe exterior of history to reveal the fun monarch behind the duty. Graham Chapman, as a chuckling Prime Minister William Gladstone, stooging like a pro, allows Terry to rip through this vintage romp. Terry lifts up the royal skirt and playfully sets up comic moment after comic moment. Ironically perhaps, in this black and white throwback amidst the show's other, more colourful sketches, Terry ends up with a bucket of white paint over his head and delivers a well-placed kick to the pants of the PM before a moment of custard-pie madness fades into a framed photograph and segues into the next sketch. A snapshot of affectionate cinematic send-up within a cutting-edge, inspirational collage of craziness. That Terry's first burst of energetic Python comedy that blazing day in the summer of '69 is so rooted in his passion for slapstick is history having its finger on the pulse of a comedy mind, totally by luck rather than judgement.

The following day, 9 July 1969, Terry, John, Graham and Michael were driven to the Church of St Mary Magdalene, in Boveney, near Windsor, for the Walter Scott sketch. The day after, Terry was in Bournemouth, billeted at the Durley Dean Hotel, in order to film on the beach and, by default, attract a huge crowd of onlookers and sightseers – who would see a great deal more than they had bargained for as he skilfully and amusingly took off his trousers in public! Friday 11 July saw the death of Genghis Khan – in terms of Python comedy, you understand – and two men carrying a donkey past a Butlin's redcoat.

After which Terry travelled back to London in a first-class train compartment with Michael, John and Graham, where they discussed the upcoming shows four and five, and happily reflected that the past week had been most excellent and extremely productive. It had been one of the great weeks. Enjoyable and historical. Still, that there is nothing really to differentiate these filming conditions and, indeed, the comedy of the sketches from say *Twice a Fortnight* or *Broaden Your Mind* or *The Complete and Utter History of Britain* merely reinforces the fact that Python was, yes, just another sketch show. It never started as radical, something different. It very much grew organically from the many, many sketch shows, many from Terry's own fertile imagination, that had come before.

It's also true to say that Terry was still very much a jobbing writer at the BBC during this, subsequently historic, few days filming wonderfully weird skits on the hoof. Just five days after he had happily dropped his kecks in front of wide-eyed holidaymakers in Dorset, his linking material for the pilot of the Alan Price and Georgie Fame-fronted variety show *The Price of Fame* was recorded. This musical and comical spectacular closed with Georgie belting out the Everly Brothers hit 'Bye Bye Love' and for Terry, pocketing seventy quid for his efforts, it was nothing different from what he had been doing for the BBC from the very beginning. Providing gloriously silly things to say for singers of gloriously silly love songs. Georgie Fame would be back at the Beeb, and back singing that same silly love song, for an edition of *The Two Ronnies*, in June 1972. And Terry would still be writing sketches for the show at the time. The Fred Tomlinson Singers would often appear too. Ronnies and Pythons. Not really a cigarette paper between them in terms of the writing process and the treatment of them within the BBC Light Entertainment Department.

On Wednesday 16 July 1969, Terry happily joined his fellow fledgling Pythons filming in Barnes, west London. While their world-beating comedy combination was heating up, the team sat down to watch real, living history on television, as Apollo 11 blasted off towards the moon. With glorious incongruity, Terry finished that historic day prancing about and getting a proper sweat on, in a mouse costume, for 'The Mouse Problem'. The centrepiece of the second episode of *Monty Python's Flying Circus*, it was a sketch that Ronnie Barker had baulked at during the *Frost Report* days. For Ronnie B. it was all too silly. Not unfunny. Just silly.

That Python episode too, despite being bumped to the second week, was the very first to have its sketches taped in front of a studio audience. The very first Python sketch proper put before an audience saw Terry as a bowler-hatted City gent enjoying an after-noon stroll in the country. He encounters Graham's smock-wearing local yokel farmer, and after some jolly good idle banter Terry spots that the farmer's sheep are nesting in the trees and attempting to fly. The fact that they plummet rather than take to the air like birds is the first twist of Python surrealism within a standard narrative. Terry's bluster, bafflement and bemused reac-tions allow for some of Graham's best Python acting, while Terry is, more subtly, our representative in a totally mad world. Terry, dressed for a City bank and the London underground, is us, having been minding our own business, suddenly finding the wackiness of Monty Python forced upon us.

Like the character Terry plays, that first audience were probably confused, some would have been momentarily outraged, but they were not bored. They would never ever be bored. That first Python audience was of old-age pensioners, many of whom were under the misguided impression that they were coming in to see an actual circus. There wasn't much of a reaction to the flying sheep sketch – just the quiet bewilderment of pensioners on a day out. This sketch too was from a stockpile of material rejected for *The Frost Report*. Again, the reason being it was too silly. Well, silly for sure . . . but too silly? Perish the thought. It further goes to empha-sise that, rather than being consciously innovative and unprece-dented, Python was, at its inception, a database for the silliest of comedy. That was the very point.

The nation at large would be treated to the very first episode of *Monty Python's Flying Circus*, unleashed on BBC1, from five minutes before 11 p.m. on Sunday 5 October 1969. In a television landscape that also included such safe staples as *Stars on Sunday*, *Mr. & Mrs.* and *The Wombles*, the *Radio Times* billed Python as a 'satire show', inauspicious and misrepresentative from the start.

Terry's very first appearance comes rather late in that opening episode, and his performance is rather subdued. He is a schoolteacher, keeping a record of squashed pigs from the previous sketch by scratching chalk lines through them on his blackboard. His subsequent attempts and joyful amazement at his largely Italian class grasping his Italian lessons so speedily is hardly the most riveting Python sketch. It's hardly the most riveting in the series or indeed in this episode, even, but it displays, unquestionably, a talent who has, as the closing credits will scream, conceived, written and performed the material, simply finding his feet, trying out the concept, seeing just how far he can take this concentrated stream of consciousness.

That very first broadcast moment of Terry as a Python doesn't have to be riveting. It just has to *be*. For, within moments, Terry is back. In the very next sketch he is now playing Arthur 'Two Sheds' Jackson in a television interview situation, desperately trying to discuss his latest symphony with Eric Idle, who, annoyingly, seems more interested in how he got his nickname of 'Two Sheds'. And Boom!, Terry is there. In familiar off-kilter, frustrated sketch character mode. A fully formed Python character and a product of that fertile and never-still creative comedy mind that had been active and often overactive for five years.

This first burst of Python was the culmination of Terry's comedy journey from Oxford. A full stop. A new beginning. As the Sixties vanished in the rear-view mirror, Terry was dropping comic bonbons and presenting grotesque characters that would live and live and live: the managing director of Whizzo Chocolate; the enthused and overambitious athlete who is determined to jump across the English Channel; the bowler-hatted, pub-dwelling City gent of the 'Nudge Nudge' sketch, he who is a man of the world, he's been there, he's been around, he's slept with a lady . . .

The very last time Terry would pop up on screen in the 1960s was on 28 December 1969, that glorious hinterland between Christmas and New Year, when episode eleven of *Monty Python's Flying Circus* was first broadcast. Although it was hardly planned as such, it

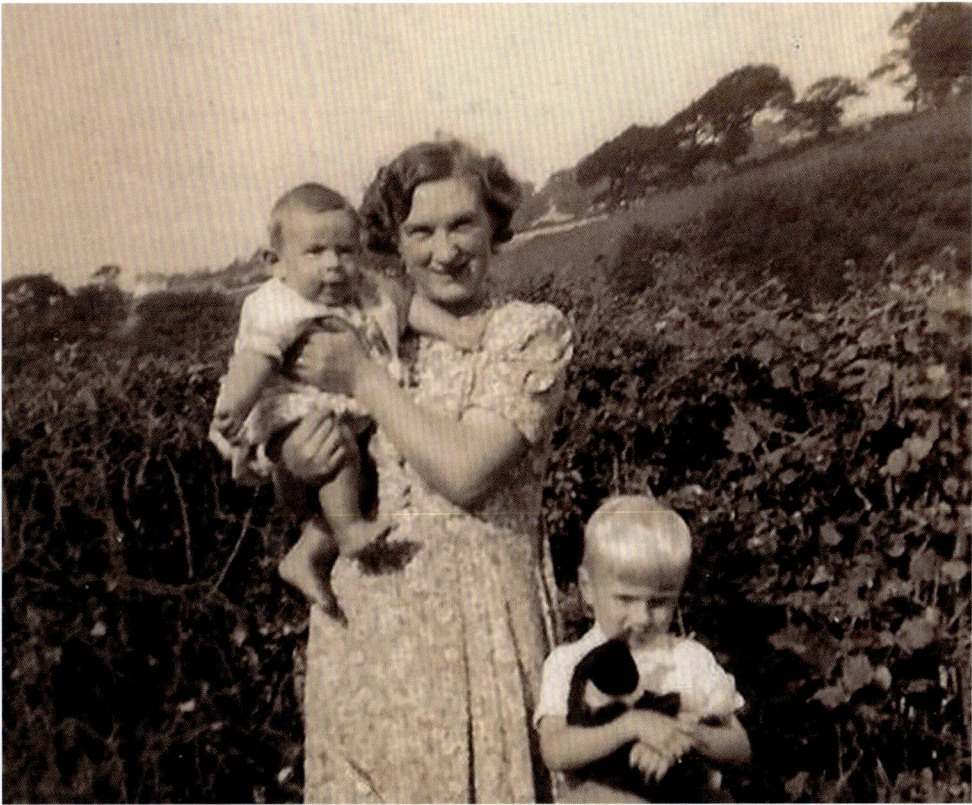

A babe in arms of mother Dilys, in the summer of 1942.
Brother Nigel clutches the family cat.

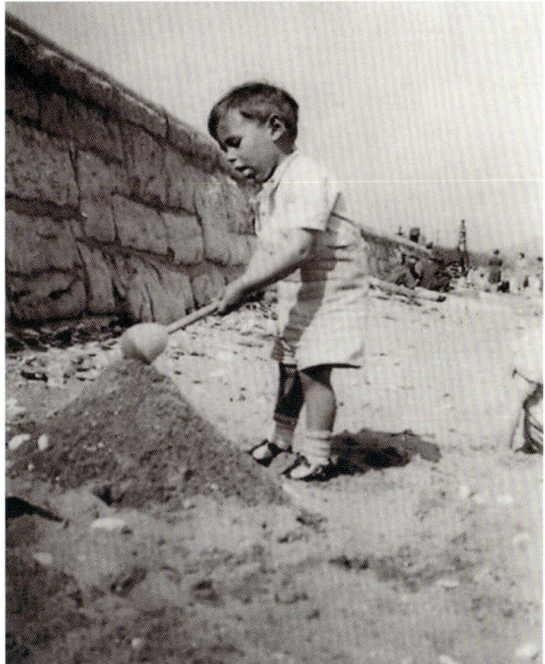

Terry's Happy Place I:
To allow Terry to speak for
himself: 'It's me in August
1944 on Colwyn Bay beach.
I'm two and a half years old.'

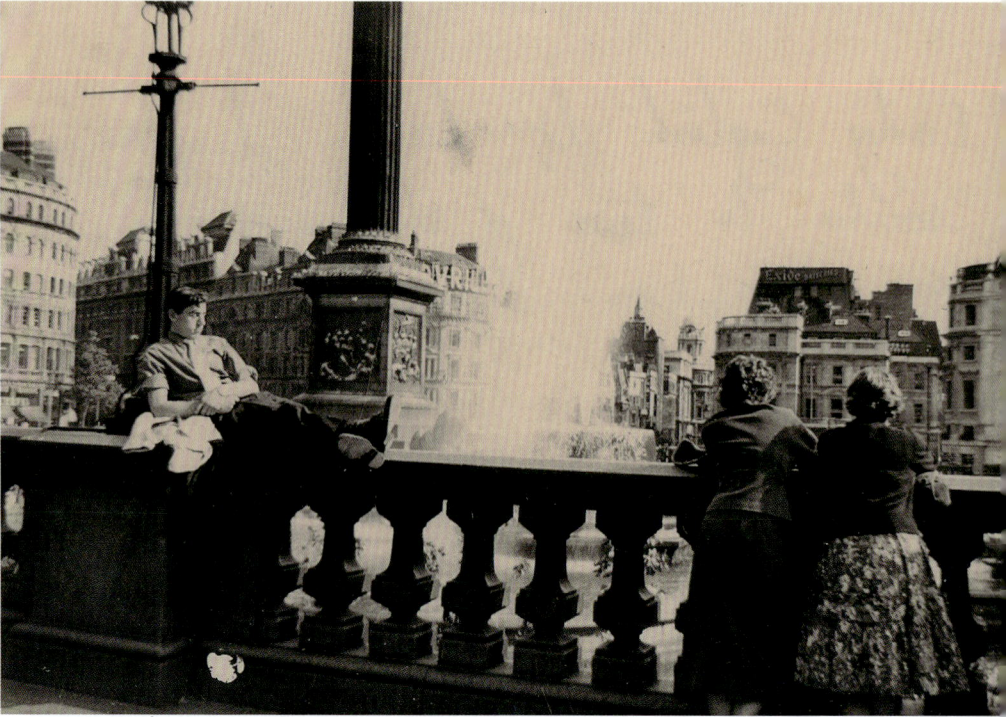

The brooding Welsh coolness already in place as a lounging teenager in
Trafalgar Square, London, in the late 1950s.

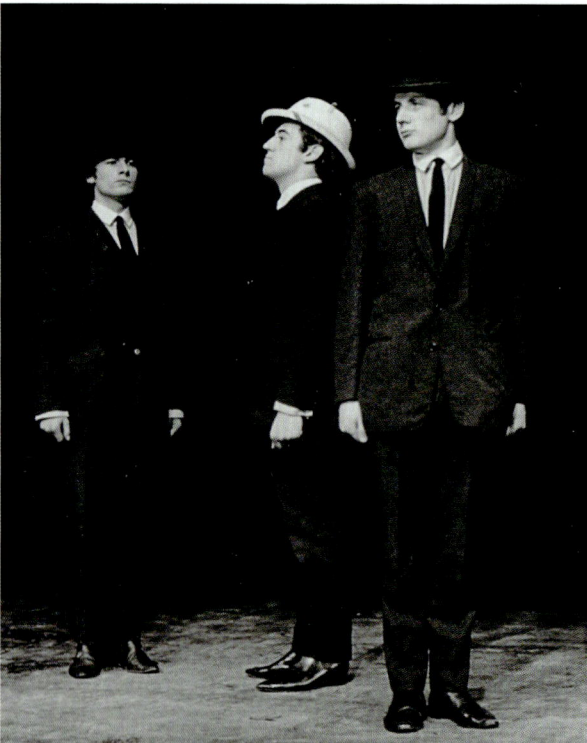

A Pith Helmet in a world
of bowler hats: with Doug
Fisher and Michael Palin in
*The Oxford Revue*, 1964.

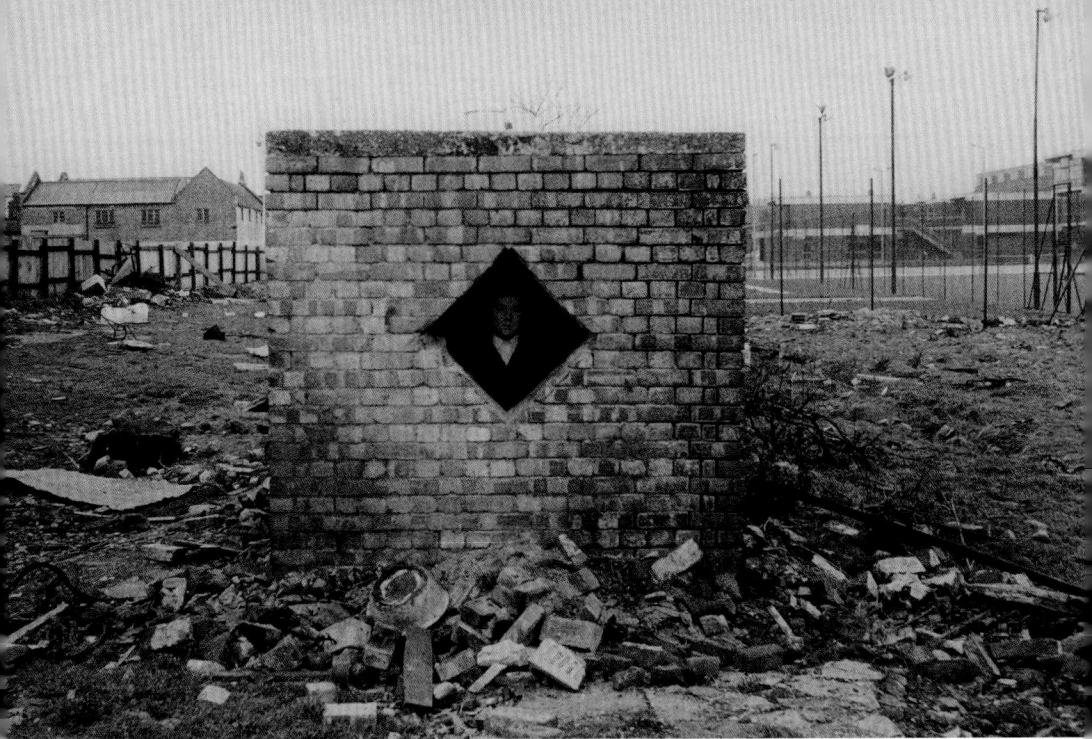

In the rubble of Lambeth Walk and with his comedy hero recently deceased, Terry channels his inner Buster Keaton, 1966.

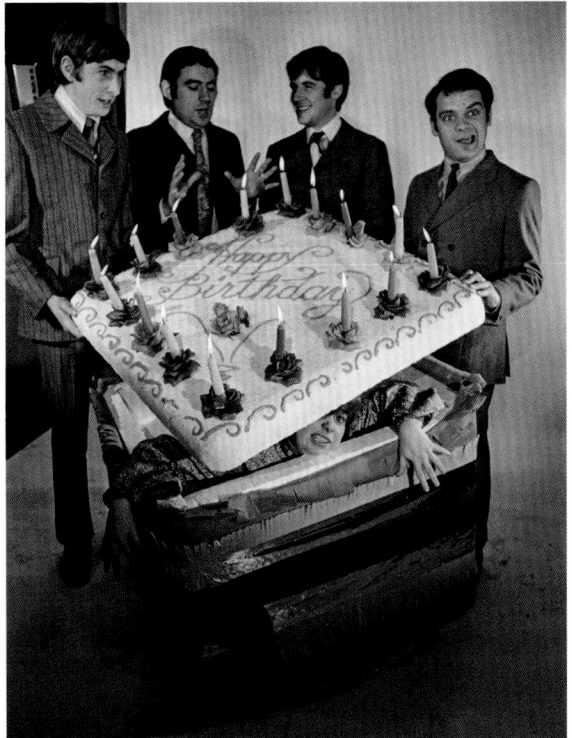

Denise Coffey's 21st birthday is celebrated during the making of the first episode of *Do Not Adjust Your Set*, on Tuesday, 12 December 1967. Denise is in the cake with Eric Idle, Michael Palin and David Jason gathered round. Terry is either warming his hands on the candles or about to grab a slice!

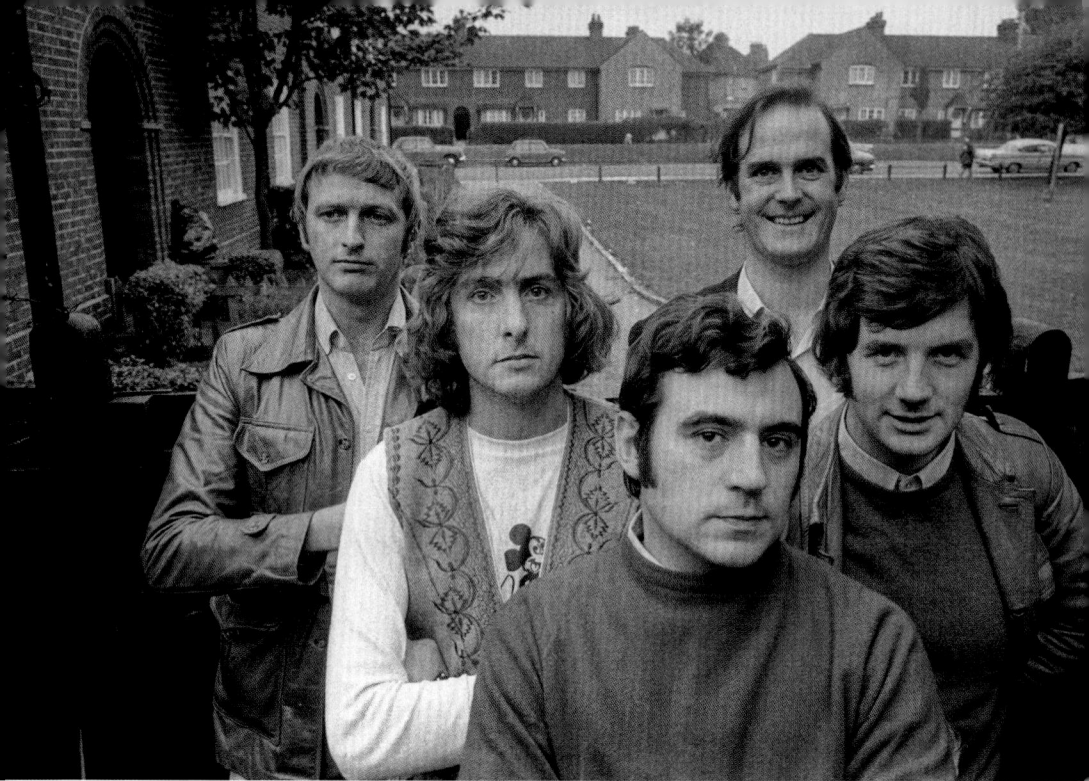

Terry, front and centre, already very much the self-assured glue of Monty Python in promotion for the second series, with Graham Chapman, Eric Idle, John Cleese and Michael Palin, October 1970.

Terry and Alison, happy and silly in the Garden of Python, at Grove Park, in the early 1970s.

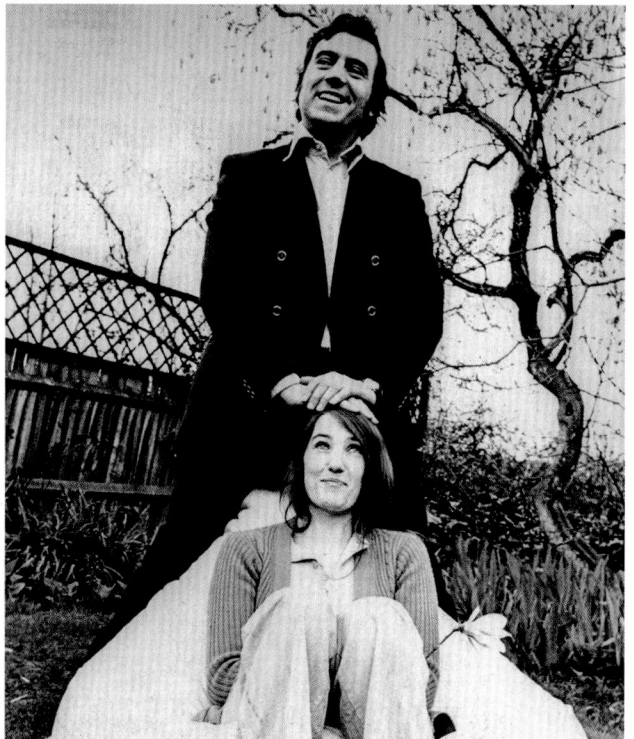

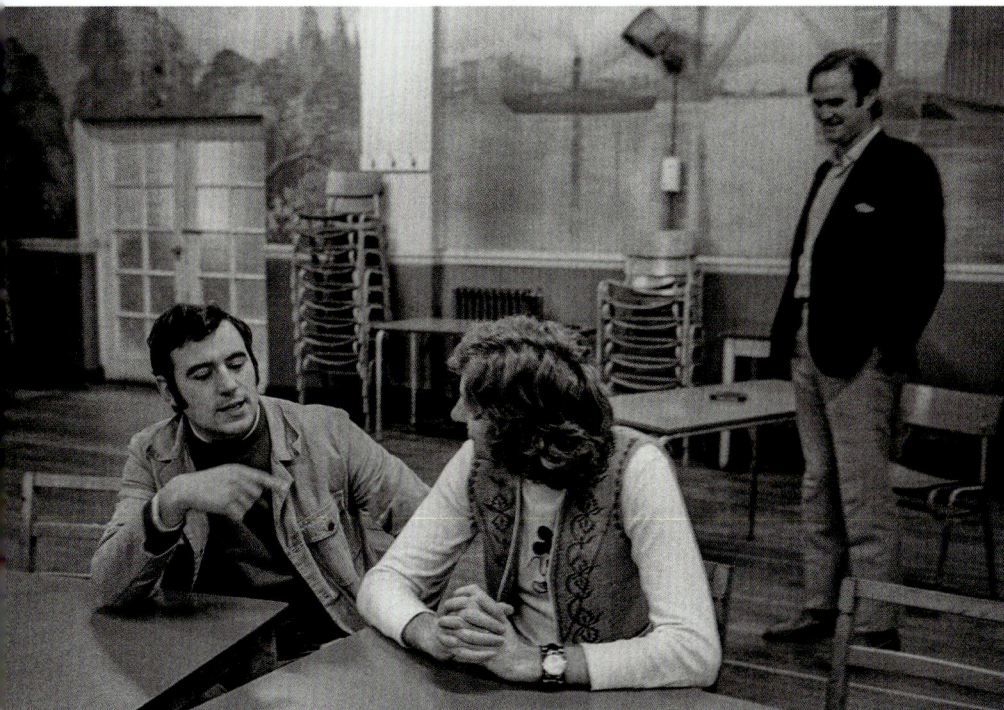

John Cleese lovingly looks on as Terry chats with Eric Idle during rehearsals for the second series of *Monty Python's Flying Circus*. Sketch show comic genius fuelled by cigarettes and coffee . . . in a room in Acton, West London.

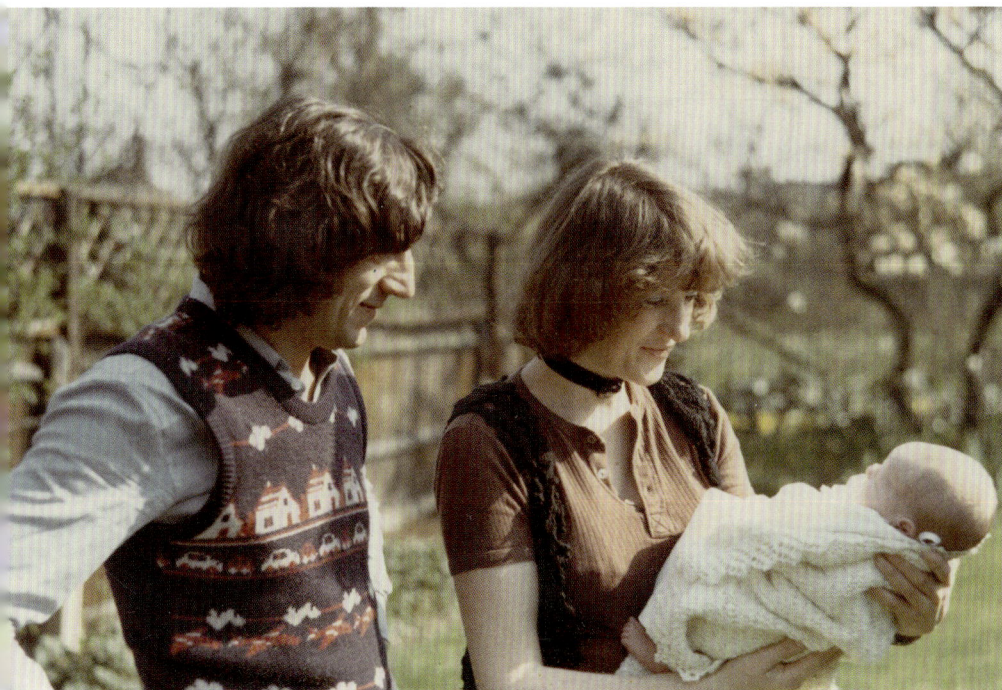

Terry and Alison, with their firstborn, Sally, at Grove Park, in April 1974.

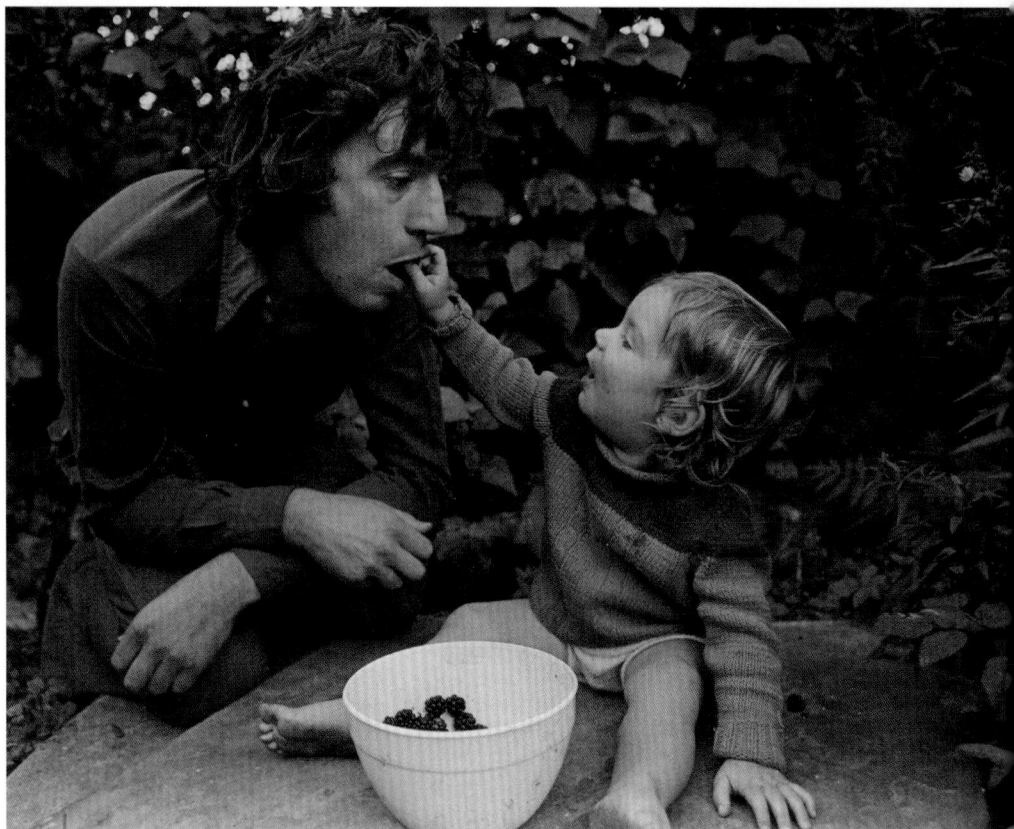

Blackberrying with infant Bill, 1979.

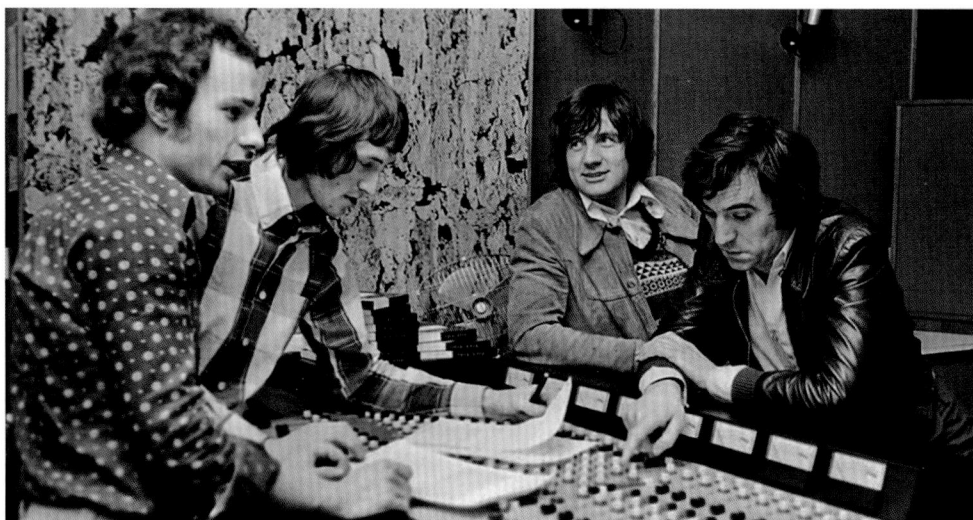

Dave Howman, André Jacquemin and Michael Palin at Sunrise Studios, Wardour Street, recording the *Holy Grail* album. Terry can't resist discovering more about the mixing desk!

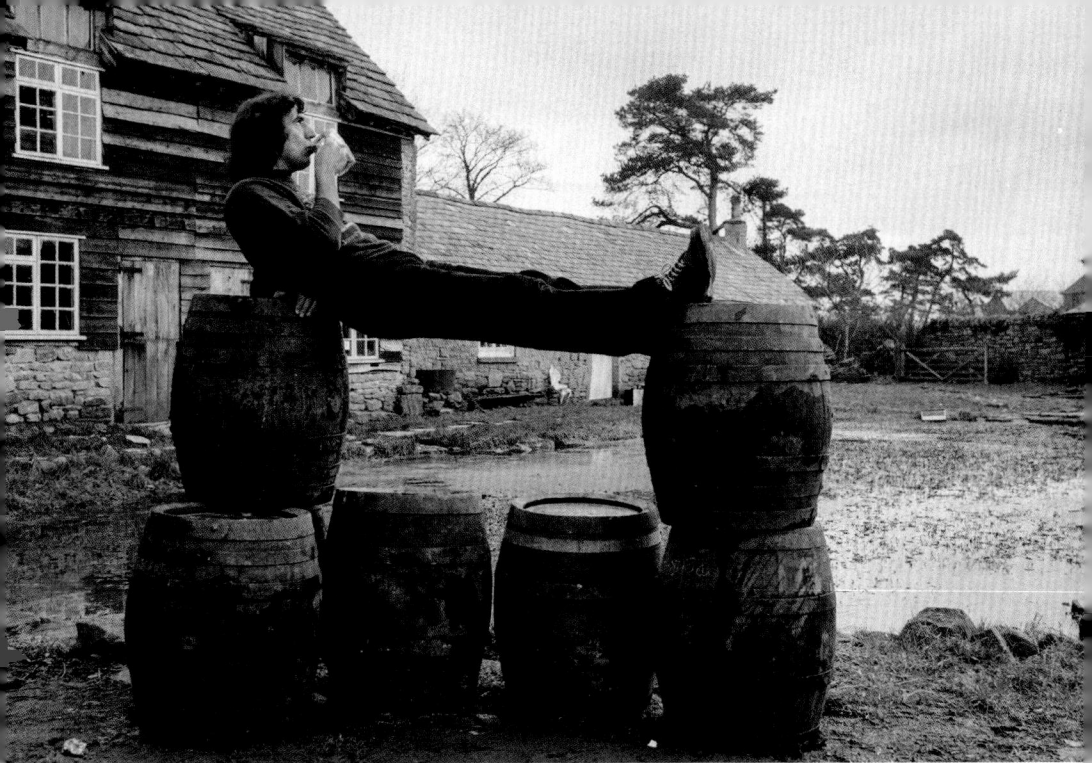

Terry's Happy Place II:
Aged 35 supping a pint of Jones's First Brew at Penrhos Court in 1977.

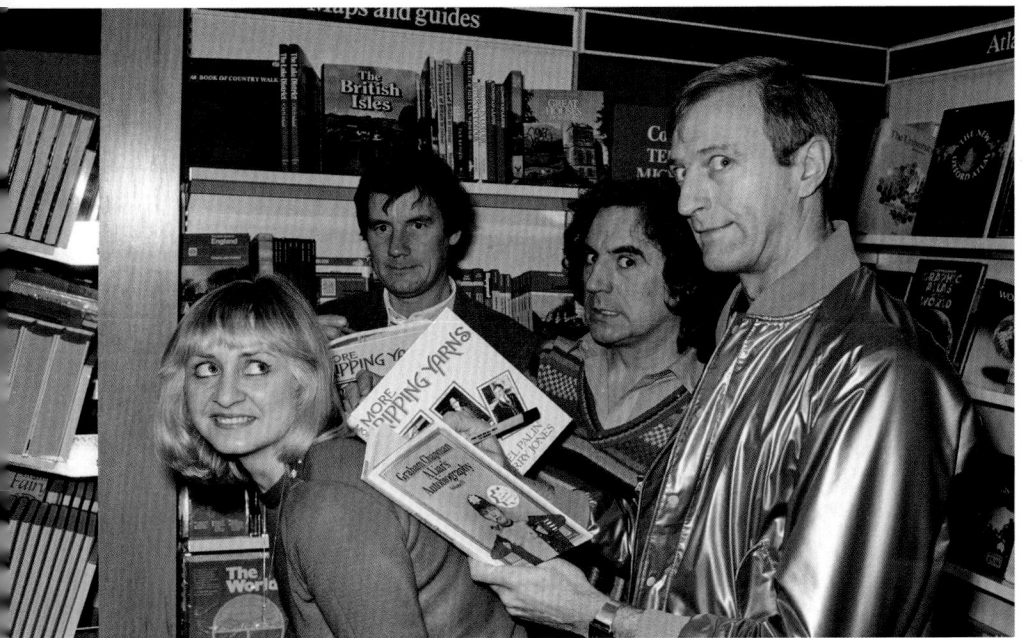

Python United: Michael Palin and Terry signing the *Ripping Yarns* script books
and Graham Chapman promoting *A Liar's Autobiography*, aided and abetted by
shop assistant and fan Jina Ristori at a signing at WHSmiths, Holborn Circus, on
Monday, 8 December 1980.

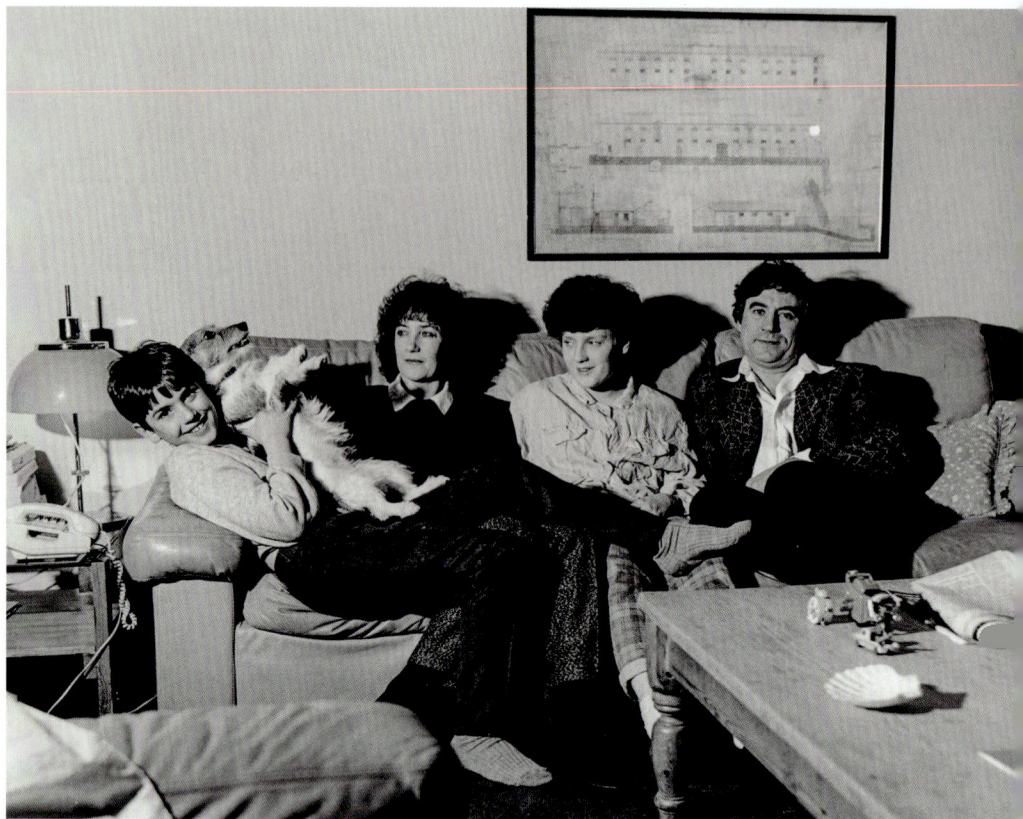

Keeping Up with the Joneses: Bill, Alison, Sally and Terry at home in Grove Park in the late 1980s.

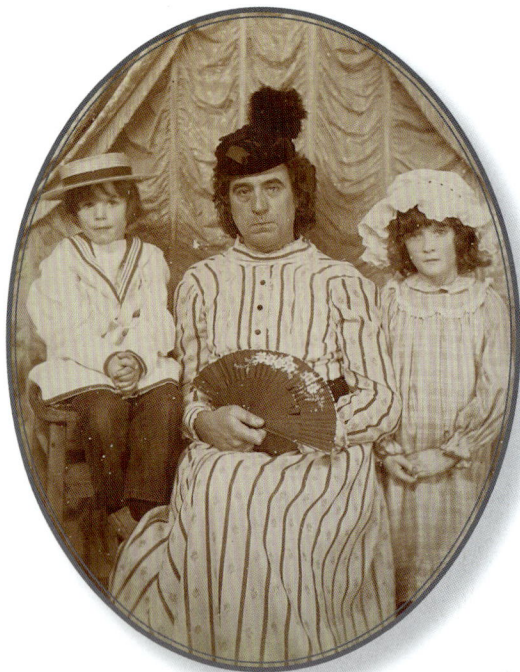

When your dad is Terry Jones and you stumble into an Olde-Tyme Dress-Up Photo Booth . . .

remains one of Terry's strongest individual efforts, with his gate-crashing and addressing of the studio audience during the 'World of History' television debate, a shattering of the studio-bound confines of broadcasting and revelation of the entire show as just that. A show. This was the core of Terry's comedy: exposing and enquiring.

Moreover, that eleventh episode includes the briefest but most bewildering of vignettes, with Terry as the wide-eyed and mysterious Mr Maniac, a heady cross between Robert Louis Stevenson's Edward Hyde and rock enigma Alice Cooper. Mr Maniac is another of Terry's characters who addresses the audience, this time the audience who are sitting spellbound at home, watching *Monty Python's Flying Circus*. Mr Maniac's shtick is an attempt to hypnotise bricks. Yes, hypnotise bricks. It's the most Terry Jones of Terry Jones comedy moments. The episode ends with Terry once again in drag, as part of the Batley Townswomen's Guild's re-enactment of Pearl Harbor (what else?). It is a madness that sums up a decade of cultural and artistic revolution, with these youngsters poking a comic tongue out at the war years – that generation who still ran the establishment and had commissioned Monty Python in the first place.

# CHAPTER SEVEN

## PYTHON! PYTHON! PYTHON!

*The only point to Python is to be funny. No messages. Just something to laugh at.*

*T*ERRY *Jones' Personal Best*, a Monty Python DVD compilation from 2006, with freshly filmed cheeky introductions from Terry, typically included a rather tongue-in-cheek although a-little-bit-in-earnest cover blurb explaining that the viewer should 'pour yourself a glass of sherry and join Terry at the piano for a silly walk down memory lane, which he calls, "How I created *Monty Python's Flying Circus*".' It was a joke, of course, but as with the best jokes there was more than a grain of truth in the statement. Michael Palin explains: 'To be honest, Terry believed he was the best judge of what worked and what didn't work for Python. Maybe he was the best judge . . . He was certainly very different from how John and Eric saw Python. John and Eric saw Monty Python as a means to an end. A way to earn money and buy freedom from work. Terry was the complete opposite. He felt Python was an end in itself. For Terry, the work was what he enjoyed doing. Python kept him from the idle pursuit of leisure!'

By the time the first series of *Monty Python's Flying Circus* was being broadcast and being discussed by the nation, in October 1969, Terry had bought the home that would soon become the House of Python. Having been living together since 1966, Terry and Alison had been looking to buy their own home since early 1968. It took them a year and a half before they could afford it but, in the meantime, *Complete and Utter History* co-star Diana Quick came to the rescue, as Alison recalls: 'We had been thrown out of our room and Diana got in touch with Terry. She was living with her then boyfriend, the actor Ken Cranham, and she said she was struggling with the rent on the house and would we like to move in and help out. We jumped at the chance!'

Although Diana and Kenneth didn't marry until 1974, by October 1969, Terry and Alison were able to buy the house that would be the Jones family home for the next thirty years, as well as the venue for scratched heads and comic innovation, as all the Pythons would gather there to write and rewrite material for the next series. 'We moved in with a bed and a couple of chairs,' Alison recalls, on Monday 3 November 1969.

With six bedrooms and just Terry and Alison living there at the time, the couple's big, old, empty house in Grove Park proved the perfect writers' retreat. As Alison recalls: 'From that point on, pretty much every word of Python was written there.' On visiting a local antique shop, the couple bought some old desks and an additional table for the top room. While Michael and Helen Palin had a house of their own, the others were all still in rented flats and apartments. Terry would play host and, somewhat by default, became the custodian and driving force of Monty Python. Alison remembers how the other Pythons would come over and sit in different parts of the house, working alone, working together, chatting about which sketch would work best in which show. In the summer, they would all have lunch in the garden, which was also used for a rehearsal space. Alison would often come home from her work as a botanist and find 'all six gallivanting round the place, pretending to be anything from batty old ladies to knights of the round table!'

Terry and Mike's sketches continued to be hallmarked by historical references and the sort of hilarious, monotonous, dull characters that had been making them laugh since Oxford. Those first sketches of 1970 could even have come straight from the stage of *The Oxford Revue*. The Second World War mentality of 'The Funniest Joke in the World'; Terry, as a train station signal box operator being attacked by a grizzly bear; the Upper Class Twit of the Year, with Terry as Nigel Incubator-Jones, an old Etonian married to a very attractive table lamp; Mike as Mr A.T. Hun, desperate to be arrested by Terry, in fake moustache. The hairy prop ultimately defeats Terry and, in mid-sketch, he makes the decision to discard it completely. Python was that kind of a show. And Terry was that kind of an actor.

It was Terry's delight in filmed vignettes rather than studio-bound sketches that saw much of his comedy start with long, drawn-out pans across desolate countryside, often with a gloriously stirring classical music accompaniment. But influences from variety theatre and the old music hall recordings he had collected as an Oxford undergraduate were as crucial to his Python contribution as his appreciation for silent comedy. The love of singalong comedy songs certainly informed 'The Lumberjack Song'. It debuted in December 1969 and remains one of the most famous of all the Python songs, in which Michael's character dreams of the life of a possibly somewhat unconventional lumberjack. Despite musical influence from the folk song 'Foggy Dew', and even a bit of Mozart's Don Giovanni, it was, fundamentally, a music hall song from the 1930s. Michael says of its genesis: 'We came up with the rhythm to it, a sense of the tune. But then we got stuck and rang Fred Tomlinson and said: "So Fred, this is roughly how we want it to sound, could you put it all together for us?" Which he did. Brilliantly. But, yes, it was sort of music hall. I'd never really thought of that before.'

The old ways were certainly the way to write comedy. For Terry and Mike, with five years of intense comedy toil together, the words would flow. And now, with four other creatives alongside them, those words would fizz with renewed energy and battle with renewed vigour for the place in that cramped half-hour slot.

Within that safe and secure Python group – a group that was now, for all intents and purposes, working together from Terry's safe and secure home space – they could do whatever they wanted. They could turn the screen upside down or present a blank screen with just voices in a kind of visual radio; they could even play with the BBC logo, dropping it into the middle of a show. The Python way was to muck about with the codes and conventions of broadcasting to such an extent that the audience would often be left wondering whether what they were watching was a Python parody or in fact the next programme in the schedule. This was joyful anarchy and a revolution without a shot being fired.

Of course, this wasn't wholly new ground. Though it was being trodden in a uniquely Python way. Some comedy greats had been there and messed with the format before. None more so and with such barmy flourishes as Spike Milligan. *The Goon Show* had been the template for anarchy in comedy since the 1950s, a time when the fledgling Pythons had first discovered and began to understand comedy. Spike was the god. He could be very, very funny from all sorts of different directions. You didn't know where it was going to come from. On television, Spike's sketch shows carried a certain danger. He would literally leave his gang of seasoned stooges and the viewers hanging; for example, by addressing the audience and asking the rather disquieting question: 'What are we going to do now?' over and over again. This was of particular interest to Terry and the other Pythons because of what they were trying to achieve. To write comedy in a different way than it had been written before.

Like Spike, the Pythons would embrace stuffy BBC authority. The Flying Circus had John, in a dinner jacket, intoning, 'And now for something completely different' as a sort of in-house and in-programme continuity announcer. And whereas Spike's sketches would often come to an abrupt and unnatural end, Python had the animations of Terry Gilliam, the very key to that something completely different that Terry Jones had spotted and embraced. And they were young. Spike, now in his fifties and having faced the trauma of war, and challenges to his mental health for most of his life, which often derailed him, couldn't compete. Michael Palin recalls that: 'Spike had broken all the rules and we always acknowledged him, always thanked him. He had gone through the madness so we didn't have to.'

On some days, Spike could be the Pythons' biggest fan; on others, he would tell everyone who cared to listen that the group had ripped him off. Spike would call them unscrupulous bastards and comment after each and every sketch that he had done that, and that, and that . . . The Pythons would always agree with him, though often through gritted teeth. Spike's bipolar disorder – then known as manic depression, and put down to those wartime experiences – was widely known. The group admired him, even when, as Michael Palin recalls, 'Spike would scream: "Ah, fucking thieves. You are stealing my material! It's daylight robbery. Daylight rob-be-rey!" He would say it in that high-pitched, sing-song comedy voice, so Terry and I never knew whether he was having us on or not!'

Within the group, Terry and John were often the opposing forces, but also the bookends. Terry had a tendency to be vague, adopting a certain nice and very affable rambling approach. However, in its quiet, stubborn way, this could be as immovable as John's sharp insistence. John would say: 'Do this!' And Terry would say, 'Well . . . maybe, perhaps we could do something slightly more like how I want to do it.' And then he would snap out: 'We'll do this! What do you think?', and John would get terribly irritated. Michael says that Terry's stubbornness would put John's back up during those early Python years. Terry would admit that the conflict was there. And yet it was a healthy one that never got out of hand. Well, not often. As Terry said: 'I only ever threw a chair at John Cleese once . . . I think!' And, besides, it was Terry's chair that he threw! More often than not, the sheer joy of writing and performing kept the unit together, despite personality differences and creative disagreements.

The first series of *Monty Python's Flying Circus* had been considered a big risk and had attracted respectable if not huge audience figures. There was a way to go before it blossomed into an internationally acclaimed juggernaut of bizarre comedy, and success was far from certain. When five episodes from the first series were repeated on BBC2, the *Radio Times* singled out John Cleese – describing him as 'the tall one' and the only team member who viewers may be familiar with. The rest were, it opined, hardly household faces. These hitherto jobbing scriptwriters had to be circumspect. Michael remembers, 'I suppose there were certain points when you thought, "Ah, we are actors. What can I do? What am I going to do after this?"' Even during the commissioning and scripting of the second series, Terry in particular – with a home to keep up – would retain that feeling of needing something else in reserve in case it all fell apart. Which is why he was still slipping the funnies to Marty Feldman and *The Two Ronnies*.

Before filming began for the second series of *Monty Python's Flying Circus*, on Saturday 20 June 1970, Terry and Alison got married. Alison explains, 'We had never discussed marriage. It was something we didn't really think we needed to do.' Still, this was a different time with different expectations. Parents could be awkward about such things and Terry's parents, now retired, were still a powerful force within his life. He would dutifully make the trip to see them each and every weekend, and, even though Terry and Alison had been living together since 1966, they would not be allowed to stay in the same room. Of course, any couple finds a way around these parental restrictions. Terry would suggest that Alison go up to his room: 'But we had to make sure to make the bed, and for me to leave before Terry drew the curtains in the morning. Just in case one of the neighbours saw me leave his bedroom!'

All these farcical shenanigans were too much for Terry's mother. Friends and relatives had been talking, and she didn't like people talking about her youngest son. 'Terry's parents, or, at the very least, Terry's mother, wasn't happy about us buying the house. Even though we had been living together for over three years by then.' For Terry's mother, that simply wasn't done: her son should not be living with a woman unless they were married. 'Terry's mother was very upset about it,' Alison continues, 'and, after one particular phone call with her, Terry said: "Look, if we don't think marriage is terribly important and my parents are getting upset about it, shouldn't we just get married? Because it doesn't matter to us whether we do or not. Why don't we just get married and make them happy?" So I said "OK". There was no engagement ring; there was no going down on one knee and "will you marry me" stuff. It was just agreed. Purely to save face for Terry's mother.'

Once the decision had been made, there was no holding back Terry and Alison. They went down to the register office and, rather naively, asked whether they could get married the following Saturday. The beleaguered registrar muttered: 'Of course you can't!' However, having looked up the following week, he noticed that, by some small miracle, there had been a cancellation for the next Saturday morning. 'That was quite astonishing. So we just got married. We organised a party and had everybody in our back garden. Terry's parents were very happy. My parents were very happy too. And we were very happy.' In the wedding photograph Alison is dressed in a long, flowing gown, every inch the medieval babe. Every inch Terry's ideal bride.

Not long before the wedding, on 2 May 1970, Terry and the gang were at the Camden Theatre to record the *Monty Python's Flying Circus* album, the group's first, for BBC Records. Before such modern marvels as the video recorder or Betamax, buying a record was of course the only way that members of the public could actually own and enjoy these precious comedy moments at home at a time of their choosing, unbeholden to the whims of the BBC repeat schedule. Still, the Pythons, being innovators, wanted to reference and include the pitfalls and technology of recording an album into the album itself. An entirely new section of the Barber Shop sketch was written and performed in order to show the scope and spectacle of a stereo recording. The only snag being that the promised stereo recording equipment was not forthcoming (the BBC recorded and released the album in mono). Despite knowing the equipment wasn't available, the Pythons recorded the stereo demonstration anyway. Simply because they found the complete redundancy of the joke even funnier.

At least the team's offering was now heralded by the BBC as 'super zany comedy' rather than 'satire'. Also, an American audience had sat up and taken notice. Or, at the very least, the New York publishing executive Victor Lownes had sat up, taken notice and decided the Pythons could go down well in the States. Lownes, who was the London-based representative for *Playboy* magazine and Playboy Clubs at the time, funded the venture: a feature film presentation of the best of Python's television sketches. It was called *And Now for Something Completely Different*. But Lownes was not completely honest with the group, as Terry often bemoaned. 'The agreement was that the film would not be shown in Britain at all. It was simply to launch us in the States. As far as I remember, none of us were that bothered about being launched in the States, but I liked the idea of a film.'

Ironic to think that it was this influx of the huge back catalogue of Python into America by the mid-Seventies that made the group financially and creatively powerful. For America, it really was something completely different. And, in the end, *And Now for Something Completely Different*'s film compilation of Series One sketches, including 'Nudge, Nudge' and 'The Lumberjack Song', would be released in British cinemas in September of 1971 – actually ahead of a summer 1972 release in America. Terry was incensed. He was angry that the general public in Britain were traipsing to the cinema to see Python repeat material that had already been seen on television: 'particularly as the film was called *And Now for Something Completely Different!*'

Still, by that autumn it had been nearly two years since those sketches had first been televised, and British audiences were well-versed and very keen to revisit familiar television comedy at their local cinemas. Big screen productions of *Till Death Us Do Part* and *Up Pompeii!* had proved extremely profitable in the previous couple of years. No, the real issue with Terry, when the brisk five-week shoot started on 26 October 1970 – just ten days after completion of the recording for the second batch of television episodes – was the restrictive filming conditions and the limited budget. Never completely satisfied with Ian MacNaughton's direction of the television series, Terry was rather miffed when MacNaughton was assigned the film too. It was a fait accompli that entrepreneur Lownes had insisted upon. Moreover, because the budget was a very modest £80,000, the sketches for the film were shot in an abandoned United Dairies dairy in Totteridge. The metallic echo of discarded milk urns was intrusive and distracting and, as Terry remembered: 'it was hardly the ideal place in which to try and be funny!' For all its faults, though, *And Now for Something Completely Different* was Terry and Michael's first feature film, though the initial excitement of that had been countered by the makeshift nature of the film's production.

Far more ideal was the stage. For, while television audiences were enjoying the second series, Colin Richardson, the enterprising talent booker for Lanchester Polytechnic's art festival, had been in touch. Having secured such diverse acts as Elton John and Arthur 'Big Boy' Crudup, Richardson wondered whether the Python boys would be available and willing to take part. You bet. Thus it was that a three-day residency was agreed. The date on the ticket was 31 January 1971, but in actual fact it was after midnight before the Pythons got to the stage. So it was Monday 1 February 1971 when these seasoned revue comedians made their stage debut as a team. It was Terry's twenty-ninth birthday.

Soon after, he was hard at work on *Monty Python's Big Red Book*, which was published, with a bright blue cover, by Methuen in the November of 1971. So now, having seen 'The Lumberjack Song' on television, bought it on record and seen it again at the cinema, you could sing along with confidence from the lyrics reproduced in the book. This was Monty Python as a multimedia template, producing brand new material while at the same time lovingly wallowing in old sketches. Within just two years, Python had become a profitable, self-aware comedy franchise. That attack on the norm, and attack on authority, had resulted in the team being not just very clever comics but very astute, albeit accidental, businessmen too.

For Michael Palin, this was all part of the process: 'we were six very different comedy brains. But six brains thinking as one comedy brain. At least, some of the time.' Certainly, Terry's brain was quite extraordinary. He wanted other people to share his thoughts, somehow, and that was through his comedy. The Pythons were not anarchists by any means, but when they got together and started assembling material the most fertile ground for their comedy was the foibles of the people they saw around them. The comedy was even more productive when the Pythons felt that those people were in a superior position over most people and yet more stupid, pompous or pretentious than the average man in the street. For, as Michael says, 'If we feel that, when somebody unsuitably in authority is telling people to do something, it is gratifying to be able to deflate them by the power of comedy!'

The Pythons had also been emboldened to seize power themselves. Still smarting at the disappointing, although successful, BBC record, in the June of 1971 the team decamped to the Marquee Studios in Wardour Street to record another Monty Python record called, surprisingly enough, *Another Monty Python Record*. However, this was not for the BBC's label but for Charisma. For better and for worse, Terry put himself in charge. The record was sold in the cover for Beethoven's Symphony No. 2 in D Minor, with that title scribbled out in crayon and the Python title added. It appears pure Terry Gilliam and, indeed, Terry G. claims ownership of the idea and the artwork. Terry J. always insisted it had been his idea! And with his history in design and his leadership on this project, it's highly possible. Listen, this is Terry's book. Let's give him this one, with a Gilliam assist, not to mention some invaluable input from his sister-in-law, Kate Hepburn, studying at the Royal College of Art and already helping the team with their graphic design. And that's just it. It's a team effort.

They were all about fully embracing the media in which they were working – the vinyl revisiting of the 'Ethel the Frog' sketch includes the specially written line 'Sorry, Squire, I've scratched the record!', which, skilfully engineered, does indeed result in a seeming scratch and jump and repeat of that line. Unsuspecting listeners might think their disc really had been scratched. The Charisma team were indeed skilled at such trickery, although Terry did comment that 'all the studio guys were high on dope!' This, if true, presumably didn't help the impractical situation of the control room being at one end of a long corridor and the studio being at the other. With no video contact between the two.

The engineer recorded everything the team performed in the studio, running the tapes continually. Unfortunately, Terry had assumed that the engineer was making notes of when a sketch began and ended, and if it was a good take. The engineer assumed Terry was making the same notes. In the end, Terry was faced with a big pile of about 300 tapes and absolutely no record of what was on which. Having assumed responsibility for the project, he sat and listened to every single tape. In the end it was well put together . . . but studio time being expensive, the whole process cost Python £40,000.

All was forgiven though when *Another Monty Python Record* was released in the October of 1971 and promptly sold 20,000 copies in the first ten weeks. A further print run of *Monty Python's Big Red Book* was published the following February, and the first batch of 55,000 copies was a complete sell-out. A number one bestseller in London, this archetypal comedy book was a critical success too. While the film, which Terry in particular had been so unhappy with, was doing great business across the country. By the end of 1971, the Columbia Cinema in London had held *And Now For Something Completely Different* over for eleven straight weeks. During which time it had already pulled in box office profits of £50,000, nearly two-thirds of its production costs. In Oxford cinemas, huge public demand to see the film extended its showing time from the intended one week to a month.

Moreover, in the April of 1971, a Python television special had won the Silver Rose of Montreux. It had been quite a year. A year of looking forward but, more often, looking back. The future looked bright, although rumblings within the group and disquiet within the BBC would not make the next few years easy.

For Terry personally, life would certainly never be the same again. Off the back of the win in Montreux, Python had been seen for the first time by some influential broadcasters across the world. Although the Italian delegation – of all people – thought the show was too obscene to screen and they walked out. The sketch that shocked was the one with Terry and Carol Cleveland's supposed sex scene, with black and white footage of torpedoes and submarines and explosions suggesting foreplay, copulation and orgasm. The pay-off, of course, is that the suggestive black and white footage is simply an excited Terry showing genuine newsreels to the uninterested and sexually disappointed Carol. Perhaps it was Terry's lacklustre sexual display in the bedroom that so upset the Italians. A real man wouldn't behave like that. Not even for a joke.

Regardless, it certainly didn't put off Alfred Biolek, a television producer from Bavaria Films.

The original plan was for the Pythons to join forces with a Dutch comedy troupe for a cross-country comedy collaboration. Terry vetoed that idea straight away. They all did. Biolek was undeterred though and a meeting was set up for Ian MacNaughton at the Bavaria Studios. The idea for a Python show especially for the German market was floated, and appealed enough for Terry and the team to go along to the second meeting, which led to a German Monty Python TV special being agreed upon. Never one to willingly cede creative control, Terry, in particular, was not keen on his voice being dubbed by a German actor. So the Pythons decided to perform the sketches themselves. In German.

Terry reflected that: 'looking back, maybe that wasn't such a great idea. I remember being very cavalier in those days and saying: "Oh, we'll learn it phonetically . . ."' Stan Laurel and Oliver Hardy had done it for their Spanish versions of a few short films, and if it was good enough for them it was good enough for Python. In the first sketch, filmed on the first day in Bavaria, Michael Palin was playing an Australian discussing the rectum of a kangaroo. In German, of course. Terry suddenly had some serious doubts. 'I kept asking the translator: "Is this all right? Is this funny?" But we had to do it. In the end, it just sounded like us, attempting to speak German. Which is just right, really. It's what they wanted. It's what we wanted!'

It was just right enough to warrant two episodes of *Monty Python's Fliegender Zirkus*, although only the first was broadcast in German for the German audience; in January 1972, the second, screened that December, was shot for the German market but in English. Terry had clearly got cold feet about their clodhopping attempt at speaking German. Even so, as usual, the Pythons had written the sketches for the two shows to make themselves laugh, with absolutely no concessions to the German audience at all.

Terry later explained that they just wrote the shows in the exact same way they always had done: 'I suppose we stuck in the sketch about sixteenth-century German artist and theorist Albrecht Dürer on purpose . . . or did we? No, not really. That could have been in the BBC shows quite easily. I mean, we did German-type sketches on the BBC all the time. I suppose the Bavarian Restaurant sketch didn't have to be in Bavaria but it was.' They were in Bavaria when they shot it, so you could just as easily call it the Restaurant sketch: 'I mean, you don't call the Dirty Fork sketch the Wood Lane Restaurant sketch, do you? The Bavarian Restaurant sketch is just a restaurant sketch. In Bavaria.' Well, yes, Terry. (I'm smiling as I write this because, quite frankly, it was like being in a Python sketch when Terry related it, with a glorious twinkle and a laugh in his voice. We were in a north London public house at the time, so if you wish you can dub that the Highgate Boozer anecdote. Or just the boozer anecdote. It doesn't matter where it was set. Does it, Terry?)

Filming in Germany, trying to remember lines learned phonetically without a clear idea of how they were translated, sounded both hilarious and somewhat stressful, the way Terry related it. However, filming abroad put an extra pressure on Terry, as his mother, having now been in poor health for several years, would get terribly upset whenever he had to travel for filming. She would worry that something would happen and her huge concern was that she would die while he was away. The filming in Germany was pretty much more than she could bear, and she worked herself up into such a state about it that she almost brought herself to a fever pitch. She had been like that before, when he had been filming on location in Norfolk or West Yorkshire. Admittedly, the German gig was a flight away rather than a train journey, but Terry couldn't turn down work. Comedy and work came first. While the Pythons were in Bavaria, Alison was on her way to a scientific conference in Italy (where they were perhaps still discussing Python in heated tones) and so she joined Terry in Munich en route. She remembers: 'That night, just after midnight, we had word from home that Terry's mum had had a heart attack and was in hospital. We rushed home the next day but she had sadly died before we got back.'

The show, however, must go on, even though the strain of being a very active Python was taking its toll on John Cleese. In the months before signing up for a third series of thirteen episodes of the Flying Circus, John was very vocal in his opinion that the team were already beginning to repeat themselves. Despite, or perhaps because of, their creative battles, Terry was very keen to keep the six-man group together. In the end, it was the reassurance and enthusiasm of Michael Mills that proved the deciding factor in John staying. Cleese admired and trusted his judgement, and was grateful for his initial faith in the show. When Mills advised him to stay for the good of the group, John listened. The times were a'changing, though, for Mills was on the verge of relinquishing his role at the BBC and heading for Thames Television. The BBC's director general was still Sir Charles Curran, who had been in the post since the beginnings of Python in 1969. Still, with the departure of Mills, that established practice of allowing the individual producer of a given show complete control over that show was beginning to flounder. Now, more often than not, internal unease about the content of a proposed programme was passed directly for comment to the head of the BBC, Paul Fox. Certainly, the corporation was getting more and more anxious about some of the material in Python.

It was felt that the Pythons had pushed the boundary too far with the 'Undertaker' sketch, in which Graham Chapman suggests that, rather than bury or cremate the youthful mother of John Cleese, they eat her. Groans of disgust on the soundtrack are heightened as if to highlight that even the people making the show were just a little offended. Certainly in the wake of the death of Terry's own mother. However, self-awareness wasn't enough. The Pythons had overstepped to such an extent that Duncan

Wood, who had been appointed Head of Comedy at the BBC in 1970, was now requesting to see and, let's not beat around the Shepherd's Bush here, vet the episodes before they were passed for transmission.

The reports from the Audience Research Department may insist that Monty Python was as popular and as subversive as ever, with viewers in December 1972 delighted that 'the nearest thing to a visual *Goon Show*' was back on their screens 'as wonderfully peculiar as ever' – you can almost hear Spike Milligan screaming 'Daylight rob-ber-ry!' even now. However, an internal memo from Duncan Wood to Ian MacNaughton, of 18 September 1972, had already shown that the writing was on the wall. Not only did he:

> think we've had enough of cartoon figures with Paul Fox's head on them. It really is a house joke, and although I'm sure Paul will take it in good part, it seems silly to chance your arm that he won't when 99% of the viewers won't know who it is anyway.

It was a private BBC joke that the Pythons wanted to make, certainly in light of the shifting regime in which Fox could now wield the power to halt their freedom in cracking any joke they wanted to crack. As the often humourless face of BBC authority, Fox was the ultimate authority figure for the Pythons to attack. When they, invariably, got their way, they would snigger behind their hands, and consider it a good day's work. More damning and interfering was a polite but firm request to remove the phrase 'silly bunt' from the 'Travel Agent' sketch. The Pythons won this battle too, but the requirement to remove one offending word would defeat them. The word was 'masturbating'.

The sketch in question was the 'All-England Summarize Proust Competition' and the offending line was uttered by Harry Baggot of Luton, played by Graham, when he listed his hobbies as 'strangling animals, golf, and masturbating.' For Terry, in the thick of the sketch as the smarmy host Arthur Mee, the offence was: 'very bizarre. Apparently "strangling animals" was fine.' The fact that it was also Terry and Mike who had written the sketch naturally set off the warrior hell-bent on protecting the work. Terry remembered that he went to Duncan Wood – then head of comedy – and said, 'Duncan, what's wrong with masturbating? I masturbate, you masturbate, don't you, Duncan?' Whether Duncan Wood admitted to masturbating was left unrecorded. Regardless, the word was omitted from the episode.

For Terry it was a frustration, if not the final straw. The second Charisma Records release, *Monty Python's Previous Record*, was recorded in October 1972, exactly a month after the Duncan Wood masturbation debate. The Proust sketch was re-recorded for the album, which was released for the Christmas market of 1972. Needless to say, it retained the controversial word.

The album also introduced eighteen-year-old sound guru André Jacquemin to the Pythons. Michael said he was making a record and asked André to come over to his house for a chat. André went to Mike's house and everybody was there apart from John Cleese. Terry was playing with Mike's kids, as André recalls: 'It was like a party. The place was just a lot of fun. Terry was lovely. Maybe he saw my fear of taking on this crazy project.' Terry was keen to avoid repeating the costly misadventure of *Another Monty Python Record* and the hours he had spent trying to find and put together the best takes of the sketches from among the many hours of recording. Terry felt relieved that there was somebody who could cope with it all – or, at least, someone who they could blame if it all went wrong! André had never done a job like that and admits now that, 'To be honest I didn't really know what I was doing in those days. It was my first act of bullshitting. I agreed to do it, and I was paid two hundred quid!' Which turned out to be a great investment as his expertise saved the potential loss of another £40,000 – as well as Terry's sanity.

Jacquemin – who hadn't realised it was the Pythons before John joined the meeting, late – provides an interesting outsider's perspective on the group dynamics and work ethic. Such was Terry's commitment to the rightness of his comedy, and even the rightness of the comedy of the Pythons as a unit, that any threat to it could cause him to explode with frustration. 'The only time I really thought Terry lost it with the group, despite it all going terribly well, was when we were recording something that Eric had written, and Mike said, "Let's change this line round . . ." For some reason, Terry went ballistic. He was swearing and shouting: "No, you can't do that!" He screamed and stormed out of the room, slamming the door behind him. The whole building shook. I turned to Mike and said, "Is he going to be all right?" Mike said, "Ahh, don't worry, he'll be back in a minute. He'll be absolutely fine."'

André wasn't so sure because Terry was red in the face and furious. He had never seen anybody so angry. Anyway, sure enough, five minutes later, the door opened and in walked Terry and said: 'How's it going, boys?' As if nothing had happened. It was just his way of getting over his anger – very quickly. The passionate Welshman. What's more, he was completely all right about the changes they had made too. Apart from that one flare-up, according to Jacquemin the recording sessions were a breeze. André kept notes and kept the budget tight, while the Pythons were a jolly, happy, matey team, playful and fun and dedicated to getting everything right. Particularly Terry.

This jolliness was retained throughout 1973. The BBC put out a repeat season called 'The Pick of Python' in the spring, *The Brand New Monty Python Bok* was written for publication in the November and *The Monty Python Matching Tie and Handkerchief* album was recorded for release that Christmas. There were awards too – a BAFTA for Best Comedy Series and an award for Best Light Entertainment Programme from the Society of Film and Television Arts. The team were buoyant; there was a feeling of something like a seasoned rock group when they went on the road with a package of their greatest hits. *Monty Python's First Farewell Tour* covered the United Kingdom before tackling the wide-open spaces of Canada, filling 3,000-seaters in Winnipeg, Edmonton, Calgary and Vancouver. They then returned home to London's glittering West End to perform the familiar, chant-a-long sketches at the Theatre Royal, Drury Lane.

For Terry, it suddenly all clicked into place in his head. This was exactly what Python was all about. As a creative unit, it should never fester, it should always move forward, ideally in as many different directions as possible. But they had now amassed a back catalogue of sketches that were swiftly – and lucratively – seeping into the comedy subconsciousness. Audiences wanted to see the sketches they knew, and Terry was still performing 'Nudge, Nudge' and 'The Lumberjack Song', which had been part of his personal repertoire for five years. Now this return and revision and repeat of the familiar not only fuelled his synapses, but also: 'bonded us as a team of performers. That tour was the most joyous of times.' And Terry had become a father – Sally was born during the Drury Lane shows, in March 1974. Her birth was even announced on stage!

The passion knew no bounds. And Terry's commitment to Python as an ongoing comedy force was almost frightening in its intensity. As Michael Palin maintains: 'Terry just seemed more personally attached to Python than any of us. It was and always remained very important to him.' Terry *was* a team player. He had always enjoyed that team spirit but, like at school, when he was rewarded for being the brightest and the best at every sport, he instinctively felt that he knew exactly which way Python should develop. Terry loved the camaraderie of a match well played, the discussion of the highs and lows of the action afterwards in the communal shower room. And if comedy was like a football match, then Terry saw himself as the team captain – never compromising on any strategy of play, never wavering on any word of a well-honed, oft-performed sketch. Michael Palin explains that: 'Terry was someone you wanted on your side, on your team. It could also be a drain on the team. Terry would argue and argue a point, even when he was the only one who felt so strongly about something.'

That creative conflict at the heart of Python – those six comedy brains thinking as one comedy brain – could overpower and over-shadow the huge achievements of the group. Certainly, for Terry, when our conversations would turn to Python in the dawning years of the twenty-first century, he would at first seem jaded. After all, he had by then spent decades repeating the same 'funny stories' to journalists and interviewers and avid fans like me, ever eager for more about Python. He could even at times be dismiss-ive: 'Honestly, you know, a lot of what we did just wasn't very good!' But in those early interactions in various pubs in the West End, my youthful enthusiasm would conquer my natural shyness. I would bluster and garble but the point I would make, time and time again, was that *all* the Python sketches were good. It's just that some bits were better than other bits. In response to that, Terry would smile his crooked smile and visibly shed a skin of slight irritation and negativity. In those moments, I could see that Terry was transported back to those halcyon twenty months or so, when Python was rewriting the rule book, winning awards, selling loads of books and records, and, most importantly of all, playing to packed houses of people who simply wanted to have a good time. I got the impression that, then, the Pythons were having the best time of everybody. It was fun. Pure and simple.

Once, during that peak of Python, at the end of an evening at Terry G.'s West Hampstead apartment at the top of a mansion block, Terry J. was preparing to go home to Camberwell. It was the days when everybody drove everywhere, even when everyone had had a little bit too much to drink. But still, someone a little less drunk than everybody else said, 'Are you sure you are all right to drive home?' to which Terry said, 'Yes!' and proceeded to roll down the entire curving flight of stairs. All five flights. Alison was witness to this feat of derring-do: 'Terry just curled himself up into a ball and rolled down! Someone said: "He can't go home in that state!" and I said: "Well, the fact that he's now stood up at the bottom, without a hair out of place, I think he'll be fine!"' Indeed, there was Terry at the bottom of the stairs, at the end of a fun and silly night spent with his friends and comedy compatriots. Hands outstretched, almost in a 'ta-dah!' moment, his gymnastic dexterity and *joie de vivre* on display for all to see.

That spirit, energy and fun was and is what Python is all about. It's a glorious summer; it's those picnics on the grass at Oxford and Cambridge; it's a time of youth and good humour. So, in those moments, when I insisted that Python *was* good, Terry would find a contented place. A place where he was young and brilliant. 'You know,' he would say, 'Mike Palin said something once. When Python was good, it was really, really good. We were making comedy that was "almost glum-proof". I like that. A cure for the glums. That makes it well worth doing.'

# CHAPTER EIGHT

## ONCE A KNIGHT'S ENOUGH FOR ANYONE . . .

*I'm not sure I like being called a 'Serious
Historian'. They laughed in the Middle Ages,
you know. They laughed all the time!*

TERRY *was* a serious historian, of course. Or he would certainly become one, his typewriter recommissioned to ponder upon Chaucer and Richard II, Romans and Barbarians. In later life, Terry lived and breathed his period of expertise – the Middle Ages – but it all started with a joke. A 600-year-old joke – a joke that was almost as old as the title of this particular chapter. A joke in which Terry's twin passions of comedy and history converged.

Whenever Terry was assigned a place on a soft sofa to chat about his latest history publication or documentary, the conversation would invariably be preceded by a clip from Monty Python. Terry knew it; the presenters knew it; the researchers and the talent bookers knew it – Terry was on the show or in the magazine because he was a Python with a project to promote. Everybody was also in on the in-joke that Terry would happily play along with it, on occasion gently chiding or mocking the host or the journalist who had lazily spun out the same old line about this renowned Python, this well-loved funny man, now embracing his studious side. The fact was Terry had always embraced his studious side, particularly when being a funny man. Though it all started as a joke, historic truth was at the heart of Terry's best-loved work.

Terry had read Geoffrey Chaucer at school. Chaucer has been dubbed the 'father of English literature' and the 'father of English poetry', but it was as the father of English satire that Terry warmed to his wit. Terry was less impressed by his stories. He baulked at the tragic tumble into misery within 'The Monk's Tale' and the head-strong heroism of 'The Knight's Tale'. At university, Terry's studies took in Beowulf to Byron, via Shakespeare, Spenser and Milton. A history of literature and language from 1475 until 1824, but nothing beyond that. Not that Terry cared. His passion was for the medieval. He wrote a thesis on Chaucer's Knight at Alexandria and came to the conclusion that it wasn't Chaucer who was dull and uninterest-ing, it was the misinterpretations of misguided literary scholars he was studying that were dull and uninteresting. For Terry, the prob-lem was that Chaucer's stories were being read as po-faced caution-ary tales and not as the parodies they were. This distrust of scholarly works was the seed that initially deterred him from wanting to write about other people's work and, instead, write his own material, create his own jokes. Perhaps this view also helps to explain why, when Terry had written his own sketches, he then wanted to perform them himself – he did not want other actors to misinterpret his jokes as literary scholars had misinterpreted Chaucer's.

Still, Terry's fascination with Geoffrey Chaucer and, in particu-lar, the first thirty-six lines of 'The Knight's Tale', was his passion, his hobby, his obsession. All through Oxford, on to his fledgling days at the BBC, and even when he was chatting to women he fancied, the conversation would invariably turn to Geoffrey Chaucer, as Alison Telfer can testify: 'Pretty much from our first date onwards, Terry would talk about Geoffrey Chaucer, and certainly from the first few weeks we were living together. If he had any spare time at all at the weekends, he would be down in the library, reading up about Geoffrey Chaucer.'

Life and work and the need to earn a living continually got in the way, however. When Monty Python became popular enough to guarantee reasonably steady finances, Terry found he was more at liberty to go back and study Chaucer. He had read 'The Worthiness of Chaucer's Knight', an article by American academic Charles Mitchell. Moreover, in 1971, Italian film-maker Pier Paolo Pasolini had been in Britain shooting *The Canterbury Tales*, an orgy of burnt oak and buttocks. The satire of Chaucer was the very spirit of the times. His hedonistic, carnivalesque sense of fun was very much in synchrony with the last half of the Sixties and the first half of the Seventies. More pertinently, Chaucer was in tune with Terry's own sense of freewheeling comedy success. To him, Chaucer and Python were inextricably entwined.

While Terry's personal passion and ambition had to function within the larger group, the medieval authenticity of the feature film that would become *Monty Python and the Holy Grail* is certainly very much his individual vision. The idea for the film flourished during early 1973, when Python was enjoying a break from television and tackling the fresh challenge of book publishing and relishing the gleeful bonding of live performance. Although the film *And Now for Something Completely Different* had proved a surprise commercial success – certainly it was a surprise to Terry – the group still considered cinema to be the ultimate medium to conquer. With the Pythons never tighter as a unit, the move to the big screen was a deliberate decision to grow the Python brand. Moreover, for Terry's personal gratification, a combination of comedy and the Middle Ages would be the ideal project with which to make the leap to film director.

The original concept was that only half the film would be set in medieval times, while the other would be set in the 1970s. The grail was to have been discovered in the department store Harrods, for, as Terry joked: 'you can get anything in Harrods!' However, that the vast majority of the final cut of *Holy Grail* would be historical is very much down to Terry, and Terry's desire to make a Middle Ages romp. It's Python does Chaucer, basically.

And while the palpable excitement of Terry directing his first film was slightly counterbalanced by the fact that Terry Gilliam also wanted to direct *his* first film, it was only slight. Half a film was far better than nothing and *Holy Grail* had, after all, been conceived as a split plotline. Healthy disagreement and debate within the group had always proved invaluable in any case, and Terry was the director, on behalf of the group. Whatever anybody else may have thought.

Film production was, of course, a costly business. Even if *Monty Python and the Holy Grail* was to be made on a relative shoestring budget of £229,000. Notwithstanding that the sum was fairly typical of a six-week British film comedy shoot, the *Holy Grail* script was something a little more ambitious; something completely different. In the end, rock 'n' roll saved the day – or, at the very least, wealthy rock 'n' roll fans of Monty Python did. Producer Michael White had secured investments from Pink Floyd and Led Zeppelin. A Stairway to Comedy Heaven, indeed. Not that Terry was overly bothered about where the money came from, as long as they had the money. And he was directing. At last!

Ever since those fledgling days of making short films at home in Surrey, and throughout those nagging days in television when he felt he was the best judge of how his comedy should look, Terry had wanted to call the shots. He wanted to have full control. Gone now was the mad Scottish direction of Ian MacNaughton.

The jokes were as mad as ever though, and now they were being played out in Scotland too. In a very very cold, very, very dark Scotland, as it turned out – for five weeks in the May and June of 1974. Shooting in wide open spaces rather than a costly studio was cheaper, for one thing. What's more, that desolate countryside looked right. Terry stuck to his belief that a joke had to look right in order for it to reach its maximum hilarity. While his creative master plan is laudable, it did mean shooting conditions were decidedly bleak. As Terry once told me, with a wry grin, 'We were all cold and wet and miserable. All except Graham. He was very cold, very wet, very miserable, and very drunk!' Still, as Alison Telfer remembers, the joy of the team was very much evident. With a six-week-old Sally in tow, Alison took the overnight train, 'and stayed for three weeks. As part of the unit. The Pythons were all having a ball. The only dissent I ever saw was within the crew, but the two Terrys worked wonderfully well together.'

Although, creatively, they would often knock heads and disagree, Terry G. and Terry J. had a similar fierceness of vision. A desire to absolutely get what they wanted. Their way or the high-way. On the *Grail*, it would appear, they shared the same vision, and the on-the-hoof, day-by-day, very piecemeal, very Python scouting of suitable locations was a joint effort. Alison says, 'Myself and Maggie Gilliam and our two Terrys would traipse round the Scottish landscape looking for ideal places for them to shoot. They got on very well. Maggie and I just tagged along. With Sally tucked under my arm.'

Alison and Sally were to appear in the film, and even made it as far as donning costumes. But Sally's director dad changed his mind. Alison says, 'I was dressed up in dirty rags for a crowd scene but the trouble was I had to have Sally with me and she was very, very pale. Terry just couldn't bring himself to put mud on her. There I stood, as a muddy old peasant, with this bright white baby in my arms!' The historian Terry Jones could only have King Arthur striding around the place in clean and elegant clothes in that scene. Everybody else had to be covered in shit. If a joke looks right, people will laugh! Even if Terry the Historian would be continually undermining certain elements that were perceived history rather than actual history. As well as being covered in filth, the crowd artistes were given blackened teeth. For Terry this was a step too far: 'in actual fact people in the Middle Ages had pretty good teeth. They hadn't discovered sugar as yet and so hadn't discovered tooth decay either!' Still, he accepted that the audience at large would expect these peasants to look as bad as possible. Anyway, if the joke looked right to the viewer, it would be funny.

The location had to be steeped in the correct history too. Even though the Scottish governmental department in charge of protecting the environment was not happy. The thought of Terry and his crazy Python crew gallivanting all over some of their precious castles was considered not only potentially damaging but moreover an act that would undermine the dignity of the buildings. Terry pointed out that, for over half a millennium, it had been the site of bloody battle, family feud and terrible torture. But a few blokes singing silly songs and whacking coconuts together and dragging and catapulting a wooden 'Trojan Rabbit' all over the place was clearly too much for them. These people were not Python people.

The search across the width and breadth of breathtaking Perthshire turned up the derelict Doune Castle, just eight miles north-west of Stirling. This was history. This was authentic. And, although this was always a comedy first and foremost and a history lesson second, the sharp focus of Terry's passion for Chaucer's Knight was part of the film's palette. For the building of Doune Castle was contemporary with Geoffrey Chaucer. That coursed stone had been overseen, in the late fourteenth century, by Robert Stewart, the Duke of Albany, the 'Uncrowned King of Scotland', and laid while Geoffrey Chaucer lived and breathed and wrote. If you believed in fate and signs and that, then this was it. With the imposing backdrop of Doune Castle and the surrounding landscape, Terry's film became something of a medieval epic with loads of very silly things going on within it. There's Michael Palin as the bolshy Dennis citing republican doctrine in the face of Graham Chapman's stoic King Arthur. Terry himself, as the filth-collecting mother of Dennis, joins in with the militant diatribe, screaming, 'Well, I didn't vote for you!' Terry's vast array of comic cameos ranges from the squeaking left-hand side of the three-headed knight to the wan and effete Prince Herbert, who only wants to avoid his fate of being married off in order to increase the wealth of his father – Mike as a northern swamp magnate. Terry's skill at mime is deployed as Prince Herbert surreptitiously scribbles a note begging for help to escape his imprisonment in his father's castle. Graham and Eric are the idiotic guards, happily watching Terry secretly scribe, and not stopping him as he gingerly fires the missive out of his barred window.

That Terry was making his feature film directorial debut here, and giving several delicately comic performances, and coaxing lots more hilarious turns from his fellow Pythons, is admirable to say the least: these included, unforgettably, John Cleese as the demonic Tim the Enchanter, and the foolhardy Black Knight who fights on as his limbs are chopped away, and the taunting French guard who will fart in your general direction. John is Sir Lancelot the Brave too. A fresh-faced heroic bumbler. All the knights are cut from this same armour. Enthusiastic, unquestioningly brave, and just a little bit stupid. All apart from Eric Idle's Sir Robin, who is not-quite-so-brave-as-Sir-Lancelot. In actual fact, he's an utter coward who, as the song goes, is: 'bravely taking to his feet . . . and pissing off home!' Terry's central role is that of Sir Bedevere, one of King Arthur's Knights of the Round Table, sporting a huge moustache and played like a pseudo-intellectual, with pompous, matter-of-life observations, memorably as the very logic of burning a witch if she hasn't drowned in the ducking pool is questioned and debated like a lesson in a public school.

Terry gladly professed that the majority of the books in his library: 'are of or about the fourteenth century. I think I can reason why that is. In a way, I like that distance between myself and my own world and the things I'm reading about. I think I'm a bit naive about the world as it is now. When I put my nose in a book, I have that need to distance myself from what I see and feel each and every day. You can see things much clearer when they are in the past or a fantasy on reality or abstracted from what's going on around you.' This passion, when Terry was face to face with Doune Castle, was made, if not flesh and blood, then tangible stone. Directing *Monty Python and the Holy Grail* had consolidated his desire to write an academic work.

The overriding thing that really rankled with Terry was that literary scholars didn't seem to like 'The Knight's Tale' very much and, as far as he was concerned, they didn't like it because they didn't understand it. Terry now had the drive to write his book. Years of research was about to become a few years of actually writing the thing, but he had the title. *Chaucer's Knight: The Portrait of a Medieval Mercenary*. History is all about interpretation, and Terry had a passionate interpretation he needed to share. For Terry, Chaucer purposefully retold the historical truth of a dreaded and disastrous battle as a triumphant victory. For, far from Chaucer's gallant hero, Terry's interpretation of the Knight is that he is a cunning, despicable figure. Chaucer is satire. It's just that the joke, the pastiche of this 600-year-old text, had been lost to a modern audience.

Every time Terry had caught a glimpse of his valuable and treasured library of scholarly works on Chaucer, the conviction that he was right would niggle away at him. It was impossible to ignore. He had an uncontrollable desire to put the record straight. Terry Jones, comedian, comedy writer, comedy film-maker and funny man, took on the challenge to reinstate the comedy within Chaucer's misinterpreted prose. This was a Knight in Tarnished Armour. What's more, Terry saw Chaucer's work as a direct spoof of *Teseida*, the epic work by fourteenth-century Italian poet Giovanni Boccaccio.

Over an extensive ten-year period from the late 1960s, in between writing, editing and shooting Python, Terry grabbed every opportunity to decamp to the sainted portals of the British

Library. As he would often say, the historian never stops learning. Even about his pet subject. Indeed, even while writing the book that would become *Chaucer's Knight*, Terry was still learning, forever going back, unpicking and ironing out details, and adding fresh discoveries about medieval Prussia to the paperback edition. What resulted from all those hours of research and rethinking was a weighty 300 pages, in his contemporary, uncluttered and cohesive style, which seemed to him, on the face of it, unpublishable. Even though Terry valiantly restricted his academic leanings to extensive footnotes, figuring that only the dedicated scholar would bother reading those! He happily admitted that these were: 'a kind of cry out for respectability, but I didn't do it because I wanted to be respectable.' This wasn't Python. It was a Python, on the surface of it, trying to be serious. Yes, that oft-repeated amazement of a comedian having a serious side was there from the outset. Of course this particular comedian, like so many comedians, had always had a serious side, and within Terry's historical research he found his catalyst, his protagonist, his baddie.

Terry's historical villain was Sir John Hawkwood. This was no Python knight from *Holy Grail*. Bedevere the Wise, the rather po-faced knight Terry cast himself to play in the film, was, unsurprisingly, based upon a character from the legend of King Arthur as told in Wales. A one-handed warrior, Bedwyr Bedrydant was Arthur's loyal marshal, one of the most respected personages in court in medieval Europe. In the English retelling of the Arthurian adventure, he was the trusted knight who returned the fabled sword Excalibur to the mysterious Lady of the Lake. Sir John Hawkwood was the very antithesis of the brave knight. Terry's historical thesis cast Hawkwood as a mercenary, providing his services as soldier and killer to the highest bidder. A blaggard, in fact. As if to emphasise Terry's heartfelt belief that history was a contemporary thing – it was a living history – he could get severely worked up over the dastardly exploits of Hawkwood, this fourteenth-century assassin for hire, who found fame and fortune in Italy. Such was Terry's anger that when visiting Florence he would make a beeline for the cathedral and enjoy giving a disgruntled stare to the much-respected fresco of Sir John Hawkwood there, painted by Paolo Uccello. The portrait is the work of art from which his reputation as a heroic knight had been based upon since it was painted in 1436. It hangs there to this day, side-by-side with a monument dedicated to Italy's favourite poet, thinker and religious authority-baiter, Dante.

Terry's research convinced him that Sir John Hawkwood was the inspiration for the illustration for Chaucer's 'The Knight's Tale', in the Ellesmere edition of *The Canterbury Tales*, the earliest surviving manuscript of Chaucer's tales, printed in the early fifteenth century. For Terry, the similarity between this fictional knight and Hawkwood was clear to see.

This was the 600-year-old joke that *Chaucer's Knight* exposed. 'The Knight's Tale' was a lampooning of a callous mercenary, not a celebration of a brave warrior. Terry's book set out to analyse and disentangle this satire, though in his preface he admitted that this was a tall order. Six hundred years is, after all, a long time, particularly when satire, by its nature, relies on a certain amount of established knowledge on the part of the audience. Terry beds this thought within the point of reference his reader would associate him with. That of broadcast comedy. He believes that 'it is hard enough now to explain why "I.T.M.A." made us laugh a mere twenty-five years ago.' That Terry references a BBC radio comedy show from his own wartime past anchors his book in his mentality as a comedy writer and a historian of comedy. In this attempt to highlight how, although the context of jokes may be lost to time, the principles of how they work stay the same, Terry even references one of his own jokes. Rather modestly describing Monty Python as 'the TV show in which I have been involved over the last ten years', he recounts the 'Wrestling Epilogue' sketch, from episode two, in which 'instead of debating the existence or non-existence of God, a bishop and a humanist philosopher fought each other for it. It seems to me that Chaucer made this same joke almost six hundred years ago.'

Terry's book also sets out his stall as a theorist who holds a personal opinion, and – aware that it will ruffle academic feathers – one that has its 'shortcomings'. Terry's spearhead attack was to immerse himself in it until he had a full understanding of the actual history of the Middle Ages and the mercenary knights as opposed to the rather fanciful and creative history of literary scholars. They had got it wrong because they had merely read Chaucer rather than trying to understand the time in which Chaucer lived – the context needed for satire to work. Chaucer wasn't writing fact, of course. This was fiction. But, being satire, it was a reflection of reality, and, above all, Terry believed, it was a comedic commentary on Chaucer's own abhorrence of the commercialisation of warfare. It was considered one of the great evils of Chaucer's age. Regrettably, in the second half of the twentieth century, it still was.

So, Terry Jones, that young student at Oxford who had been incensed, was now Terry Jones, a thirty-something man, still incensed but with a celebrity profile. That celebrity clout was then, as it is even more so today, honey to the bee of the publishing industry. And Terry found a champion in the form of Colin Webb, who would steer his literary ship for many years. As often as not through uncharted waters.

Colin was working for Hamish Hamilton at the time, having been charged with pepping up the list with books on cinema and comedy. There he published a collection of Richard Boston's humorous *Guardian* articles, titled *Baldness Be My Friend* – his lack of hair being an amusing grievance that he wrote about often. It was Boston who mentioned to Colin that his good friend, Terry Jones, had a book he wanted to publish but, surprisingly, simply couldn't place. Methuen, the home of Python in print at that time, had passed on it. As Colin Webb recalls, 'the Pythons were remarkably loyal to certain people'; but with Methuen off the table, Terry decided to actively look for a willing publisher. 'As I recall, the majority of publishers had turned it down, simply because they didn't see how it had a connection with someone who had become known for comedy and humour.'

Colin met Terry and: 'I got on with him very well. Immediately, as it happened, because we had a background of various things in common.' Colin had started in publishing in 1964, at Woburn Press, where he had overseen the publication of books dedicated to Morecambe and Wise, Barry Took and Marty Feldman's *Round the Horne* radio scripts, and the first collections of Spike Milligan's *Goon Shows*: 'As a result of that first meeting, I published Terry. *Chaucer's Knight* was our first book together.'

Although Colin had total faith in the book and, in turn, Terry had total faith in Colin, it must have been egg on the faces of several commissioning editors when *Chaucer's Knight* did so remarkably well: 'it sold very nicely but, even more importantly to Terry, it was remarkably well reviewed. It even got a fabulous review in the *Wall Street Journal*.' Colin and, indeed, Terry knew that the publicity machine and the far and wide stocking of the book was largely down to his Python fame, but they knew too that hardened book reviewers would be dubious about this funny man off of the screen trying to cut it as a serious historian.

The distinguished Dr Reginald T. Davies, having joined as an assistant lecturer in the Department of English Literature at Liverpool University and then become reader and public orator, wrote on behalf of many, in the *Times Literary Supplement*, on 22 February 1981:

*One who lives off his study of literature may, perhaps, be forgiven for approaching this book gingerly: Terry Jones of the Monty Python team may have written an ingenious send-up of proliferating scholarship! But not so. Enjoying a secret second career as learned medievalist, through three hundred serious pages he develops, with sure professional foot, a thoroughly documented, single-minded thesis, new in literary studies, but consistent with its primary commitment to reductive satire.*

Davies went on to confirm that several other historians shared Terry's interpretation that this knight was, to quote the book, the most ruthless of a gang of mercenaries 'swarming across Europe' at the time, with no 'family background, no coat-of-arms . . . [and] no manorial estates'.

According to Terry, Chaucer's Knight lacked pity as he slaughtered and morals as he purloined. Concluding that the knight was a disreputable figure instilled even more respect for the satirist at the heart of Terry's book, reasoning as it does that it is scarcely credible that Chaucer – as both humourist and Christian – would glorify such a bounder as a hero.

That his findings were filtering through to respected reviewers and, moreover, distinguished historians, meant everything to Terry. This was vindication of the highest order. Here was a funny man and a serious historian. The two were one and the same, and he knew exactly what he was doing. Having said that, Terry was forever playful throughout the publishing process, and in a euphoria of happiness. You could never take the Python completely out of the historian, and he dedicated his publisher's prized copy of *Chaucer's Knight*:

*To Colin who made this book possible,*
*love from a grateful author\**
~~*Nevill Coghill*~~ *Terry 28 Jan 1980.*

*\*Also willing to do odd jobs + complete Baby-Minding Service (details on request) and now incorporating the 'Benidorm' School of Spanish Dancing (applicants should be under 21, female and scantily dressed if possible).*

As Colin reflected, over forty years on, that was: 'Very Terry!' It was also the culmination of a very good time. Colin and his wife Ann spent lots of time with Terry and Alison. Much fine wine and good food was consumed and a real friendship and relationship between author and publisher was forged. As a result, Colin maintains a rather lovely thought: 'it was Terry's work which, in many ways, defines his personality.' This is a summing up that many of Terry's friends agree with. The man and the work were so tightly intertwined, so complete, that conversation would invariably lead back to history and books.

*Chaucer's Knight* had long been a burning passion project for Terry. It was also one he knew would upset certain pretentious academics, but, as Colin Webb believes, 'it was all done with such determination and enthusiasm and, above all else, sheer glee, that most so-called serious historians took it in their stride.'

Of course, not everyone agreed. Some serious historians, like children in the playground, argue and fight and taunt each other. There were some who disagreed with Terry's argument, but, though he might have felt a little battered by these counterclaims and, indeed, counter-books, with a weary shake of the head he would be his usual philosophical self and mutter that when he was dead, in twenty years' time, maybe then, and only then, the naysayers would admit he was right. In actual fact, twenty years and more after *Chaucer's Knight* was first published to critical acclaim and high sales, Terry was still dutifully and merrily ploughing that self-same field of research.

Indeed, history is not only a subjective thing but also a contemporary thing, open to multiple interpretations. That Terry stated that Chaucer's Knight was not only a villain but a funny villain, a pantomime baddie in many ways, was a very Terry-like stance to take. That he proved his theory, over and over again throughout the book, was undeniable, and praised accordingly. As Terry explained: 'My pathetic political convictions of the present directly

stem from my readings of the fourteenth century and the controversy between the Lollards and the Church back then.' The Lollards
were the radicals who were intent on reform. In contrast, the reac-
tionaries of the established Church were slow in registering the
threat these radicals posed. And when the Church did react, it was
in the extreme. So extreme that they were burning people in
barrels! Terry would draw comparisons with the communist
movement of the 1930s, when terribly respectable Cambridge
undergraduates were flying the red flag.

He also enjoyed pointing out that jokes are recycled down the
years. At the time he began writing, older, traditional commentators enjoyed claiming that the trends for long hair and less rigidly
gendered clothing meant that they couldn't tell what sex the
young people of today were. That same joke, observed Terry, had
been published in a cartoon in *Punch* in the 1880s and, what's
more, it had been a comic observation in medieval times too.
Terry would often quote a favourite Middle Ages joke: 'The way
that people do dress you cannot tell who are the boys and who are
the girls.' It was the same reaction to changing fashions, passed
down the ages. Perhaps it was Terry's love of comedy, and love of
contemporary parallels, that went some way to, on occasions,
dulling his clear reputation as a learned historian with a great
deal of sense to say.

Terry had another niggling theory regarding Chaucer: a dark
suspicion that Chaucer's death in 1400 was so mysterious and
so undocumented. Even that date is uncertain; it was etched
onto his tomb some hundred years after his death. There was no
will, nothing. And this was a very famous man, an important
public figure: a famed writer, considered the country's finest
living poet, a respected public speaker, a scholar and diplomat,
as well as brother-in-law to John of Gaunt, one of the most
powerful men in the kingdom. And for such a person, so well
known at the time of his death, to leave behind no record, no

clue to the cause of his death, seemed deeply suspect to Terry. To conjoin the past and the present, as we must, this was a celebrity, or, as Terry referred to him, 'the pre-eminent intellectual superstar of his time', and yet his sudden and unexpected passing left absolutely no trace. For Terry the historian, this was all too bizarre. This greatest of English writers didn't even leave any manuscripts behind. As Terry pondered with incredulity: 'How could this be?'

It was an intriguing question for any historian. However, for a while, Terry's polymath, butterfly brain was consumed by many other pressing projects. He was intrigued by the end of Chaucer but felt that it was such a vast task, he would have to set aside far too much valuable time in order to do it justice.

Then, in the late 1990s, he was invited to attend the Chaucer Congress, a symposium of Chaucer scholars in Paris. As part of Terry's lecture, he wanted to use his session to summarise his suspicions about Chaucer's death, to momentarily scratch this itch. Terry Durland, senior lecturer in literature at Trinity College, Dublin, suggested that instead of a talk they hold a coroner's inquest. It was to be a living, breathing, contemporary investigation into Chaucer's death, with Durland acting as the coroner and Terry as the chief accuser alongside three other academics, Juliette Dor, Alan Fletcher and Robert Yeager. It swiftly proved that this fascinating hypothesis could be best explored by a hive mind of experts. It would also mean that Terry would have some heavyweight assistance in compiling his book. Thus it was that this collective of historians, under Terry's headline name, found a publisher for their findings.

Twenty-odd years since turning down *Chaucer's Knight*, it was old Python faithful Methuen who published this voluminous and well-crafted criminal spin on the passing of Chaucer, *Who Murdered Chaucer? A Medieval Mystery*, in 2003. It was, as the title suggests, more of a detective yarn about the writer than another reappraisal of his work. Terry set up this crime fiction-cum-historical debate, suggesting murder or political assassination, based on the idea that Chaucer's work had become awkward and inconvenient as the reactionary Henry IV expunged the liberal legacy of Richard II. It was all to do with the maelstrom at the heart of English politics at the beginning of the fourteenth century. By the dawn of the twenty-first century that was a field of expertise Terry was well respected for and a topic that, as the publisher's blurb put it, combined his usual: 'revelatory scholarship with the flair for narrative that marks all [his] work . . . an absorbing synthesis of history and literary analysis.'

It was pure serendipity, but Terry's delving into Chaucer's final chapter came hot on the heels of the BBC's high-profile dramatisations of eight of his *Canterbury Tales*. Terry, who dutifully sat through one of these – 'The Sea Captain's Tale' – saw exactly what the series was doing. It wasn't really Chaucer but it was what Chaucer would have done with a twenty-first-century BBC film crew, a contemporary reimagining of a Chaucer theme, which, in turn, he had borrowed, maybe from our old Italian chum Boccaccio or maybe from some other even earlier writer. However, Terry's real frustration over the series was that, as a result, the BBC refused to commission his own Chaucer documentary. With the drama series, in tow with a run of animated adaptations, Terry was told, in no uncertain terms, that 'the BBC thought that was enough Chaucer!'

In January 2004 the Beeb did broadcast Terry's major TV series *Medieval Lives*, though, an ambitious documentary travelogue in association with Professor Alan Ereira. Who 'had read *Chaucer's Knight* long before I met Terry, and thought that what he did was very clever. And original.' Alan wasn't 100 per cent in agreement with everything Terry had written, but that is always the way with historians and he was, in the main, with him pretty much all the way.

As Terry explained with regards to the purpose of *Medieval Lives*: 'it was my way to get my own back on the Renaissance!' He had a historical bee in his bonnet again, and it was a frustration that historians and art critics would light up at the merest mention of the Renaissance, as if the human race had no sense of individuality before it. In fact, Terry would argue, the Renaissance was a retrograde step in how it not only celebrated the learnings of Ancient Greece and Ancient Rome as the ultimate in enlightenment but urged the population to return to writing and conversing in classical Latin. As a result, it killed spoken Latin stone dead. This was the very reason why Terry championed the writings of Chaucer and Dante: they energetically wrote in the vernacular and, thus, 'celebrated the vitality, exuberance and individuality of ordinary men and women.' These were writers who wrote in a very modern way, and, as Terry argued, the Middle Ages was a very modern place to live!

He would revolt when historians would condemn the Middle Ages as some sort of uninspiring era of stagnation and ignorance. Nor should one ever – even in jest – suggest to Terry that people in medieval England were convinced that the world was flat. They really didn't believe that. It was an invention – aimed at the legacy of Christopher Columbus – by the American writer of *Sleepy Hollow*, Washington Irving, in 1828. It was a myth that endured all the way through to a debunking of the Middle Ages in a millennium opinion piece in the *New York Times*. A piece that added fuel to the fire of Terry's aim in writing *Medieval Lives*. He would talk delightfully about his favourite medieval writers, with Chaucer front stage and central, of course. To Terry, the voices of these 600-year-old scribes rang in his ears on a daily basis, and they were, genuinely, 'just as alive as we are today'. It was his historical mission to share this passion. To share his knowledge and understanding of Chaucer, simply as a way to know and understand more about ourselves.

And that's exactly what history is. What history meant to Terry. It was a way to connect the present with the past, a way to sprinkle some wonderment over those long, often misinterpreted voices. And, for Terry, the straightest way to get his message across – the swiftest arrow to the heart of the matter – was comedy. And if that meant wallowing in yet another screening and post-screening discussion of *Monty Python and the Holy Grail*, then so be it.

Thirty summers after it had taken Britain and then, rather wonderfully and rather surprisingly, America, by storm, the film itself was now history. A living, breathing, laughing, but accurate, history of Terry's Middle Ages. Terry was chuffed to talk about *Grail*. At any time. Not only was it a film he was inordinately proud of – achieving, as it does, a very funny celebration of medieval history – but it was a blessed relief that people still loved it as much as they did. For many it is *the* Python document. The Holy Grail, if you will.

Even as the twenty-first century rattled on remorselessly, Terry could give you a cold stare and shiver at the memory of the uncertainty and unsteadiness of the pre-production and filming of *Monty Python and the Holy Grail*. Despite their apparent confidence and ease in embracing books and the stage, the Python group were well aware of the bigger, international arena that cinema opened up. After much cajoling and rewriting, many within the group voiced concerns that the final shooting script just wasn't funny enough. Terry, as lead director, had faith in the material, although even that began to wane during the making of the film. The script was far too ambitious for the budget. The money certainly couldn't stretch to the planned battle sequence that was the original ending of the final shooting script for the film. This medieval massacre was, therefore, scuppered before it even began, by the appearance of extras, dressed as contemporary police officers, breaking up the fight: like the law of 1975 stepping in and dispersing an overly keen historical re-enactment group.

But even the constraints of the limited budget added charm to *Monty Python and the Holy Grail*. The Middle Ages meets the mid-Seventies. The invasion of the now into the past at the film's end is one final, self-aware acknowledgement of the reality of Python comedy within not only history, but in the act of making a film. However, Terry's initial dilemma about covering up the shortcomings of the money at his disposal was compounded by the reaction of the audience who sat and watched the rough cut of the film. This was a crowd of investors and, as Terry recalled, sure enough: 'they laughed for the first five minutes, then absolute silence for the whole rest of the film. It was one of the worst nights of my life.'

Things could only get better – and they did. *Monty Python and the Holy Grail* holds some of Python's most treasured and oft-quoted characters: Eric Idle crying out, 'Bring out your dead!' and even accepting those who aren't quite dead yet; Terry Gilliam's moronic jailer who has 'got lumps of it round the back!'; and that most charming of Terry's performances, our beloved, pale and pathetic Prince Herbert, of Swamp Castle, who rather than marrying a princess with huge tracts of land, just wants to sing, sing, sing . . .

The Charisma record, *The Album of the Soundtrack of the Trailer of the Film of Monty Python and the Holy Grail*, was around half soundtrack and half fresh material recorded in March 1975, ahead of the film's release across America. And it was Terry, along with Graham Chapman, who journeyed to the States in order to promote the film. They attended the New York screening, which attracted a crowd of people desperate for a ticket. Such was the buzz of popularity that, when Terry and Graham arrived for the screening in Chicago, they found a young Python devotee there already; he had got to the cinema early in order to guarantee himself a seat. This was 'Professor of Python' Kim 'Howard' Johnson: 'Monty Python had been running on PBS – the Public Broadcasting Service – firstly in Dallas, and then across the country. I had got obsessed with the show. A lot of America had got obsessed with Python. So much so that the queue for the *Holy Grail* screening at the Carnegie Theatre in Chicago was right round the block. I had been there for hours and hours in order to get a front row seat. And I had a couple of carved coconuts as gifts for Graham and Terry.'

As with almost everything Terry did, the coconuts were not just comedy, they were comedy history. Their use on location was a handy and cheap way to suggest horses, but the self-same comic trick had, typically, been used by Spike Milligan and his bunch of crazy cronies in *A Show Called Fred*, in 1956. In that televised attempt at a *Goon Show*-styled sketch, Peter Sellers and Graham Stark had performed an entrance, on 'horseback', with nothing but a coconut each. Suitable then that it was the Goons – well, Sellers and Spike with Dick Emery – in *The Case of the Mukkinese Battle-Horn* that Terry had selected as the support short film for *Grail's* American release. Daylight robbery, I tell you!

Although none of the Pythons expected American success, particularly Terry, in light of the fact that *And Now for Something Completely Different* had only done moderate business in the States, he did readily agree to add an appearance on PBS to his promotional tour across America. It was ostensibly to urge audiences to go and see *Monty Python and the Holy Grail*, but Terry's expectations were low: 'I went on the channel to bring in some cash. If only to raise enough for our fares home!' In the end, it was a push that helped the film make a profit of $50 million over the next decade.

A whole lot more money was added to the *Holy Grail* coffers when, thirty years after the film was made, Eric Idle turned the whole romp into the musical *Spamalot*. Terry was supportive, reflecting that 'eventually we all got a little percentage and a credit on the poster, for writing the original film.' He even attended the Broadway premiere, and the West End one too. It was all glorious grist to the mill of a mini epic that has seen Holy Grail Ale, computer games, action figures, furry bloodstained rabbit slippers and, yes, even collectible coconuts.

And even though he wasn't around to enjoy the fiftieth-anniversary re-release of *Monty Python and the Holy Grail*, it is a joyous film that remains instrumental in solidifying and rarefying Terry's hard historical researches. If people watch the film and then read *Chaucer's Knight*, that's as wonderful a historical legacy as Terry could have hoped for. It is also wonderful that, for Terry, history remained a source of magic and amazement. His final academic job was a translation and reappraisal of the General Prologue to Chaucer's *The Canterbury Tales* for a proposed website and, most innovatively, an educational mobile phone app. It was eventually launched just a few months after Terry's death. The app's creator, Professor Peter Robinson, in Canada, said at the time: 'Terry's work and passion for Chaucer was an inspiration.' The historian never stops learning indeed. And while that is true, for Terry that learning could never start early enough in others. Hence why he would gleefully accept children's films and children's television assignments that were oozing with comedy and tinged with history.

At the end of the twentieth century, Terry had a hand in the adapted English script for the French, German and Italian co-production of the live-action comic strip movie *Asterix and Obelix Take on Caesar*. A typically humorous assault on authority, within Terry's translated screenplay the oft-repeated and lacklustre orders issued by bored military officers end up simply being vocalised as the same old: 'Blah! Blah! Blah!' He also voiced Obelix, the hulking sculptor and deliveryman, in the English version of the film. As played, in the blockbuster flesh, by Gerard Depardieu.

This subversion in comedy and cartoons was a very Terry way of introducing kids to history. Even if that meant reimagining the folk of the Middle Ages as dragons. Yes, as dragons! *Blazing Dragons* was a popular animated series, a co-production between Nelvana Limited in Canada, and the animation studio Ellipse, in

France. Screened in Britain on the commercial station Carlton Television and in America on Toon Disney, it was a rollicking success that, although it only ran from the September of 1996 until the February of 1998, generated and indeed generates a very vocal cult following. While the idea of humanised dragons may sound like the fevered cheese dream of a serious historian, it was, as Terry would tell me with a chuckle over a few pints, the simple result of a very drunken lunch with Emmy-Award winning broadcaster and writer Gavin Scott. He had met and befriended Terry when he was script editor and developer for *The Young Indiana Jones Chronicles*. Terry was employed as actor and director on the series, and enjoyed the company of Scott. So much so that the gloriously nutty notion of *Blazing Dragons* was hatched. That initial boozy banter was pretty much Terry's sole contribution to the franchise. As with much of his life, he regretted never having the time to further develop the idea because he always had something much more pressing to occupy his mind. He couldn't even slip in a recording session here or a voice-over session there to play one of the key dragons, although: 'as far as I remember, they wanted me to play the king. It would have been good to be the king. King Allfire of Camelhot. Oh dear! I just couldn't do it! Not because I didn't want to. I just didn't have the time.' Brooklyn-born actor and artist Aron Tager obliged in Terry's stead, although Terry did prove available to voice a few characters for the video game based upon the series. He is the 1st Uncouth Revolting Peasant, Trivet the Jester and, most pleasingly of all, Sir Burnevere, a dragon-twist on his Welsh-inspired *Holy Grail* character. The cartoon television series – in which Burnevere was Scottish and would cry 'Hoot McGregor!' when things went wrong – and the computer game it inspired led to a frantic and very vocal online fan club called Blazing Dragons Revolution.

Terry would look, with mock concern, over his pint glass when I mentioned that this dedicated group were continually calling upon

Terry and his co-creator to bring the series back. 'Don't tell them that I haven't even ever seen an episode, let alone that I have absolutely no power in bringing it back. Well, maybe I have, but I'm not entirely sure I want to. Is it any good?' Although no expert, I had seen enough to reassure Terry that it was decidedly Pythonesque in its knowing comedic twisting of history. What's more, the spirited song and dance opening credits, with colourful dragons having a ball, was very *Holy Grail* in its singalong quality.

Having returned, with Michael Palin, for a location report for the 30th anniversary DVD of *Holy Grail*, a few years later Terry, alone, made his own personal pilgrimage back to Doune Castle. Unannounced and unrecognised, it was Historic Scotland employee Catherine Mason who recognised him and gave him the guided tour. There and then he agreed to record the attraction's audio commentary. Catherine remembers: 'we provided him with the script but he added and adlibbed that material.' Sure enough, as you would expect, Terry is always funny and never boring. He even instructs you to press the green button for more on the Python connections from when 'me and some friends made a very silly film here!' The only stipulations for Terry were that he would not receive a fee for his services and that the castle must never, ever charge visitors for his guiding narration. As Catherine Mason remembers: 'it was Terry's gift to the castle.' It still is. Terry may be long gone, but his historical passion and comic memories still thrill tourists, with his final lapse into the swallow debate as real swallows swoop over your head!

There's something fitting that the weird and the wacky and the wonderful kind of bookend Terry's professional life as a historian. It was a lifelong odyssey, and, while many profiles and even some obituaries called Terry a professional funny man and an amateur historian, Terry always claimed: 'it's actually the other way around. It's not hard to put on a frock and squawk some silly lines! The hard work is getting to grips with Geoffrey Chaucer. That's something I'm still working out. I think it always will be.'

# A MIDDLE WORD

## A QUITE UNNECESSARY INTRUSION INTO THE NARRATIVE STRUCTURE OF THIS BOOK BY ERIC IDLE

HEY, sorry to intrude like this, popping up here in the middle of this book completely uninvited, but I'm far too late for the foreword and I'm not sure I will survive long enough for the afterword, so I thought it best to nip in here to say just how much I loved Terry and how much I still miss him.

I first saw him on stage in 1963 at the Edinburgh Festival, where he was part of the Oxford revue, I was part of the rival Cambridge crew, and Graeme Garden and I popped along to see what they were up to. What they were up to was being very funny, and it was a surprise therefore a few months later to see Terry acting extremely seriously in the West End, in *Hang Down Your Head and Die*, a polemical play protesting the barbarity of hanging. At that time, I remember, he resembled Anthony Newley, but as he aged he reminded me more of Robert De Niro. He was a handsome bastard anyway, but always a very kind man.

We first worked together after Oxbridge as writers for David Frost on the BBC's *The Frost Report*, amidst some of the finest wits in television, including the irreplaceable Marty Feldman and the irrepressible Barry Cryer. We were only callow youths and new to the trade, but they made us very welcome and encouraged us. Terry had cleverly partnered up with Michael Palin, whom I had seen the following year at the Edinburgh Festival and who was funny enough for a brigade of comics, so that when Humphrey

Barclay invited me to write and star in a children's television show to be called *Do Not Adjust Your Set* I agreed, *provided* I could have Terry and Michael help write and perform it with me. So they were co-opted by Humphrey and away we went, joining David Jason, Denise Coffey and the Bonzo Dog Doo-Dah Band, winning awards for our kids' show, and garnering a large audience of adults who would race home to watch us at five twenty in the evening. We were extremely popular with waiters, I recall, and two people who stopped work every week to watch us were John Cleese and Graham Chapman. From this grew *Monty Python's Flying Circus*, which was a collision between our kids' show and *At Last the 1948 Show*. What followed could not have been predicted by any of us – a collaboration that lasted from 1969 until 1983, and grew from a late-night TV show on the BBC to a world-renowned comedy troupe that segued from television into four movies, three of which were brilliantly directed by Terry.

My finest time with Terry was playing Ratty to his Toad in his movie of *The Wind in the Willows*, which he also wrote and directed, and indeed for the rest of his life we emailed each other as 'Ratty' and 'Toady'. In fact towards the end, as his memory of who people were faded, I asked his son to say hello from Ratty, and to my joy they told me he lit up and beamed.

I have so many happy memories of him, but this isn't the middle of my book and I have intruded quite enough in this one, so I must make my excuses and leave.

I miss you so much, Toady.

Love,

Ratty

Eric Idle, California, May 2025

# CHAPTER NINE

## TALL TALES AND REAL ALES

*If society is making good beer, then it's a healthy*
*society. Real ale is a civilised drink.*

DESPITE the financial security and comedy greatness that Python and, in particular, *Monty Python and the Holy Grail* had bestowed upon all of them, Terry was still contributing skits and sketches to other funny men. There was still the occasional filmed slapstick interlude for Marty Feldman and the odd reheated party scenario for *The Two Ronnies*. There was even an aborted – albeit paid for, in full – storyline for *The Stanley Baxter Show*. The item, entitled 'The Doughnut in Granny's Greenhouse', never resurfaced, although, decades later, Terry threw open a challenge to the handful of writers and other creatives gathered in the garden of his north London home one brilliant and bright Sunday lunchtime. It was to be a short-story writing contest. The title of the story was to be 'The Greatest Doughnut in the Galaxy'. I never finished mine. Neither did Terry. The story, that is, not the doughnut. Although I'd like to think that Terry might have gone back to the Stanley Baxter plot for inspiration.

Michael Palin wasn't there that Sunday lunchtime, but he was at Terry's elbow in those glory days of the 1970s, and Terry had never been more productive, as Alison Telfer recalls: 'at one point he was writing Python in the afternoon, doing a show in the evening and writing something else in the morning.' Juggling three projects at once was rather like having a scriptwriting repertory theatre company in his head. And that's not to mention the pantomime. Wait, what? Terry wrote a pantomime with Michael Palin? Surely not. Oh yes, he did. Two, in fact.

The shows in question were versions and variations on the themes of *Aladdin* and *Beauty and the Beast*. *Aladdin* was commissioned and staged for the Civic Theatre in Watford, for the 1967/68 season, with Oxford chum David Wood as Wishee Washee; *Beauty and the Beast* played the Colchester Theatre, for a month from 21 December 1971. Michael Palin remembers the pantos as another challenge, another fun way to be funny: 'we saw them as clearing the decks, in a way. We loved writing together. It was fun, in those days, and we enjoyed putting little bits of subversive into the tried and tested pantomime style'. They created a very boring leading man, called Prince Fong. He had a very boring song that went something like this: 'My name is Fong and this is my terrible song. And although it won't be long, my name is still Fong . . .' Half the audience liked that, as a concept of a joke on a joke – the leading man of a pantomime is dashing and brave. You don't have boring heroes in pantos. The other half of the audience just thought it was rubbish! Michael reflects that certainly for *Beauty and the Beast* it was 'a privilege to be writing for the stage and for kids, again. Having written Python, Terry and I had been really spoiled. To return to pantomime after that experience was a great exercise in writing something exciting while staying – just – within the boundaries of convention.'

Terry would once again gently send up the art of pantomime-writing within his book *The Curse of the Vampire's Socks and Other Doggerel*, in 1988. An example of relentless poetry was 'A New Attempt on the World Rhyming Championship Record', in salute to dogged panto scribe Harry Hyam, whose final effort was staged in Burgwindheim . . . The poem goes on for a long, long time in a similar vein. It was all grist to the comedy mill, these cheeky little bits of silliness within a rather conservative structure of pantomime.

Like the BBC days of old, such silliness would make Terry smile. They still had to write that conservative, structured pantomime, though, as Michael Palin remembers: 'I'm embarrassed to say, but we just couldn't bring ourselves to write the really soppy love stuff. It wasn't our thing . . .'

Silliness certainly was their thing, and they kept ploughing that hilarious field within and without Python, as Michael explains: 'Terry was very stimulating to work with, and very honest about things. We didn't say what the other was doing was good because we felt we should. We were very, very honest with ourselves about the material. It didn't spoil the friendship at all. If anything, it built it up into something stronger. There was a trust.'

In the midst of Python's third series, on 3 November 1972, Ben Travers, assistant head of copyright, alerted agent Kenneth Ewing that:

> we should like to commission Michael Palin and Terry Jones to write a treatment for a 60 minute episode [which was crossed out and the word 'farce' added] in our television drama series 'Black and Blue', for delivery by 17 November 1972.

By December the theme of the 'farce' was apparent. An employee of a chocolate factory falls into a mixing vat of the sweet stuff. Undetected. The consignment of chocolate goes out to the shops; the public love the taste of meat with their cocoa beans; and the bosses calculate just how many people they can spare in the name of rising sales. The play was called 'Secrets' and was indeed screened under the auspices of the *Black and Blue* series. 'Secrets' was very much more black comedy than blue comedy. This was deliciously black. Dark, in fact. Dark Chocolate, to be precise. Warren Mitchell would star as the factory owner in this sweetly sick spin-off of the basic concept of Python's 'Crunchy Frog' sketch in which Terry, as the owner of the Whizzo Chocolate Company, adds amphibians – bones and all – to his confectionery. 'Secrets' simply took this idea to cannibalistic extremes. The closing advertising sting in the play tells you all you need to know about it: 'Only the Best People Go into Our Chocolates'.

Internal correspondence concerning the commissioned script of 'Secrets' was positive, with Richard Broke writing to Ben Travers on 3 January 1973 that:

> we are accepting the farce by these writers, and they are currently engaged on rewrites because the script makes some fairly complex technical demands, and because this is their first full-length play, [Mark Shivas] and I would be glad if you could accept on condition that the writers make themselves available for any further rewriting which the Director might require. This may well not be necessary, but is a precaution we would like to take. I would emphasise that the relationship between the writers and ourselves is an excellent one!

Terry and Mike were delighted with the results too. 'Secrets' went out to strong opinion, both positive and negative, and, in their quest to spread the delights of bad taste comedy, each and every complaint the BBC received made them more and more pleased. The play was a success. A sick success. Even fifteen years later, the idea of 'Secrets' was controversial and cutting-edge enough for Euston Films Limited and The Samuel Goldwyn Company to turn it into the feature film *Consuming Passions*. Jonathan Pryce was the hair-flicking boss, Vanessa Redgrave the eastern European landlady and Tyler Butterworth the hapless hero. The soft centre, if you will. Terry and Michael enjoyed a nice little payday for the 'Based on ...' acknowledgement of their screenplay, which was adapted for the big screen by Paul D. Zimmerman and Andrew Davies, and shot at Pinewood Studios.

It wasn't all sweet though. In the wake of Python's second place success at the Montreux Festival, Terry and Mike had, once again, been called upon to tinker with the 'Secrets' script. The BBC considered it strong enough as their competition entry that year and so commissioned the writers to polish and rework 'their existing ninety-minute film script to see if it would make a viable entry' for the Montreux Festival of 1973. In the end this project fell through, although the writers picked up a nice 'once-for-all joint fee of £250'.

All this activity outside of Monty Python was a healthy distraction from the cold fact that the group was fragmenting. For Terry, it was slightly disquieting that the most damaging cracks were still coming from within Python itself. In the face of increasing interference from the BBC bosses, he felt the group should be even more strongly united. Still, John Cleese, reluctant to play in any case, continually gave his unenthused reaction to that third series of *Monty Python's Flying Circus*. He boiled it down to the fact that, in his summation, the only wholly original sketches had been 'Dennis Moore' and 'Cheese Shop'. In retrospect, as with *Monty Python and the Holy Grail* being far, far more than the group's filming experiences of cold and mud and misery, *Monty Python* series three is far, far more than a jolly highwayman song and a list of dairy consumables. There was Sam Peckinpah's 'Salad Days', a cultural juxtaposition from the school of *Twice a Fortnight*; there was that censored but still relentlessly funny Proust sketch; and there was Terry, centre stage, as the desperate bowler-hatted businessman who can't help but make everyone laugh hysterically. It's the comedian's curse in sketch form. However desperate he is to be taken seriously, all those around him are convulsed with laughter. So desperate is he that he contemplates suicide. Terry's performance alone is testament that Python still had something seriously silly to say.

Still, even after the Python tour of Canada and ahead of their taking of Drury Lane, Michael Palin recorded in his diary entry of 23 September 1973 that time seemed to be running out for Python. As usual, a conversation was needed. And it had to be in a pub with his closest ally within the group: 'Terry and I went up to the Flask in Hampstead and had a good air-clearing talk about the future.' The crux of the discussion was twofold. Firstly, Michael reasoned that Python had to be the six of them. Together. Even with an agreed concession for John to opt out of performing any more Python on television but still 'writing a regulation three and a half minutes per show'. Terry was enthusiastic about the idea. He cited the strong and funny material that the group had written for *The Monty Python Matching Tie and Handkerchief* album as proof that, together, the group had limitless potential, but Michael's diary wonders whether it was: 'worth doing, currently at present, if at all . . . I think we may be straining to keep up our standards and, without John, the strain could be too great.'

While Terry seemed keen to continue with Python, however forced the process may have to be, his passion could be contagious. Moreover, Python was still very much a vibrant commercial concern. Even so, Michael was more interested in maintaining the productive writing partnership between the two of them. He and Terry, he reflected in the diary, 'have another direction to go in, with a play in commission and another on the stocks. We work fast and economically, and still pretty successfully together.'

Indeed, three days after that conversation, Terry and Michael were commissioned by script editor Richard Broke and producer Mark Shivas to write an, as yet untitled, comedy about childbirth. This project, for the same team as was behind 'Secrets', never came to fruition. The following month, on 5 October 1973 to be precise – exactly four years after the broadcast of the first Python episode – Terry and Michael were in talks for another play, this time under the *Group One* drama series banner. Mark

Shivas was to produce again. While the childbirth scenario was to be treated comedically, this new commission was to take Terry and Mike into fresh territory: a thirty-minute serious drama for late-night television. The script was contracted to be delivered by 26 October 1973, by which time the overall series title had become *Run Through*. Call it what you will, the playlet never made it to the screen.

More fertile, and safer, and far, far easier to write, was a couple of quickies for *It's Cliff Richard*. On 30 August 1974 Terry and Michael were commissioned, and paid a joint fee of £20, for a twenty-second joke called 'Image of His Father', and a nineteen-second gag entitled 'Yards of Ale'. The Peter Pan of Pop played it perfectly. It was like *The Frost Report* days all over again, with Terry and Mike being happy to accept these jobs alongside much more challenging ventures.

The Cliff gig came just after the shooting of *Holy Grail* and before its release. In that window of madness, the Pythons were back at the BBC. Well, five of them were. The majority of the group had made a decision about the future and accepted John's terms of contributing written material to the proposed fourth series of television episodes. John would still be very much part of the process, albeit, in the main, contentedly contributing scripted leftovers from the writing sessions for *Holy Grail*. John did, however, stick to his guns about refusing to get up at silly o'clock and wear a silly costume in a silly location.

With one of the engines gone, the five Pythons were given just six episodes, as opposed to the previous thirteen, and stripped of the Flying Circus status. The series was simply now entitled *Monty Python* and all had to do a little more heavy lifting – particularly Graham, who was still drinking heavily – and now, with John out of the group discussion, had to write with others. None stepped up to the plate to keep Python going more than Terry Jones, whose favourite sketches, like the monotonous post office and the Royal

Air Force banter and the Most Awful Family in Britain, undoubtedly ranked with any of the best material from the previous three series. In performance, too, Terry was on fire. His earnest, ever-questioning judge in the courtroom remains an oft-referenced pinnacle of bluff and bluster. Python 4, or Monty Python 1, if you prefer, is awash with literary and historical bonbons of an extremely high standard.

Front and centre was Terry Jones: as thin as a whippet and twice as energetic. A streamlined Python team captain who was keen, nay desperate to continue with the five-man performing television group, as well as joint projects on film, on stage and in print. Besides, Terry had been in sketch teams since Oxford. People joined; people left. That was the nature of sketch shows. Terry wasn't quite so cavalier as to think that Python could be a free-for-all, a comedy pop group with ever-renewing personnel, but he was confident that the brand was strong enough to withstand changes. Sketch performers may not be indispensable but they could be interchangeable. Interestingly though, the most doubtful of this attitude within Python was Terry's own writing partner, Michael Palin.

The fourth series is a treasure trove, although it was deemed only a BBC2 treasure trove. Its first episode, on the last day of October 1974, did warrant a *Radio Times* cover and full-spread interview with the team, which tried to answer such taxing questions as were the Montgolfier brothers the first balloonists? Was Louis XIV a Glaswegian? And should you vote Norwegian at the next election? But everybody could see it wasn't quite the same. Everybody except Terry Jones, of course. Even threats from within the group to split asunder didn't deter Terry from plotting and planning further Python shows for television. In the end, the individual members just got on with their own thing regardless.

By the end of 1975, the writing was on the wall for Monty Python as a cohesive television comedy team. They all stayed at the BBC, just not in each other's pockets. From the May, with *Holy Grail* heading to cinemas and record players, Eric Idle was running his very own channel – well, a comedy sketch show on the BBC at least, called *Rutland Weekend Television* – while from the September, John Cleese was checking problematic guests into *Fawlty Towers*. January 1976 saw Graham Chapman star in *Out of the Trees*, a very Python-like sketch show, which went uncommissioned as a series, while Terry and Mike still stuck together with the pilot for *Ripping Yarns*. Terry had to face the fact that, simply through logistics, it was going to be pretty much impossible to get all six Pythons into a room together on a regular basis to work on new material for television. Whether all six were willing to do so was immaterial. Terry's consolation for not having as much Python as he had had over the last five years was to have a lot more exclusive writing time with Michael Palin.

Clearly, the Jones and Palin writing partnership was still strong and spirited, as they soldiered on with ideas for a series of *The Boy's Own Paper*, *Union Jack* and *Roy of the Rovers*-styled adventures of derring-do and sporting achievement, an affectionate send-up of the stories Terry and Michael had loved as children. This gentle poke at old-fashioned, stiff-upper-lipped British heroism in a series of humorous half-hour plays would come to define them within cult comedy circles forever more. However, it was also the breaking point. Although the association and the friendship would remain vital until the end of Terry's life, *Ripping Yarns* marked the loud, final crescendo of an exclusive creative partnership of over ten years' standing.

As far as the Corporation was concerned, *Ripping Yarns* was a showcase for Michael Palin. It had been Terry who had been the first in to attack, vehemently complaining over the BBC's tinkering with Monty Python. As a result, he had got himself a reputation as a troublemaker. Moreover, Terry was very vocal about his objection to playing the corporate game. He wasn't keen on attending press parties and placating the powers that be. For Michael Palin, all that was simply part of the job! As a result, the BBC was keen to promote *Ripping Yarns* as the Michael Palin show. And it showed. The official *Ripping Yarns* press release explained that:

> in the wake of the immensely successful Monty Python series, its creators are each engaged in individual pursuits in television comedy. Michael Palin, with his writing partner Terry Jones, has opted for a tale set in the Edwardian era – the heyday of school stories.

Michael's writing partner. Not Terry and Michael, or even Michael and Terry, but Michael with Terry. Indeed, the missive went on to say:

> *Michael Palin plays Tomkinson, our hero, and doubles as the Headmaster who runs an establishment steeped in such trad-itions as St Tadgers Day, upon which day boys who had been at the school for less than two years were allowed to be nailed to the walls by senior prefects. Terry Jones plays Ellis, a weak and ineffectual housemaster. Gwen Watford plays Tomkinson's mother and Ian Ogilvy plays Grayson, the School Bully – he had twice won the Public School Bullying cup.*

Weak and ineffectual, maxims for Terry's character, not Terry himself. But those are negative words; damp words. In the end, 'Tomkinson's Schooldays' would be the only Ripping Yarn in which Terry acted. He co-wrote the lot, of course, but, for those who didn't bother reading the credits, *Ripping Yarns* would be seen as Michael's starring vehicle. Exactly as the BBC had wished it.

Whatever the BBC wanted to think, though, *Ripping Yarns* was a culmination of threads that ran throughout the Jones and Palin writing partnership. Terry himself was always very keen to credit his elder brother Nigel for the basic idea – that of a mockery of the stereotypes of Imperial Britain that still lingered in Seventies society – but there had always been elements of this within their work. Even in collaborations that Terry and Michael hadn't written themselves.

For even on these rarest of occasions, Terry was a keen team player. The most Terry and Mike of these fringe projects was *Funny Game, Football,* a comedy album for Charisma, which was unleashed just ahead of *Monty Python's Previous Record.* Terry, as a whining woman – what else? – faces brutal conversion to the beautiful game. On the record, he also plays a contestant with a baggage of football trivia on the game show hosted by Michael Palin and delivers a wistful torrent on football's glory days: 'I Remember it Well'. As well as Terry and Mike, the writers Joe Steeples, Bill Tidy and Michael Wale also performed, alongside comedy actors Arthur Mullard and Bryan Pringle, with music from Neil Innes completing the squad. It's a fairly rare, rather minor little tickle of the funny bone, but, in essence, it's a comic finger towards the Ripping Yarn 'Golden Gordon' and the frantic cry of Gordon Ottershaw: 'Eight–one! Eight–bloody–one!'

Certainly within the Pythons – an arena of some freedom but still one with six, very different and increasingly individual comedy brains at play – elements of *Ripping Yarns* had also emerged, notably in *The Brand New Monty Python Bok,* which included Terry and Michael's 'Biggles is Extremely Silly', an apparently previously unpublished 1938 story of aerial derring-do. The flying ace created by Captain W.E. Johns, whose thrilling adventures had him see action in both the First and Second World War, would crop up again as a comedy reference point in the fourth series of Python on telly too. Not to mention Python perennial the 'Spanish Inquisition'. Nobody expected Terry as Cardinal Biggles. Not at first. All very Terry and Mike. Very *Ripping Yarns.*

Also published by Methuen, and so connected with the franchise that first editions were adorned with a sticker reading, 'A Monty Python Educational Product', came *Bert Fegg's Nasty Book for Boys and Girls*. In the book, for nasty children of all ages, Terry and Michael not only adapted some of their Python material, but resurrected panto memories – oh yes, they did – with 'Aladdin and his Terrible Problem' (the terrible problem being Pisso, his alcoholic dog sidekick). There was even further foreshadowing of 'Golden Gordon', with football tactic instructions related through a comic strip, with, of all things, the Motown group the Supremes displaying ball control! Most revealing of all, within the pages of *Bert Fegg's Nasty Book for Boys and Girls* was a story called 'Across the Andes by Frog', pointing directly forward and away from the Python group. This indeed was very much a parody in print of a *Boy's Own* tale, one which would be extended into a television Ripping Yarn.

And this long-form narrative comedy was the key to the *Ripping Yarns* series. It was an extension of insanity that Terry and Mike would also explore on stage. *Their Finest Hours* was a double bill of plays, first presented at Sheffield's Crucible Theatre. It was home territory for Michael Palin and Terry was on very friendly terms with David Leland, the actor and writer who had in 1975 been appointed director of the theatre. *Their Finest Hours* was Leland's commission and was a theatre experience of two halves: 'Underwood's Finest Hour' was a reworking of the 'childbirth' play that had stalled at the BBC. Derek Underwood's wife is expecting a baby, although the doctor is more interested in cricket, intently listening to the Test Match with England still requiring sixty-four runs to beat the West Indies. Despite the recorded voice of respected commentator John Arlott relating the score, in a specially recorded voice-over for the play, Ned Chaillet, theatre critic of the *Daily Telegraph*, thought it was 'not unamusing [although] more a tribute to cricket ... than a try at theatre.' 'Buchanan's Finest Hour', the second offering, was a much more absurdist parable of the British spirit. Buchanan, a disgraced

Member of Parliament, agrees to be consigned to a large packing crate – on stage – in order to prove that British-made is best. Buchanan remains within the crate for the duration of the play – a crate in which, as it gradually transpires, a whole wacky community also resides, including the Pope. Throughout the play the crate is moved, cajoled and generally mucked about with. It's the perfect Venn diagram between the stoic determination of *Ripping Yarns* and the utter bonkersness of Python.

Indeed, Terry and Michael had already experimented with the long-form surreal sketch within Python itself. As much from necessity to fill a series as a strong desire to move away from the sketch show format, Terry and Mike had offered up a self-contained half-hour during series three of *Monty Python's Flying Circus*. Reg Pither, on a cycling tour of north Cornwall, was the ultimate showcase for the very English dullness that had been at the core of Michael Palin's funniest performances since Oxford. And although that loving send-up of the monosyllabic bore was a creation of both Terry and Michael, it was Michael who played it to perfection. Terry, as an actor, was brilliant at screaming eccentrics and ponderous dullards, and, while any one of these characters could have sat at the centre of a comedy situation or, indeed, a situation comedy, it was Michael's playful mixture of the endearing and the boring that stood out. Reg Pither was a very British failure and although the other Pythons pitched in with material, and played roles within the comedy journey, it was a very Terry and Mike script too. Michael says: 'I loved playing him. I enjoy those gullible characters who are stronger than they first appear. He's a mild-mannered chap but he simply won't let you get away. He's rather aggressive in his niceness. Persistent, infuriating, but relentlessly cheerful with his lot. His aim is to bore you to death, and he's loving it.'

'The Cycling Tour' was an experiment in long-form Python. 'Mr Neutron', in Python series four, was cut from similar cloth, albeit it slightly more ragged, slightly more constructed along the old line of interlinking sketches.

As far as Terry was concerned, 'The Cycling Tour', in particular, was the way forward. It had started as a Terry and Mike half-hour and been embraced within the ever hungry-for-material Monty Python collective. The fact that it worked struck a chord with Terry. Perhaps he and Mike could write a series of these and simply use the other Pythons as actors. It could be the best of both worlds: editorial control over the comedy, with trusted cohorts to play the other parts, and play them in a way that would never, ever miss the joke as written. As Terry fantasised: 'Ideally, *Ripping Yarns* would have been written by us, and performed by us and the other Pythons. Initially I saw the show as a way of keeping Python together and hiring John and Eric and Graham as actors. They were far too busy with their own projects though and I don't think we even got as far as asking them.'

Rather than being a reimagining of the Python circus with Terry and Mike as the ringmasters, *Ripping Yarns* saw some very distinguished actors drafted in, notably Denholm Elliott, Bill Fraser, Roy Kinnear and a brilliantly befuddled teaming of Richard Vernon and Joan Sanderson. Although sibling Python rivalry had Terry ruing the fact that John Cleese had secured Sanderson as the hard-of-hearing and argumentative Mrs Richards in the *Fawlty Towers* episode 'Communication Problems': 'John got her before us. Not in a petty way, but we were all working on different things at the same time, trying to prove ourselves away from the group. Obviously we wanted all our fellow Pythons to do well. Just not that well!'

Moreover, for Terry, despite the quality of the casts, *Ripping Yarns* was something of a retrograde step: 'I had a few pre-Python moments of doubt and frustration with *Ripping Yarns*, in that we were writing for other people again and not all the actors in the shows were quite getting the jokes. Mind you, in the end Mike played all the best characters. Brilliantly, it must be said. So I found myself writing all the funniest lines for Mike.'

And there hangs the crux and the shivering of the Jones and Palin foundations at the very heart of *Ripping Yarns*. For someone who had hoped to be an actor since his schooldays, the irony of not acting in the *Ripping Yarns* series would not have been lost on Terry. Perhaps even more so since, long ago, he wrote that he was 'hopping' to be an actor, a central surreal element of 'Tomkinson's Schooldays' is a hopping competition: the Thirty Mile Hop, against a Buddhist public school. Irony of ironies, it is Michael's character who wins this hopping race and is subsequently promoted to School Bully.

There really were no hard feelings – or, if there were, the following decades were a balm. When Network DVD repackaged the complete collection of *Ripping Yarns*, the release was promoted by a special hopathon, on Saturday 3 March 2012. Michael Palin was in attendance. As was Terry. Both dressed in schoolboy attire to support the venture and take part in not one but two attempts to break Guinness World Records: the largest group gathering 400-metre hop and the 400-metre relay hop. Terry was hopping with the best of them. But not hopping mad. Our conversation that day returned to the question of *Ripping Yarns*, and his complete lack of appearances in the series that 'Tomkinson's Schooldays' inspired. Terry was as stoic and good-natured as ever. It really didn't matter to him, he assured me.

But as far as Michael remembers it, back in the Seventies 'it was quite tense, to be honest. An extremely awkward situation.' When reminded of Terry's attitude to it all, Michael 'still feels that awkwardness even now. All these years later.' The brutal truth of the matter was that Michael was, like every other Python apart from Terry, trying to prove he could do something good on his own: 'part of it was that I wanted to try out my own kind of humour, and something alone, just to see how that worked.'

Indeed, 'Tomkinson's Schooldays' had been very much Palin's idea: 'I had grown up reading stories like "The Ducker of Denbigh", all about life in this posh school, Rookwood, where the greatest dramatic tension seemed to be whether the rotters who attended Belltowers school could be bowled out before tea! Terry tapped into those memories, of course, but it was something that was very much me.'

As far as Terry was concerned: '*Ripping Yarns* was Mike and me writing historical comedy again.' This was very much Terry's comedy safe place. Indeed, the parallel with great swathes of their previous work was recognised in a March 1975 interview, ahead of filming 'Tomkinson's Schooldays', in which Sheridan Morley chatted with Terry and Michael about the future. 'The Complete and Utter Palin and Jones' headline had one big foot very much in the past of *The Complete and Utter History of Britain*. *Ripping Yarns* wasn't so much a comic history of Britain though, it was a way to lovingly send up a shared fondness of Agatha Christie and Rudyard Kipling and *Tom Brown's School Days* by Thomas Hughes.

Despite wrangles with the BBC, with Python, and this desire to prove himself, Michael still didn't want to write the series alone and, moreover, couldn't break away from the writing partnership with Terry. In terms of writing and acting, *Ripping Yarns* would have the Palin stamp all over it, but it would most definitely be a Jones and Palin product: 'That was very difficult with Terry, because Terry always had a very strong and a very intense idea of how things should be done. And that was fine most of the time, but just occasionally it had to be done his way or not at all. I found that a little bit stifling at times.'

It wasn't so much the difficulty between Terry and Mike that rang the changes, as much as that determination within the BBC. Early ambitions for Terry to direct the pilot show, 'Tomkinson's Schooldays', were quashed within the BBC immediately. The show was assigned to the safe pair of hands of Jim Franklin, from *The*

*Frost Report* days. The *Ripping Yarns* producer would be Terry Hughes, who had previously been Terry's boss in the *Two Ronnies* writers' room. Despite Terry's name on the script and his, admittedly lowly, supporting position in the cast, the publicity machine for 'Tomkinson's Schooldays' was very much to be focused on Michael Palin as the star turn. Within internal BBC memos throughout the middle of October 1975 it was being discussed as 'The Mike Palin Revue'; by November, it had become 'The Mike Palin Special'. Now, regardless of these being very much working titles and sounding more like the show should have dancing girls and guest stars in it, the point that looms large is that nowhere, ever, was it referred to as The Palin and Jones Half Hour or anything similar. It was a reality that both angered and disappointed Terry. And, admits Michael: 'Frankly, the BBC wanted it to be my show. It was a very difficult situation, but we compromised. In the end, Terry was terrific about it really. We had some very difficult chats and he never could get used to not being in the series, but we wrote all the Yarns together.'

And the topics and targets for parody within *Ripping Yarns* were all of interest to both Terry and Mike. To that end, it is impossible to improve on the catchy synopsis of the first series that, alongside the episodes themselves, Terry and Mike wrote, rewrote and reworked for official BBC publicity purposes. It is important to note that, even with *Ripping Yarns*, very much a pastiche on classic literature, the writers are still using contemporary television as a point of comedy reference. The first series of *Ripping Yarns* was broadcast from 27 September 1977 and began with 'The Testing of Eric Olthwaite', 'a 1930s all-action spectacle which makes *Starsky and Hutch* look like a driving lesson'. It was filmed in Durham and set: 'in the dark days of the Depression before *When the Boat Comes In* had started bringing jobs to the area.' It revelled in 'a cast of thousands all talking in Yorkshire accents ...' Contemporary television was clearly still in their sights with the next episode for, although not directly name-checked, the early 1970s prisoner-of-war drama *Colditz* was heavily echoed in 'Escape from Stalag Luft 112B': 'The heroic story of a Major Errol Phipps, a British officer who escaped over 500 times in the First World War'. This is the story of how 'the Germans attempt to break him of the habit. He is sent to a top-security prison where there are four Alsatians to each bed . . .' Broadcast a little under two years since the death of the queen of crime fiction, 'Murder at Moorstones Manor' was teased as: 'the story Agatha Christie never dared to write', with enough 'strange deaths, clues and suspects to fill at least 23' novels. The *Ripping Yarns* press release also promised, with tongue firmly in cheek, that 'anyone who guesses the ending will be given a free ticket to the BBC canteen for life.'

'Across the Andes by Frog', extended from the printed word of the Bert Fegg book, was 'an heroic story of courage, resolution and endeavour in the face of almost overwhelming odds. In 1927 one of Britain's least-known explorers, Captain Walter Snetterton, set out with six hand-picked frogs for the first amphibian assault on the Andes . . . A ripping story of one man and a bucket of slime against the world. Shot in Scotland and just behind the brand new James Bond studio at Pinewood.' Last and arguably the plum in the whole *Ripping Yarns* pudding was 'The Curse of the Claw', a Gothic thirty-minute Hammer Horror film, set in Maidenhead, and 'definitely not a story for the squeamish or those with no sense of humour.' It tells 'the terrifying story of a man who dabbled in the dark mysteries of the Orient, and lived to tell the tale. Or did he . . .?'

Inevitably, the first batch of *Ripping Yarns*, broadcast in September and October 1977, built up the marquee value of multi-actor Michael Palin, although Terry and Mike were still very much as one with regards to what these perfect pastiches were trying to achieve. As Michael explains: 'The key to a lot of the stories is that people don't grow up in that sort of society. The public school bully simply became an officer in the regiment, where he could bully his men, and then an MP where he could bully the world at large. So you actually got a sort of institutionalised bullying which was instilled in people from a very early age; from schooldays. In the same way, manners and discipline and restraint were instilled from a very early age. Now we may think they are wonderful things, but the point is that they have to be looked at and questioned in every time and every period.'

There is a sense of being forced to conform and forced to grow up that was the very antithesis of Terry. He was not someone who relished having to wear a jacket and tie in order to enjoy a meal in a restaurant. He was not a person to see injustice and fail to react to it. He was not a person to suppress his enthusiasm and passions and ambitions. All of these mini dramas and more were lovingly explored and developed within *Ripping Yarns*. In reality, Terry may not have had the opportunity or the unfettered bravery to expose society's unfairness. Within *Ripping Yarns* he could write down the witty putdown or the cutting comeback and, by doing so, not only make the audience laugh at their own foibles but also make them reflect. If only for a short while. For Terry, that window of comic exposure at the BBC was slowly but surely closing.

While his fellow Pythons were spreading their wings on television, Terry Gilliam was in pre-production for *Jabberwocky*, his horror fantasy riff on Lewis Carroll. In cinemas for the spring of 1977, between the pilot and the first batch of *Ripping Yarns*, it once again put Michael Palin centre stage, as the hapless hero Dennis Cooper. Although it was never conceived as a Python film, Gilliam cast Jones as the ill-fated poacher, who is literally ripped asunder by the fearsome creature of the title. This happens in the first reel; in the first scene. Dudley Moore, an Oxford graduate from the 1950s, had originally been cast in the role, but Terry was a mate, and a shoo-in for the memorable cameo role. Even so, it reinforced the BBC's shifting of emphasis on Palin as the star of the Palin and

Jones partnership. Despite Terry's eagerness to help out, *Jabberwocky* followed 'Tomkinson's Schooldays' in casting Michael as the star and Terry in a minor supporting role. Besides, the scene was to be filmed on location in Wales!

Terry couldn't resist offering a word of advice on the directing of the film. The brief but savage attack on his poacher character was filmed, at Pembroke Castle, in Pembrokeshire, from the Jabberwocky's bloody and very high point of view and thus necessitated a crane shot. With the light fast fading, Terry J. suggested that perhaps the shot would work better from that little corner of the forest over there. Terry G. knew that the spot he had sourced and selected was the right one. Terry J. insisted. He insisted so much that producer John Goldstone stepped in and gently nudged Terry G. into just trying the other spot, as urged by Terry Jones. The crane was dismantled, moved, reassembled . . . and the shot didn't work! Terry later admitted: 'I did rather piss Terry G. off that day. All I can say, in my own defence, was that it was more than apparent that Terry wanted to direct his own movies and I wanted to direct my own movies.' The Terrys remained firm friends though, as did Terry and Michael Palin, of course, although Mike concedes that 'Terry just wanted to direct. Both Terrys did.' And Terry Gilliam would team up with Michael Palin to write the box office winner *Time Bandits*. Terry Jones was no part of it.

It is unsurprising that, despite this mild playground-like squabbling and falling out, 'Tomkinson's Schooldays' remained one of Terry's favourite achievements. Not only was it the only Ripping Yarn episode that went some way to capturing what he hoped the whole series would be, but it was also appreciated enough by a living, breathing comedy hero to provoke a fan letter, sent to the BBC and passed from pillar to post and back again until it ended up on the desk of Michael Palin. The Goonish surrealism of 'The School Leopard' had particularly tickled Spike Milligan. His message read simply: 'Ripping Yarns are Super – more please!'

The fact that Spike's missive of praise ultimately found its way to Michael and not Terry is yet one more indication that the wheels within wheels at the BBC were under no illusions as to who they considered the main attraction of *Ripping Yarns*. A note from Bob Gilbreath, Light Entertainment Organiser (Comedy) Television, of 22 February 1978, added fuel to the fire when he flagged up the fact that: 'Michael Palin's *Ripping Yarns* are at present scheduled to repeat . . .' Ouch! At least Spike Milligan would get his wish. More *Ripping Yarns* would come. And the fact that *Ripping Yarns* was named Best Comedy of 1977 at the Broadcasting Press Guild Awards certainly helped, although the second batch of episodes was slightly delayed and much truncated. Alan J.W. Bell was drafted in as producer and director for a run of just three episodes, transmitted in October 1979. Michael Palin admits that not only was *Ripping Yarns*: 'always looked upon as a showcase for me, really, and not necessarily Palin and Jones, but the BBC were not so keen on Terry as an actor, or as a writer in actual fact. It was all very difficult.' With the BBC, their place of employment, actively pushing Terry aside somewhat, it was simply friendship and loyalty that saw Terry and Michael collaborate once more on the new episodes. Michael, indeed, insisted. *Ripping Yarns* was both him and Terry; and memories of Terry insisting that Michael be part of *Do Not Adjust Your Set* a decade earlier must have been strong. This was a writing unit. The resolve of the Jones and Palin team had been powerfully at work, once more, within the extended Python group, during a writers' retreat holiday to Majorca for what would become *Monty Python's Life of Brian*, although even here the team was largely writing a lot of material on their own, or, most intriguingly, experimenting with different writing partners.

The final three *Ripping Yarns* that were broadcast that October of 1979 are both special and typical: 'Roger of the Raj' is a saga of British Imperial India; 'Whinfrey's Last Case' is a thrilling adventure of a German plot lurking within a Cornish fishing village; while the aforementioned footballing farce 'Golden Gordon' is the only series episode that gets a little way towards being what Terry had always hoped the show would be: the Pythons performing in a series he and Mike had written. For John Cleese, adopting the acting alias of Kim Bread, does make an appearance. Only just. An anonymous cameo as a passer-by. Still, it was a sure sign that the Pythons had been back together again. And it was a favour. John would go by the name of Kim Bread again when, in 1993, he popped up, post credits, in another Alan J.W. Bell comedy half-hour, in the UFO-spotting *Last of the Summer Wine* episode 'Welcome to Earth'.

And, if Terry didn't quite achieve what he wanted with *Ripping Yarns*, then neither did Michael, not quite at least: 'we were constantly up against a very tight budget with *Ripping Yarns*. Both Terry and I felt what we were doing could have been done by the Drama Department at the BBC without batting an eyelid. But because it was done by the Light Entertainment Department, we were always having to cut corners. I felt *Ripping Yarns* always just missed what I wanted them to be.' As far as the rest of us are concerned, *Ripping Yarns* is near perfection in nine episodes. As a glowing review in *The Times* had it, they 'transcended mere parody'. Still, within those wonderful scripts is a hurt that never completely stopped aching. Terry put a brave face on it but he was no fool. He had slowly but surely been ever so slightly edged out of his own series.

Undoubtedly, *Ripping Yarns* was the catalyst for Terry and Michael to begin writing more and more apart. Those final three *Ripping Yarns* scripts were very much collaborations, but the day-to-day, sitting at the same desk, and formulating plots and puns, was gone for good. Although as well as plots and puns there had also always been pints, and Michael says: '*Ripping Yarns* never ever broke our friendship. Not at all. We had worked together for a long time. Nearly twenty years. It was just the right time to try something new, something on our own, but we always had Python to bring us back together, and there was always a pint or two to share, and memories to unpick.'

If Terry was angry at the BBC, and worried at breaking up the partnership with Michael Palin, then he never showed signs of anxiety. Terry was always far too preoccupied with other projects to get anxious. He also had a young family to keep him happily busy. Daughter Sally had been joined by son Bill in 1976. What's more, Terry had blissfully reconnected with the Land of his Fathers. He had a little piece of Wales to call his own. A long, bracing walk through the valleys, ideally en route to a cosy public house for a few ales and a hearty lunch . . . that was pretty much a perfect day for Terry. It was all thanks to Alison's parents, who, as well as a lovely abode in Hampstead, had had a tiny cottage in mid Wales since 1960. From 1967, Terry was a regular visitor there. Over the years, the cottage would become Terry's haven: away from London, perhaps, but never really away from work. He just couldn't help being creative. Sally Jones remembers that: 'we would go to Wales for holidays at Easter and Christmas.' Christmas Day would be spent at home and then, on Boxing Day, the family would make the long, arduous journey to Wales: 'Dad would love his big walks to the pub and, as often as not, just invite a whole bunch of people he met there to come back to the house for dinner!' A typically gregarious gesture: 'one New Year's Eve, Dad brought back about fourteen very thirsty students. Lugging a huge box of booze!'

The cottage served as a writers' retreat, where Terry and Alison would often escape the pressure and persistence of work that Camberwell embodied. The cottage may well have had a terrible electric shower and a bucket for a toilet, but it was a place to regroup, mentally and physically. It was also a place that Terry adored. In all weathers. He would often return from Wales with a heart full of pride, gushing enthusiastically about what a wonderful time he had had: 'It *really* rained!' he would say. Nothing, but nothing, about Wales could get him down. Mind you, very little about *anywhere* could get Terry down. He was the only person any of us knew who booked a trip to Iceland in December, returning to enthusiastically report that 'It *really* snowed!' Well, it would, Terry. It would. These holidays would be leisurely. The ones in Wales would be a few weeks, a month or more. Even in the 1980s, at a time when Terry was putting himself out there as a film direc-tor for hire, his intense desire to get away from it all meant he had neglected to install a telephone in the cottage. Still, Terry being his usual contrary self, he couldn't turn away from work for that long. Many an hour in Wales would be spent in the public call box on the corner, phoning Los Angeles and trying to secure a film deal, at their lunchtime and his six o'clock, as yet another home-cooked dinner by Alison got closer and closer to ruination.

Unlike Terry, who simply couldn't wait to get back to the valleys, Terry's mother, of course, had never wanted to return home. In later life, and in increasingly poor health, she and her husband had moved to a property in Midhurst, in West Sussex. Terry, ever the devoted son, would make the trip to visit them regularly, particularly during those last few years when his mum had become an invalid. However, when Terry's mum died in 1971, Terry, his brother Nigel and their father made the decision to take her cremated ashes back to North Wales and scatter her there. The site was the church in which Terry's parents had got married.

As soon as she was finally at rest, Terry's father pretty much imme-diately packed a bag, stuck the family cat on the back seat and drove to Terry's house. As Alison recalls: 'there was something about Wales pulling him home, niggling at him. He came up to see us, plonked the cat with us to look after, and drove off to North Wales. He never did pick up that cat.' As the cat's name was Geronimo, one can only surmise that he rather relished the adventure!

Arriving 'home', Terry's dad tracked down some relatives who were running a boarding house just outside Colwyn Bay. He stayed with them, on a temporary basis, and made himself indispensable by running the guest house bar for them. Eventually he moved back to the Clwyd Valley and, once there, looked up an old girlfriend. Nora was her name. She used to live in a house across the way from Denbigh Castle, an imposing fortress that crowns a rocky outcrop above the Vale of Clwyd. Still holding a torch, and with hope in his heart, Terry's dad knocked on Nora's door. And she answered. All those years later. Nora, who had never married, eagerly invited him in for a cup of tea and the rest was pure romantic fiction. She was living with her widowed sisters and needed a man about the house. As was his way, Terry's dad made himself very useful, moved in and then, as Alison remembers, a phone call came through: 'it was Terry's dad. He said: "I'm thinking of getting married again. Do you think the boys would mind?" And I said: "No, I think they'll be really happy." Although as Terry was just about to go off to film *Monty Python and the Holy Grail*, his dad may have timed things so as Terry was busy in Scotland and didn't go along and stop him from marrying Nora!' Not that Terry was going to do that. He was genuinely delighted for his dad, and very happy that it was a hop and a skip from the cottage in Wales to see his surviving parent and lovely stepmother.

The sheer majestic beauty and rugged wilderness of the Welsh valleys stirred within Terry a dormant passion for nature and the environment. Typically, with the money and freedom that his comedy work had afforded him, he wanted to do something about it. And he did.

The year was 1977. Having returned from a lucrative New York stage run with the Pythons at the City Center, in the spring of 1976, and with that very good first batch of *Ripping Yarns* in the can, Terry had money to invest.

Over a few pints and a few jokes with his old journalist pal Richard Boston, who had introduced him to publisher Colin Webb, Terry formulated the idea for an ecology journal with a light-hearted attitude. The original working title, *The Questing Vole*, was inspired by a quotation from Evelyn Waugh's 1938 satirical novel *Scoop*, in which the earnest nature columnist William Boot writes: 'feather-footed through the plashy fens passes the questing vole.' For ease, Terry eventually shortened this title to simply *Vole*. The magazine was to be a fun but forceful look at self-sufficiency, green politics and climate change; and printed on 100 per cent recycled paper.

*Vole* launched in September 1977, with Richard Boston in the editor's seat. The Britain of the 1970s was becoming increasingly concerned about environmental issues. The science-fiction television series *Doomwatch*, which had run on the BBC from 1970 until 1972, had, rather terrifyingly, flagged up the issues; while *Doctor Who* of the Seventies had the Time Lords of Jon Pertwee and Tom Baker facing the threat of atomic grubs and plants gone rogue. Britons' concerns were not only focused on the nuclear threat but the fundamental fear of the cleanliness of the air that we breathed and the water that we drank. The Department of the Environment had been the Conservative government's initiative to appease the panic, but, by the time of devising *Vole*, Terry felt Prime Minister James Callaghan and his year-old Labour government needed a hefty push in the right direction. *Vole* was devoted to environmental issues and the protection of the countryside and country ways in general. By November 1978 *Vole* had adopted the very official-looking but totally unauthorised government stamp: 'Magazine of The Environment', with a cover design by Terry's sister-in-law, Kate Hepburn. With Terry's deep and determined involvement, it not only spread the word in an engaging and, for a short time at least, high-profile manner, but it was also very, very funny. In its ridiculously ambitious way *Vole* became a self-proclaimed Campaign for Real Life, reflecting Terry's determined view that every aspect of the British way of life should be healthy, natural and progressive. *Vole* was a humorous, on occasion silly magazine with serious things to say. Very Terry, that.

Terry was the chief financier for the venture, although naturally he also had a big hand in the design of the magazine and pitched in with pen pictures, silly drawings and the occasional fictitious reader's letter. From the second issue, he was contributing many upbeat and informed articles, starting with, unsurprisingly, a study of fourteenth-century pictorial representation of Chaucer, and the Peasants' Revolt in his opinion piece 'Terry Jones reads John Ball's hands'. That same issue also included a wry, positive review for the *Monty Python and the Holy Grail (Book)*, praising the comedy troupe for recycling old jokes in the name of ecological awareness. Nice. *Vole* wore its serious side on its sleeve too, of course. Richard Adams, the respected naturalist and novelist, most notably of rabbit saga *Watership Down*, brought real gravitas and intensity to his contributions; while Bill Tidy, a much-liked teammate from the *Funny Game, Football* album, offered pithy cartoons. Tony Benn, at the time serving as Secretary of State for Energy, was on hand for the political ramifications of countryside erosion; Paul Foot brought his skills as an investigative journalist to the table; while singer-songwriter and record producer Pete Atkin regularly wrote on environmentally friendly do-it-yourself. Bryan McAllister and Bryan Reading, the satirical political cartoonists, created 'The Belchers' for the magazine. The comic strip featured Nigel and Fiona Allbran, countryside-obsessed townies moving out of the metropolis and integrating with the locals. It was the rather more biting flip-side of something like the suburban antics of Richard Briers and Felicity Kendal in the BBC sitcom *The Good Life*, which – with the exception of an upcoming Christmas special and belated Silver Jubilee royal special – had come to an end in May 1977; or the eternal radio soap *The Archers*. Indeed, the subtitle for 'The Belchers' was 'an every-month story of Country Folk'. The references and pastiche were clear to everybody. 'The Belchers' was the most scathing and hilarious of *Vole*'s little jokes. It was short-lived, though. Under a new editor, American Charles Alverson, in the summer of 1980 *Vole* survived a format change to a less distinguished-looking tabloid. The changes caused mild disquiet within the writing team and the magazine died a rather ignoble death in September 1981.

That was a pity, for it was a valiant effort at something worthwhile and good. *Vole* made its point though, and left its mark. A pet project for Terry, which, like the most glorious summers, flashed, incandescent and impossible to ignore, for the shortest of times. One of Terry's most important achievements, it is fitting, though sobering, to think that, nearly fifty years later, Terry's beloved Oxford abode, St Edmund Hall, is still campaigning to be the Greenest College of all. That would get a wry grin from Terry. No doubt. Not least of which is my use of the word 'sobering' in that last sentence.

Once those early-Sixties days of frequenting tea shops and coffee houses as a poor, hard-working student were behind him, the lure of a public house was one that, once Terry could afford it, he indulged with alacrity. The income from theatre in that final year of Oxford, and the regular pay cheque from the BBC, would financially open up the door of the pub. Terry could happily and regularly satisfy his thirst for real ale.

By the time of *Ripping Yarns* and *Vole*, Terry had channelled his interest in beer into the short film *Henry Cleans Up*. A fourteen-minute instructional manual for pub landlords, it was written by Peter Fensom and Michael Palin, with Palin starring as the cack-handed Henry, who is losing customers because of his inability to pour a decent pint of Guinness. Python credentials were added with Carol Cleveland as Henry's glamorous wife and Terry as a bloke who can properly pull a pint. Terry's character knows every trick in the book and coolly explains the process of cleaning the pipes, maintaining your equipment and, thus, serving great, well-kept beer and building your pub clientele. There was no acting required here, as loving a decent pint just wasn't enough for Terry. He needed to know everything about it. And once he knew everything about it, his personal mission was to improve the quality of beer throughout Britain. Well, on the England/Wales border, at least.

Those long and lovely walks from the cottage to the pub were Terry's happy times. Even up steep hills and down slopes so slippery and sheer that Terry would stumble, slide and, as often as not, somersault down them, he was determined to get to the pub. And, because of the effort, Terry really wanted and expected good quality beer when he got there.

That very good financial year of 1976/77 was the time to do something about it. Concurrently, Hay-on-Wye, the fledgling Book Town, with forty-something bookshops, had seen the self-appointed 'King' Richard Booth declare 'home rule' from Hay Castle. Typically of Terry, it wasn't so much the book-buying tourists that he was concerned with. He wanted to satisfy the Welsh sheep farmers looking for a decent pint.

Terry had become very fond of Martin Griffiths, a local entrepreneur who became very fond of Terry too. Martin had bought Penrhos Court, a fifteenth-century manor at Lyonshall. Once owned by the nineteenth-century farmer and horse breeder Mr F.S. Blakely, the site was the first in Wales to gain the symbol of the Soil Association, an environmental charity active since 1946.

Terry, whose cottage was a nice little walk away, was a frequent diner at the Penrhos restaurant, run by Griffiths. Terry loved the place. Between them, they cooked up the idea for the Penrhos Brewery, based on a handshake and a scrap of paper mapping out the plan. Griffiths also owned a home recording studio, which attracted local superstar Mike Oldfield, who lived nearby in a house at Hergest Ridge, an area that inspired his 1974 album of the same name, and which fair drips with the dreamy nature of

Penrhos. Bands such as Queen, and Python-mad rockers Led Zeppelin, would also record at the Martin Griffiths studio.

Thus, Penrhos was a venture with celebrity clout, but before anybody else got involved in terms of money and outside investment it was agreed, between Terry and Martin, that Martin would provide the premises and Terry would pay for the equipment. Terry had secured Peter Austin, the soon-to-be Father of Microbrewing, who was thrilled to be involved with this first real ale revival and converted the cattle byre at Penrhos Court into the Penrhos Brewery. Set next to a ruined twelfth-century monastery as it was, it all seemed very Terry. Naturally food would be needed too, and chef Daphne Lambert was brought on board. She remembers: 'money was never ever part of the conversation. Never. All Terry and Martin – and everyone involved in it – wanted to see was this idea work.'

As if to bask in the vibes of *Vole*, Terry's plan was to make every-thing real. Real good companions would drink real ale which would wash down real food. To that end, Daphne Lambert's expertise won the establishment a certificate in honour of its organic ingredients. The pigs were fed the spent grain from the brewery and then, when they were slaughtered, they were cured and marinated in the beer. Only then was the meat deemed ready to serve in the restaurant. It was a circular process, from field to plate, that Terry absolutely adored. This completeness of it all was very much part of his ideal plan.

Nothing was wasted. It was always fresh. In an era when prawn cocktail starters, steak for the main, all followed by lemon sorbet, were the staples of most restaurants, Penrhos was something completely different. Daphne would never really know what she was cooking until the evening of that day because she didn't always necessarily know what she would have. It was an exciting gastro-nomic adventure. And not just for the skilled chef. Diners got no menu from which to choose. They ate the one dish that Daphne had cooked, and it was served up to them while they sat, not at intimate tables for two, but at long tables of many. A communal experience that echoed Terry's days at Oxford. Very Middle Ages too. Terry loved the conviviality of large groups, enjoying good-quality food and drink. Naturally, Terry would often visit the restaurant and eagerly chat about everything and nothing with the diners and the drinkers. He was recognised and admired but few would be fazed by this famous Python in their midst. He was the genteel host. The provider of the feast. They were happy days.

Outside of the personal fun for Terry at the restaurant, the wider aim was simple. To brew and deliver quality real ale to the Llanthony Priory Hotel, twelve miles south of Hay. It would be Terry's gift of good beer to the local people. Indeed, Terry was heartily sick of the stranglehold keg beer had on the industry in the 1970s. He saw it as a stranglehold over the consumer – the proper, dedicated drinker. So much so that, half-joking but also half-serious, he claimed that Penrhos should sue Watney's Red Barrel for deformation of the public's taste buds. Watney's Red, as it had been unskilfully rebranded in 1971, had already been the target of Monty Python humour. It was the epitome of bad beer in the Seventies. Penrhos was Terry's battle cry against it. One pub at a time.

The first brew of Penrhos took place on the seventh of the seventh 1977. That glorious July day was followed, just nine days later, by the official launch. Daphne Lambert recalls: 'the launch party was one of the most exciting summer days of my life. Richard Boston was there. Graham Chapman came with his partner David Sherlock. I baked fresh bread and cooked the evening meal for around a hundred guests, and then they all went down to Lyonshall Park and stripped off and swam in the river to celebrate. Then they all ran around to dry off!' For Terry, it was any excuse to get naked, and this was as good an excuse as he could have. His own beer.

Daphne Lambert recalls that: 'I suppose it was quite revolutionary but it was organic, in every sense of the word. Terry wanted something good to drink when he came to the restaurant. And, as a result, he brewed his own beer. For everybody local!'

At one point, Kington, in the Welsh borders, had twenty pubs, but with the Welsh forbidden to drink on Sundays many establishments felt the pinch. Still, what else would all those thirsty quarry workers want to do on their Sunday off but drink beer? Lots of it. And the good stuff too. Daphne still feels: 'it was the right place to have a brewery. The Railway Tavern, one of our locals, was still run by an old landlady, who would have been ninety at the time. She was so excited that Kington had got another brewery.'

And Terry was the ideal champion. He was a generous person. He had a generosity of spirit about him. And he loved what he drank – but did he have an expert's palate? Well, according to Daphne Lambert: 'I suppose pouring beer over his head made him an expert!' Yes, Terry would do practically anything to promote the Penrhos Brewery.

The occasion was the Great British Beer Festival, held at Alexandra Palace, in 1979, when he accompanied Martin Griffiths to the event. Terry was not going to behave like you would at a wine-tasting. Sniffing and whirling the drink round in the mouth and spitting it out. He was going to test the beer by pouring it over his head! Martin thought this was a crackers idea but didn't say anything. The festival organisers had lined up ten beers for tasting, and, when Terry was introduced and started going through the brews, he systematically poured each and every one over his head. He would comment as he went, saying things like: 'Hmmm . . . this one is quite slippery. I think this is Ruddles.' The only one he really disliked was, of course, Watney's Red Barrel. He said, 'Uggg, this one smells disgusting!' and then, proceeding to pour it over himself, concluded: 'Ooh, and it's greasy on your skin. Horrible!'

The beer from Penrhos was deemed the finest. Naturally. Even so, although some beers are very good for washing your hair in, those from Penrhos in particular, Terry, having grabbed some headlines with his comic antics, then swiftly zipped off for a nice long shower – in hot, clear water. But what an opening to a beer festival! Unsurprisingly, his chum Richard Boston gave the brewery a major, positive write-up in the *Guardian*.

From the outset, Penrhos had three brilliant cask beers made from British malt and local hops: Penrhos Bitter, Jones's First Brew and Penrhos Porter. But even with positive feedback on the beers themselves and Terry's celebrity well to the fore, the problems with Penrhos began almost immediately. The issue came when the brewery started to ship the beers further and further afield. It had become difficult to stay local because many of the nearby pubs were tied up in stranglehold deals with other, more established and more financially viable breweries. And although the turnover, from cask to customer, was quite quick, it was a hard time to make a living from real ale. Taking beers to Newcastle, and all over the country, quickly proved that Terry's ambitions were not sustainable. Many pubs at the time simply weren't looking for real beer. They were just used to kegs. Moreover, many of the landlords who did experiment and take on Terry's real ale weren't used to keeping it properly. Even if you can transport your good beer successfully, it has to be well kept once the landlord starts serving it. And the Penrhos deliveries were not being well kept. The instructional film *Henry Cleans Up* hadn't been made for Terry's health but for the health of good beer. His efforts had clearly gone largely unheeded!

Politically, it was a tough time too. By the early 1980s, Conservative prime minister Margaret Thatcher was at her zenith of radical, root-and-branch reform. Her policies were breaking up mining communities and making the life of a small business increasingly difficult.

An independent concern like Penrhos needed to brew beer and sell it pretty much as quickly as they produced it, because the government insisted that the business pay its duties on the beer as soon as it was brewed, rather than when it had been sold. Enter the

Royal Bank of Scotland, or more accurately exit the Royal Bank of Scotland, for its financial collapse necessitated that Martin and Daphne put Penrhos Manor on the open market. As Daphne remembers, rather than fight a losing battle and suffer bankruptcy, the couple decided 'just to close the door, and walk away. Terry was passionately angry about it all, but it was out of all of our hands. There was nothing we could have done. The RBS held the cards.'

This turnaround of the early 1980s did break a little bit of Terry's heart, if not his spirit. With *Vole* gone in 1981 and the Penrhos Brewery following suit in 1983, he saw his fresh, fun and, above all, independent ventures put to the sword of Thatcherism and commercial restraint. The years that followed proved Terry correct, of course, and he lived and drank through the glorious golden age of the microbrewery. In 'My Love Affair With Beer', an opinion piece for the thirtieth edition of *CAMRA's Good Beer Guide* in 2003, Terry proudly stated that: 'Beer, for me, is more than something I like drinking. It's a litmus of civilisation . . . Keg beer is a dead parrot.' And despite that necessary acquiescence to Python, it was a true and heartfelt statement.

Terry may have been something of an unsung pioneer, with *Vole* magazine and Penrhos Brewery, but his aim was simple. He wanted to help make the world a better place: a place of good eating and good drinking and good companions. For a short time during his late thirties, he found that place of enjoyment and peace; that place of nature and food and drink and close friends, all in his own Welsh backyard. As Daphne Lambert laments: 'Terry was such a good man. A good person. He wanted the world to be a good place and a safe place.'

# CHAPTER NINE AND THREE-QUARTERS
## SITTING COMFORTABLY? TERRY THE CHILDREN'S AUTHOR

*If I had to save just one thing I had done, it would be my copy of the first edition of the* Fairy Tales. *I'm rather proud of that.*

TERRY'S first children's book – *Bert Fegg's Nasty Book for Boys and Girls*, written with Michael Palin, using bits of scripts from Monty Python and various silliness they had concocted – was published by Methuen in 1974. The recycled nature of much of the contents was flagged up by the tongue-in-cheek back cover blurb, decrying those 'who allege that the *Nasty Book* is nothing more or less than a collection of Terry Jones and Michael Palin's old scripts'. The book was, in Terry's eyes at least, decidedly *not* a children's book. It looked very much like a children's book, from its title and cover illustration, though perhaps the sticker adorning the first edition, which read, 'A Monty Python Educational Product', was intended to appeal to Python's adult audience too. Inevitably, however, it was stocked in the children's section in most bookshops. Upon spotting it there, Terry would harrumph and immediately gather up all the copies he could see and remove them to the humour section, or the horrible odours section, or somewhere.

The origins of Dr Bert Fegg – a somewhat terrifying, fat, bald man – were in cartoons sketched by Terry while at school in Surrey, and it seems that the character never really left him: Fegg Features Limited, set up in 1975, was the name of his production company and, years later, Fegg even featured in Terry's personal email address. Bert Fegg himself seems a nasty piece of work. The author lists his interests as 'defacing bus shelters, sticking old chewing gum on nuns and frightening people on the Barnet loop section of the Northern Line'. Moreover, the publishers reassure readers that Fegg's involvement with petty thefts and larcenies in Brighton and killings in Bournemouth has never been proved. It was a delight, shared by the authors, that this totally inappropriate character should be fronting a book whose aim, apparently, was to educate the young. Fegg's message to his readership is that 'A child's greatest gift is its laughter.'

To that end *Bert Fegg's Nasty Book for Boys and Girls* was a compendium of absurdist humour, dark tales and parody. It introduced readers (young or old) to animals like the West Bromley Fighting Haddock and the Patagonian Bursting Rabbit. Some of the ideas would later find their way into *Ripping Yarns*, and Terry's love of historical humour features too. In 'The Famous Five Go Pillaging', the children, while out for a walk, witness the fall of Roman imperialism, much to the concern of their family, who are then slaughtered by quite a lot of Vikings. Mr Brown is even decapitated. Twice!

While Terry, as author, may have considered the Bert Fegg book more of an extension of his public identity as a Python comedian, its love of disgusting bodily functions and gratuitous violence to figures in authority – particularly parents – embraces the maxim of Roald Dahl's best children's fiction: that kids love cartoon-styled gore. Terry, as a comedy writer, had also relished writing *Do Not Adjust Your Set*, tapping into his own childhood highs and lows, and what he had enjoyed reading and listening to when young. It was an invigorating and satisfying process. More importantly, the show, which was written by adults for children, did, of course, subsequently appeal to an adult audience too, all of whom were encouraged to access their inner-child and laugh at utter silliness once more. This explains Terry's mild annoyance at seeing the

Bert Fegg book in the children's section. It was a fun and grue-some book for all the family!

It was this intrinsic understanding that children do not want to be talked down to from within the books they are reading that made Terry such a skilled and successful writer for the young. He was fully aware of his responsibilities but also mindful that children, like any reader, wanted exciting and engaging stories to read. He was aware too of his culpability if those stories failed to entertain the young reader. A failure that could lead to an adult lifetime of considering books boring!

In promotional interviews about his work intentionally aimed at children, Terry would, of course, invariably put himself down and comically undermine his intelligence. He would put his love for children's literature down to the fact that he considered himself: 'so naive about things . . .' but, in truth, here was a master teller of tales, a consummate orator and, by the time of his published work, a devoted father, all rolled into one.

When conversation touched upon the secret of a good children's writer, Terry would be typically modest. He would say that: 'I don't really think of myself as writing children's books, particularly. I kind of write for myself, really. Maybe I'm more compatible with twelve-year-olds!' Sounding unwitting but knowing exactly what he is saying, Terry here highlights the precise reason why his books for children were so good. He could remember what it was like to be young, and channelled that through his skill as a writer into stories that captured the imagination of his audience.

Oxford comrade David Wood muses that: 'Children's writing was certainly a thing we had in common, although we didn't often talk about it. Terry was, without doubt, one of the country's finest. His stories are so sophisticated. A brilliant mix of the truthful and the magical.'

Terry's love, knowledge, appreciation and fundamental understanding of the structure of a good and, indeed, a bad, book for children was in the very fibres of his creativity. His keen eye for an interesting historical angle and, most endearingly of all, his warm and natural storytelling skills, would inform these stories. All with one foot in the now and the other foot in Fairyland.

Terry would also eagerly accept invitations from bookshops and schools, and, as an actor of rare range, would recite his own stories and those of others with aplomb. He would retain favourite snatches and passages, and deliver them without a trace of saccharine or sarcasm and simply with pure joy.

Distant memories of his own youth notwithstanding, the key to Terry's talents as a writer for young readers was fatherhood. At that point he was hit by the realisation that the unpleasantness of his own Bert Fegg, and Roald Dahl and, yes, the Brothers Grimm, was just a little too grim for children. The first book that Terry wrote intentionally for children was actually originally written for one child – his daughter, Sally. In the late Seventies, he was reading a collection of well-established fairy tales to her at bedtime, and decided that not only were these traditional stories very unpleasant but they were also rather problematic in lots of ways. So, while reading them aloud, he began improvising, taking the written words to his own reinterpreted natural, or unnatural, conclusions. And in the end, he simply wrote his own fairy tales for Sally. Of course, Terry being Terry, it wasn't enough to jot down a few ideas with which to entertain his beloved eldest child. They were tweaked and finely honed – during a family holiday, in fact.

A desire to bring the stories to visual life became a reality when Terry discovered the illustrator Michael Foreman: 'I first met Terry at the graphic studio of my friend, Derek Birdsall,' Michael remembers. 'Derek was an absolutely brilliant man, very intuitive, and he was doing some design work on the early Monty Python books. Derek, quite rightly, thought Terry and I would get on, and introduced us. Once Terry realised who I was and my background, he mentioned he was writing bedtime stories for his young children because some of the old classic tales might give them nightmares.'

As ever, Terry valued – possibly almost needed – a collaborator. In so many ways, Michael was the perfect partner for this endeavour, and they built both a productive working relationship and a friendship that would see them through many successful books. Although that was by no means guaranteed at the time. Perhaps needless to say, Terry and Michael's discussions about the book they wanted to make together took place over a series of lunches. Quite a long series, in fact, as it would be three years before they found a publisher. Not that this seemed to matter an awful lot to start with – Terry and Michael shared an affability of nature and took pleasure in sharing good food, fine wine and interesting conversation as their ideas for the fairy tale book took shape.

Michael says: 'I had worked with lots of writers but the loveliest of collaborations was working with Terry. It just sort of grew and grew through a friendship. Terry was a chum. That's the word for it. It's a special thing. A chum is different from a friend. And Terry was a chum.' Terry's family would take holidays at Michael's studio, down in Cornwall, and the only anxiety in a very binding and beneficial friendship was apparently keeping Terry's dog away from Michael's cats!

According to Colin Webb, the instinctive publisher who appreciated the potential in *Chaucer's Knight* and would publish it in 1980, the main problem the two faced as they looked for a publisher in the late 1970s was that editors 'all had a very traditional idea about what a children's book should be'. And of course, as ever, Terry was anything but traditional. 'That is the whole point!' he would say, but to no avail. Terry's *Fairy Tales* went around to a number of established children's book publishers, but all of them turned it down flat, even though it was by a very well-known

person and you would think as a result a very commercial proposition. Terry remembered that some publishers said, 'Well, we
can't just call it *Fairy Tales*. Why don't you give it a title from one
of the stories in the book?' While others said there were too many
stories and some said there weren't enough. If any made noises
about pairing him with a different illustrator – well, there was no
question of that. Terry, a loyal collaborator as ever, would dig in
his heels and refuse to discuss it any further. In fact, any suggested
changes to the project that he was presenting would, inevitably,
put his back up. He would say: 'Well, no, this is how I want it
published!' Again, that lack of compromise was on display. It was
one of his great qualities – even if it was not always appreciated by
those trying to work with him.

Though, to be fair to Terry, Michael Foreman doesn't remember
it as being a problem in their creative partnership. 'It was a joyful
collaboration. I mean, the stories were pretty much complete
when I was given them, but, although Terry would welcome ideas
and developments as we chatted, I never had to change a thing.
They were so full of amazing and provocative ideas that I was
inspired. Far too inspired, really. I was limited to the number of
paintings I was commissioned to deliver for each book.'

Michael got to know Terry as a chum but, even more crucially,
as a writer. He understood Terry's world, his interests, his passions.
All of those qualities went into Terry's stories. The fairy tales in the
book range from the wild and silly to the strange and the wonderful to the downright spooky. Though the idea came about in the
first place because Terry had felt that the original tales needed an
update or a softening for children like Sally, he saw that a certain
type of creepiness is actually appealing to a young audience and is
a great tradition in children's literature. He still couldn't help
embracing a little of that tradition of the Grimms or Roald Dahl.
Indeed, Terry knew a chill here and a thrill there was essential to
keep the little ones nicely on the edge of their seats.

The book's roundabout route to eventual publication is an interesting one. By this point, Colin Webb and his wife, Ann, had a family of their own, and so perhaps naturally, as Terry as a father had become more interested in writing children's books, Colin had become more interested in publishing them – an area he had not worked in before. However, he was then working for the publisher Weidenfeld & Nicolson, who, rather annoyingly, didn't really have a children's list at that time. But Terry wasn't the only one struggling to find a home for an unconventional publishing proposition.

Colin Webb explains: 'At that stage, I had also got to be good pals with Tim Rice. Tim wanted to publish a children's book version of Tim and Andrew Lloyd Webber's *Joseph and the Amazing Technicolor Dreamcoat*. We had Quentin Blake lined up to illustrate it – the problem was Weidenfeld & Nicolson. It was one of those quirks of publishing that they decided that they couldn't take this on. Tim said: "Why don't we start our own publishing company and do it?" So we did!'

This was in 1981, just a little over a year since the publication of *Chaucer's Knight*. The new company was called Pavilion Books, as Colin's co-directors Tim Rice and broadcasting legend Michael Parkinson shared a love of cricket. As well as the inconceivably rejected *Joseph and the Amazing Technicolor Dreamcoat*, that first list from Pavilion Books included Terry's *Fairy Tales*. Colin Webb confirms that: 'It certainly helped that I had published *Chaucer's Knight* – so Terry came to me – but more than that, Terry instinctively knew that we had none of these traditions of established publishing houses. We were not hidebound by anything that the children's book market did, so we said: "Yes. Fantastic." We loved the stories. We read them to our kids. We loved Michael Foreman. So I could happily tell Terry that: "Yes, we will do it exactly the way you want it!" And we did. And it was a great success.'

Terry wrote everything with the same attitude, and certainly *Fairy Tales* is never condescending or fearful of tackling the big topics. The sheer grossness of *Bert Fegg* is gone, although Terry's appeal to the parents buying the book and reading it aloud is clear throughout the stories. They have modern sensibilities while also including tropes from traditional tales. Thus, the collection ranges from a cautionary story about never being satisfied with your lot – 'The Corn Dolly' – to the truth that friends are far more important than money – 'The Wonderful Cake-Horse'. There is a valuable life lesson in 'The Fly-By-Night', a story that warns against trusting strangers . . . well, only until the next adventure beckons, by which time they are no longer strangers anyway but trusted friends. There's also the home truth of 'Three Raindrops', the shortest in the collection and obviously conjured up on an evening when Sally was extremely tired! Still, in a bare few lines it packs in the punch that big-headedness will lead to ignominy. 'The Silly King' is gloriously surreal and self-indulgent and even, dare I say it, one for the Python fans. There's also an awful lot of Spike Milligan in the dotty notions of the very silly King Herbert XII strapping dogs to the royal legs and pouring custard over people. Herbert is a veritable slapstick monarch, in fact, and it is one of the funniest, laugh-out-loud tales in the book.

*Fairy Tales* also advises that one should always be satisfied with one's clear talent: in 'The Butterfly Who Sang', a cunning moth convinces the butterfly of the title to dull her beautiful wings so a frog can concentrate on her less-than-obvious musical abilities. Basically, never trust a frog's opinion is the moral here! The reader is also prompted to never tarry while making a decision, in case of missing out on something fun. That's the point of 'Katy-Make-Sure'. While true friendship being far better than untold treasure is the truth of the duplicitous goblin tale of 'Tim O'Leary'. 'The Witch and the Rainbow Cat' makes it clear that your future is in your own hands, and 'The Monster Tree' confirms that you should face up to your fears. Even the most terrifying ones. Particularly the most terrifying ones.

'Brave Molly' is about the monsters and the bullies that might, just might, be more frightened of you than you are of them! 'The Wooden City' relates the story of a kindly King who annoys his subjects by giving away wealth to the needy. The tale makes clear that kindliness is a good thing and you should never sell your soul for untold riches!

Never doubt the fact that there are more things in heaven and earth than are dreamed of in your philosophy also. That's the core of 'The Ship of Bones'.

Be true to yourself and ignore how other people see you is wrapped within the tale of 'Simple Peter's Mirror'. 'Jack-One-Step' is a clever twisting of traditional fairy-tale traits, with a schoolboy exposing the unfairness of the society of the magic folk. The unfairness is that the small fairies have fewer magic powers than the big fairies; and, in turn, the big fairies have fewer magic powers than the King. In a clear political manifesto, solidarity of the community overthrows the monarchy! Love, Laughter and Light can conquer big-headed anger and stupidity in 'The Snuff-Box'; and 'The Man Who Owned the World' drives home the thought that greed is *not* good! 'The Key' is a complex love-quadrangle that suggests that life might be better if you just leave things alone!

Take the sensible option . . . or take a gamble. Both could lead to happiness. Maybe. That's 'The Wind Ghosts'. Or, more importantly, it's a loving sugar-coat for nervous children who cannot sleep. The story is a concise exercise in how to make scary noises in the night a lot less scary. Clever Terry!

Don't change a thing about your appearance. You're perfect. Just adapt a little and life will be happy, says 'The Big Noses'. 'The Wine of Li-Po' allows Terry to embrace a subject very close to his taste buds while insisting his reader or listener should trust their own judgement, rather than believe hypocritical rhetoric . . . even over the supposed influence of the finest wine in the kingdom! 'The Island of Purple Fruit' reveals that a dream of happiness is usually just that . . . a dream, and 'The Beast with a Thousand Teeth' suggests you get to know the local bully because, you know what, you might even tame him! The idea of try, try, and try again . . . and then give up!, as lived by self-proclaimed comedy curmudgeon W. C. Fields, is the seed of reality in 'Far-Away Castle'. The parable that even the cleverest man in the world cannot outfox pure evil in 'Dr Bonocolus's Devil' is a mini episode of *The Twilight Zone*. Precise and precious and with a delicious sting in the forked tail.

'Why Birds Sing in the Morning' is a truly beautiful slice of whimsy that waxes lyrical on a glorious everyday occurrence within folklore mythology. It's concise, exciting, and breathtakingly engaging. Most inspirational of all is the consequences of extreme greed, told in a surprisingly emotive tale of ecological warning in the perfectly constructed 'The Glass Cupboard'. Travel may broaden your mind, even if you are a herring, but you can never know everything, big head . . . and you can never avoid your fate! That's the moral of 'A Fish of the World', and includes a throw-away comment that pretty much sums up Terry's gleefully over-flowing, seemingly inexhaustible imagination. 'Make soup from your stories . . .'

Even the most obvious and sensible recommendation of all – you will live to regret it if you tell lies – is at the black heart of Terry's William Blake-like abstract parable in 'The Sea-Tiger'. A feline character who inspired Michael Foreman so much that he is one of the select few who makes the cover design for *Fairy Tales*. And one can do nothing better than pull out a moment from 'The Boat That Went Nowhere' to demonstrate the sheer strength of these stories: 'I have discovered that nobody with money will part with it, unless I waste my life away, and that those whose *only* desire is wealth will never rest content, and that the only place where there is enough for all and everyone is kind and generous is Nowhere.' There endeth Terry's first lesson. For both the young and the young at heart.

The beautiful Michael Foreman paintings undoubtedly contributed hugely to the book's appeal. Each would take two or three days to complete and all were crafted with loving detail, taking in many characters and relating complex storytelling in just a handful of illustrations.

Michael's wife, Louise Foreman, says: 'The stories are so funny and thrilling. We read them to our boys every night and every night they wanted a Terry Jones story. They are fantastic.' The kids don't lie . . . and it was a freshness and drive that Colin Webb picked up on the moment he read *Fairy Tales*. And as ever, he was right. The public loved this new take on familiar old classics.

As did the critics, who appreciated not only the stories and illustrations themselves, but the dedication and commitment of the writer and the illustrator to their young audience. Much-loved children's writer Michael Rosen was effusive in his praise and Brian Patten wrote in the *Spectator* magazine that 'Jones's original tales are often as dark [as traditional fairy tales], but his lunatic sense of humour makes them unique.' Reviewing the collection for the *Daily Mail*, writer Jane Gaskell concluded: 'Terry Jones . . . has written with a golden scalpel a new Aesop's Fables . . . My favourite, if allowed to choose only one book this Christmas.'

Brian Alderson of *The Times* judged that Terry's collection 'was not a Pythonesque send-up of the real thing but 30 new-minted pieces . . . They vary from being fables . . . to being full-dress fantasy tales. Sometimes they have a pronounced moral (up with friendship, down with greed are favourite themes) sometimes they are entirely fanciful, but there isn't a single one devoid of dramatic point or lacking a nice turn of phrase, and they make for splendid reading aloud. Moreover, they have inspired Michael Foreman to some of his best illustrations ever. Lucky Sally Jones.'

Lucky Sally indeed. Of course, Terry had dedicated the book to her.

Looking back on the project over four decades on, Colin Webb is still very proud of *Fairy Tales*: 'It's a great collection of short and beautifully formed stories. And it was very well received and very well reviewed.' He also makes the very good point that Terry was doing something new that, despite the reluctance of many publishers at the time to see the commercial appeal, would go on to be an important commercial pillar of children's publishing: 'It's very interesting looking back, because the market has become saturated with books by comedians and celebrities. Terry's was the first out of that mould. Terry created that mould, because he was a name from Python, which, of course, inevitably gave it an added commercial impetus . . . but it *was* a fabulous book! It was very well written. I'm retired from publishing now but one can not help keep an eye on the industry. You can't say any of the celebrity children's books being published today are in the same league as Terry Jones. When you read some of these books, you realise just how terrible they are! Terry's have a real warmth and compassion.'

The Jones and Foreman relationship may have been developed over fun and creative lingering lunches and mutual respect, but the cementing bond came when the two discovered a shared passion for that Rupert the Bear man, Alfred Bestall. Indeed, Terry and Michael were much, much more than admirers of Bestall. They were both disciples.

Terry's humour and love of the absurd might seem to have little in common with the much-loved stories of Rupert Bear. However, while Terry's young creative mind was undoubtedly shaped by a passion for Dylan Thomas and *The Goon Show*, his affection for the inhabitants of Nutley Wood pre-dated all of this. It was the seed for his interest in protecting nature; a delight in and stories of the countryside; and while it was his earliest storytelling comfort, it was one that never left him – 'The love of Rupert Bear has remained a constant,' he confirmed. Crucially, albeit subliminally, the Rupert stories were inspired by Terry's own beloved Colwyn Bay.

Alfred Bestall drew Rupert and his friends for thirty-one years from 1935 and was very much the artist of Terry's childhood imagination. From the age of eleven, Burma-born Bestall had attended the private Methodist school, Rydal Mount, in Colwyn Bay and in those formative years, from 1904 through to 1911, he sketched his surroundings. In Terry's interpretation, Colwyn Bay *was* Nutley Wood. And, indeed, those years before manhood and a move to Birmingham would have been firmly rooted in Bestall's creative thoughts. Much as they would be in Terry's creative thoughts.

It would be Terry's own successful foray into children's book-writing that presented him with an opportunity to meet and celebrate his artistic hero. In 1981, he presented an edition of the BBC television book review programme *Paperbacks* and welcomed Bestall as a guest. It reignited – or more accurately added another log or two to – Terry's burning passion for Rupert, and, with Bestall's ninetieth birthday fast approaching, Terry set about making a documentary film in his honour. *The Rupert Bear Story* was transmitted on the fledgling station Channel 4 on 9 December 1982 with perfect timing: just five days before the illustrator's big birthday. The critical and public reaction was huge. And it was Terry's unique gift to Bestall: an affectionate, public acknowledgment of the importance of his work, not only upon Terry's own life as a writer but as a source of great joy for the entire nation. This was Terry saying, 'Thank You' on behalf of millions of us.

Terry must have been grateful for this opportunity for a number of reasons, but particularly as Alfred Bestall died barely three years after the film celebrating the artist and his work. As a fellow devotee of Rupert and Bestall, Colin Webb accompanied Terry to the funeral, in Porthmadog, in Wales, 'on a miserable and bleak winter's day at the start of 1986. Terry was determined to be there.'

Despite affording him an opportunity to visit Wales, the sombre funeral of Alfred Bestall was in stark contrast to Terry's happy place. His office at home in Grove Park. Before having children and the flair for telling children's stories came fully into focus, Terry had decided to knock two rooms at the top of the house into one big space, for a spacious place in which to write. The reason was simple. To let in the light. The bigger of the two rooms was at the front of the house but the smaller room, at the back, was the one that got the sun throughout the working day. Alison remembers that: 'Terry would be writing in the front room and open the door into the corridor, and be blinded by this amazing sunlight coming in. He would emerge, like a mole, from the darkness.' Once the conversion had taken place, the top of the house was a beautiful study. And the sunlight that was let into his working day radiates throughout his stories for children. Sally, the inspiration for *Fairy Tales* in the first place, recalls that: 'Dad would be writing up there when I got in from school. It was a sunny, magical room.' And the stories, in turn, are full of sunshine and magic.

It was Terry's second child, son Bill, who had proved the inspiration for Terry's next book for children. Though he was still young, barely seven years old at the time of publication, Bill didn't want fairy tales; he wanted adventures, derring-do, sea creatures and happy heroics. And so Terry came up with *The Saga of Erik the Viking*. A story of sunshine and magic indeed. From the stories he had read as a child, through Python and Bert Fegg and beyond, Vikings had often been a source of fun and inspiration to Terry. Although never less than exciting and engaging, Erik was a friendly kind of Viking. Just right for a story for children.

Our protagonist, Erik, is married, happily, but determined not to sleep again in his own bed until he walks upon 'the land where the sun goes at night'. With such a mission at the book's heart and within the heart of Erik himself, this rather stoic Viking gathers his crew – including Ragnar Forkbeard, Thorkhild and Sven the Strong – boards his ship, the *Golden Dragon*, and sets sail.

Terry's inspiration for the story, published, again by Pavilion Books, in 1983, was, naturally enough, the Norse legends and, in particular, those of Erik the Red, the medieval adventurer who founded the first settlements in Greenland and thus established many of the Icelandic sagas that are still told today. Terry's version is intricately involved, sometimes quite weighty, in a loving pastiche of the style of J.R.R. Tolkien and the *Lord of the Rings* books. There is real danger – the thrilling scenes at the Edge of the World will have even the most jaded of young adults in slack-jawed wonder. And the threatening characters are genuinely unsettling – the ever-laughing Old Man of the Sea is a figure straight from overly fertile nightmares. He's a renowned trickster and proves to be a cunning shapeshifter, as well as the holder – in more ways than one – of Erik's happiness. In the end, Erik realises that 'our true goal lies within ourselves and in what we do, and not in the things we think we are looking for.' It is this philosophy and this level of thinking that marks out Terry's fiction for children and is at the heart of what makes *The Saga of Erik the Viking* in particular such an enduring success. There is a level of sophistication in this good yarn well told; it's an exciting, often frightening adventure that concludes with peace, understanding and joy.

For Michael Foreman, the book was again a joy to illustrate. The joy came from Terry and the world he created on the page through his wonderful, original ideas and his interpretation of old ideas. And of course there were characters that would be a gift to any talented illustrator – spooky demons, silly kings and headstrong Vikings. Even if the Vikings did threaten to be a minor bone of contention between artist and writer . . .

Such was Michael's dedication to the *Saga of Erik the Viking* project that he actually went off to Scandinavia in order to research the locations for the paintings. The system the two had was that Terry would write the book first, then Michael would do his picture research and begin sketching – with progress of course being discussed over as many of those delightful catch-up lunches as could be arranged. Michael remembers that Terry had the power of veto of his pictures – that was Terry's privilege as the author. He says they never argued though. The only time Michael was a little concerned was with this one, which was not quite plain sailing – rather aptly, really.

The issue was that Terry insisted that Erik and his pals had to be seen in the illustrations wearing that typical headwear, the Viking helmet with horns. Michael told him: 'Terry. I've done the research. I have done much more research than was absolutely necessary! I wanted to get it right. Vikings didn't really wear those silly helmets with the cow horns. It's pure fiction!'

Terry looked at Michael and said: 'Well, the book is pure fiction! I want the Viking helmets!'

Terry knew that, like himself, generations of children had grown up with the educational Ladybird and Wonder books, as well as the 1970s British children's TV show *Michael Bentine's Potty Time*. And they always depicted Vikings in helmets with horns. Despite being a historian in heart and mind, Terry knew his audience. They would want to see the horns. Michael doggedly reiterated that they really, really hadn't worn helmets with horns.

Terry insisted! 'Look, Michael. If you don't draw them with helmets and horns, the readers won't know they are Vikings. Right?'

So, sure enough, Erik wears a helmet with horns. Michael Foreman was eventually so won over by Terry's argument that he even joined him in publicity photographs for the book, both wearing Viking helmets complete with totally historically inaccurate horns.

The book was another much-lauded success, for both the story and Michael's wonderful paintings. *The Saga of Erik the Viking* was commended for the Library Association's Kate Greenaway Medal for the best-illustrated British publication. 'You see?' admits Michael. 'Terry was right about the horns!'

Terry wasn't right about everything, of course. Though he was always characteristically intractable once he had a clear vision in his head. *Nicobobinus*, the tale of a boy called Nicobobinus who lived in Venice a long, long time ago, was a case in point. The story was perfectly fine. It related the adventures of this young lad who was so cheeky he would stick his tongue out at the prime minister, and had such a wanderlust that he determines to travel to the Land of Dragons. As Colin Webb recalls: '*Nicobobinus* is a great book. But it's another example of Terry being a little stubborn – dare I say a little pig-headed – and without a grasp on the difficult job of the marketing team when a book is published. I said to Terry: "Look! We have a problem, conceptually, in marketing, in the title of the book *Nicobobinus*. Nobody knows how to pronounce it!" I said: "Can't you call it *The Boy Who Burned Venice*?" But Terry wasn't even willing to debate the point. The book was called *Nicobobinus* and, if we weren't going to publish it under that title, he would take it elsewhere, or simply not publish it at all. I tried to reason with him. I really did. But the book had to be called *Nicobobinus* and so it was published as *Nicobobinus*. But I'm quite convinced, to this day, that it would have been much more success-ful if it had had a better title. Sorry, Terry! If people can't connect with a title or understand a title or, yes, can't even properly read your title, it puts them off.'

David Wood certainly agrees that *Nicobobinus* is a brilliant book. David was on the panel of the Whitbread Book Awards the year it was published, in 1985. 'When you are on the jury of these kinds of things, you had to read something like seventy-five books, and you had to choose one for each of the five categories: novel, biography, whatever ... Then all the judges came together to choose the coveted Whitbread Book of the Year. It was always well known that a children's book would never win it. That was a given, until Philip Pullman won it with *The Amber Spyglass*, in 2001. But in 1985, when I was a judge, Terry's *Nicobobinus* was on the short-list. I was very impressed by the book.'

David recalls telling Terry how much he had enjoyed reading it. He said: 'It was so well planned, and well structured.' And then: 'Terry stopped me and said: "Oh no no no . . . I just wrote it!" We had been talking about preparation and synopsis and knowing where your story was going. Beginning, middle and end and all that, and Terry said: "No, I just let it go where it goes. I have no idea where it's going!" Which is incredible, really. I never really believed him, but he swore that he had had the first idea and just started writing it. He was an honest man, so one has to believe him. An amazing, incredible talent. I mean, if Terry really did just sit down and write *Nicobobinus*, then that was something a little beyond brilliant!'

Indeed, *Nicobobinus* does have that natural, organic flow. A little like the flow of the Canal Grande through Venice, as Nicobobinus and his – far more easy-to-pronounce – friend Rosie embark on a stream-of-consciousness adventure. Terry's central dramatic themes of greed and cruelty recur – the children encounter bloodthirsty monks; treacherous pirates; mountains that move; and even a sailing ship that can cook a decent meal. Despite the mad intricacies of the plot, it does definitely seem that Terry was never one to over-analyse what he wrote.

Part of the idea behind the book was a very simple one. Terry thought it would be clever to set the story in a place where he could get great lunches – so, Venice! Unsurprisingly, Michael Foreman was very much in favour of this plan: 'I have been in love with Venice since my first visit in 1960. Venice was the first foreign place I had ever seen. And it is still my favourite. Thus, I grab any opportunity to go to Venice and when Terry (over yet another lunch) mentioned that his next character, Nicobobinus, might well live in Venice, I looked at him, smiled, and ordered another bottle of wine!' None of the snow and ice of *Erik the Viking*. This was going to be jolly. Though as it turned out, Terry's other commitments meant that he and Michael weren't able to be in Venice at the same time. Not that that deterred Michael. And anyway, Venice in the (loosely) Middle Ages was indeed the perfect setting for a fairy tale, for adventure. As Michael Foreman says: 'the spirit of Marco Polo' is in that 'fantastic living stage set with continual entrances stage left and right. To leave a place by boat is best because it is lingering, you leave looking backwards.'

To be a poet had been Terry's earliest creative ambition, but it wasn't until 1988 that Pavilion Books published his first, and only, collection of poetry: *The Curse of the Vampire's Socks and Other Doggerel*. The title is interesting. Apart from the fact that doggerel is a word hardly likely to be familiar to most children – the intended audience for the book – it is Terry once again publicly displaying self-doubt as a writer. Doggerel is a rather negative term, but for Terry it was an indication that this verse was to be decidedly comic in nature – very much in the vein of outrageous Scottish poet William McGonagall (who was a favourite of the Goons, and was played by Spike Milligan in the 1974 biopic *The Great McGonagall*). Terry's title promises silliness. It is certainly more Spike Milligan than Dylan Thomas.

The poems collected within *The Curse of the Vampire's Socks* are stuffed with moral dilemmas and disgusting ramifications of bad behaviour. The sort of madcap ideas and reversals that children love and most adults would never be able to think up. Like, 'what if the animals we eat could talk and decided to get their own back'. Or 'imagine if clothes withdrew their labour and ran off to the woods'. Or 'what would happen if there was an eraser that could rub out absolutely everything – even your school!'

For this collection Michael Foreman adopted a different style of illustration, that of simple pencil-line. For this particular poem, 'Bill's Eraser', even his drawing is partially rubbed out. The book's designer, Tom Sawyer, also added to the gusto of the book. Again in 'Bill's Eraser' there is a cascading typeface, causing one stanza to come to a stop as it literally falls down the printed page, while the final line is separated, alone, as you turn to the next page, for maximum impact. This is the design team working in close proximity with Terry, in order to challenge and disrupt the conventions of publishing. This is a book that, in every way, adapts itself to the silliness of the written word.

And the verse is, indeed, very, very silly, and very, very funny too. Take Laurie Oliphant, who behaves like a rabbit, nibbles dachshunds and lives in a hutch shaped like a Rover car. Or the friendly Sewer Kangaroo who pops up and grabs you when you sit on the loo. In another delightful Michael Foreman imagining of Terry's words, the 'roo in question even wears a gas mask to avoid the worst of the whiff!

Even more revolting is 'Horace', a poem that confirms the book jacket's warning that it 'will even make you squirm', for indeed Horace is a young lad who, 'much to his Mum and Dad's dismay . . . ate himself one day'.

*The Curse of the Vampire's Socks* is a proper collection: a Terry Jones Anthology of Invaluable Advice and Pointless Rhyme, which includes within its thirty-two poems several works previously printed. 'Horace' had previously appeared in *Monty Python's Big Red Book*; 'A Scottish Mystery' in *Bert Fegg's Nasty Book for Boys and Girls*; while 'A New Attempt on the World Rhyming Championship Record!' had originally been included in *Dr Fegg's Encyclopaedia of All World Knowledge*, an extended 1984 edition of the Bert Fegg book that had started Terry's career in children's books in the first place.

Terry's poems range from the Pythonesque – 'Drusilla Quill' is a catalogue of grotesque ailments – to the cheekily ludicrous – 'Moby Duck' tells the tall tale of a giant bird who terrorises the waterways. That concept tickled Terry so much that he penned a sequel, also included in the *Vampire's Socks* volume.

It's an extremely personal collection. 'The Experts' reveals the nonsense of authority in government; while typically of Terry's writings for children, there is a lot of reference to alcohol . . . Not to mention Norse fables. Here it is a rhyme, all about Algernon the Viking and his outsize nose! 'Custard Day' tells of the fun times enjoyed by the food we don't eat; while 'The Grumble-Wheezer Tree' is Terry's rather risqué pastiche of a Lewis Carroll cautionary tale. 'The Emperor's Secret' is rather cheeky too.

'Dorothy Jane' tells of the little girl who is so keen to complain that she falls out of a plane – or is she pushed? 'Soldiers' is a frank, concise and vital history lesson. Simply put, the point of the poem is that soldiers fight and kill in order to prevent themselves from getting bored. 'Mouldy Land' is a travelogue through a horrid place of bad smells and grim flavours, in which Michael Foreman drives home the unpleasantness by including the Sewer Kangaroo in the illustration. If 'Mouldy Land' suits the Sewer Kangaroo then it must really be horrible!

*The Curse of the Vampire's Socks* is an outstanding collection, with the stand-out poem being 'Extinction Day': a powerful catalogue of animal species and one plant – the Hau Kuahiwi – that have been totally destroyed by man. It is profound, thought-provoking and unforgettable. 'Extinction Day' is arguably the most focused example of Terry's practice of wrapping up a serious ecological message in his writing for children. The natural world was clearly important to him, as evidenced in his love of Wales, and his having founded *Vole* magazine. In this laudable attempt to interest children in environmental issues and concerns, his books had a valuable serious point alongside the amusingly silly. To that end, 'Extinction Day' is footnoted with the stark facts about how each and every species mentioned in the poem met their end, along with a recommendation for *The*

*Doomsday Book of Animals* by David Day, which had been published by Ebury Press in 1981.

*The Curse of the Vampire's Socks* – who, in Michael Foreman's illustration, ghoulishly emerges from an ink-well – did not necessitate an excursion to Transylvania, and the trip to Venice may not have worked out as planned, but Terry and Michael found time for a rather different adventure – a somewhat reckless and feckless road trip across France in September 1981. Sally remembers that: 'Dad adored holidays in France. We would often rent a big house, with another family, for two or three weeks. Dad would drive us all around Dordogne. These amazing stretches of countryside, packed with activities. Dad loved driving. And fun activities.'

This is something that Michael Foreman can confirm. Terry had been commissioned by the *Daily Telegraph* to write an article about a road trip that had to involve an activity of his choice. Terry chose camping and wondered whether Michael would like to go along for the ride. Hearing Michael tell the story now, it's hard not to wish a film crew had followed them . . .

They flew to Paris and hired a car. Their first stop was the town of Barbizon. Following a couple of beers at a basic bar, they located the restaurant with the best wine list. Michael remembers that Terry put on his 'wine expert' spectacles and selected a half bottle of this and then a half bottle of that and maybe another half bottle of the other. The bottles were suitably dusty and covered with cobwebs. Michael found it most impressive. They stayed at a sinister *pension* called, fittingly, the Dagger Inn, a ramshackle place surrounded by dense woodland.

The following morning they travelled by the back roads through the forest of Fontainebleau, stopping to search for truffles. Terry snuffled through the leaves like a pig. Then, he leapt to his feet and cried, 'Vines. I must see vines!' At the end of a deliciously grape-fuelled day, they realised they needed to make up for lost time and jumped on the Autoroute du Soleil, hurtling past fields of dead sunflowers and walled towns on distant hills, until the Mediterranean swam over the horizon.

They made a slight detour to visit Eric Idle, who lived in the hills behind St Tropez. Eric's hillside had been burnt out in a brush fire the week before and his swimming pool was like a rectangle of blue sky in a completely black landscape. Upon arrival, Michael and Terry played boules in the ashes and then sat in the pool and had lunch.

Then came the campsite. They had been given what they were promised was the best position, next to the shower and toilet block. This may have been very convenient but it was also muddy – because of constant use – and very noisy – thanks to swathes of holidaymakers from the north of England. Some revellers marched past Michael and Terry on their way to the loo, and, clocking Terry – who was midway through a bottle of complimentary champagne – they began to call out catchphrases from Monty Python and do 'silly walks'. Terry was not amused and decided their camping trip was over.

As dawn broke, they moved on out, and the article for the newspaper was forgotten about. Four kilometres on they found a spectacular old hotel, ringed by palm trees. Below sparkled the Mediterranean. They checked in for a week. Terry got in trouble with the campsite and the newspaper because the holiday had been sponsored solely for an article based on his break under canvas. Michael recalls, 'Terry didn't care about the job at hand. He would break rules if he didn't like what was going on! Terry drove all the way. He always wanted to be in the driving seat, quite literally. He liked to be in control. And happy. And we were very happy. We just went to the beaches. Club 55 Beach, Voile Rouge Beach . . . all the places where the people wore expensive tans and not much else. One beach was full of nudists except for one lady who wore a neck brace and a French loaf under each arm!'

One night, Terry and Michael were having dinner in the hilltop town of Gassin, with wonderful views in all directions of bays, hills, woods and mountains. They sat on a sunset terrace, sweet-smelling with pine and olives. A mosquito landed on Michael's wrist. 'Kill it,' said Terry, 'or it will go off and bite someone else.'

'Yes, but it won't kill someone else,' Michael reasoned.

Undefeated, Terry said: 'Well, bite it!'

So Michael did.

The journey concluded with an evening spent at a tiny circus at La Croix-Valmer. The attractions numbered one acrobat, one clown and Marie Claire, a talented black goat. Terry and Michael watched the crew dismantle the attraction and load everything into their transport, trucks emblazoned with a cut-out shooting star on the roof and the single, evocative word: *CIRQUE*.

'Memories of this little circus inspired me when I illustrated Terry's short story "The Star of the Farmyard", in *Fantastic Stories*, and again, later, for "The Chicken Circus", in *Animal Tales*,' Michael explained.

A potentially problematic story was originally supposed to be included in *Fantastic Stories* and once again shows Terry's determination not to compromise, much to the chagrin of Colin Webb: 'Terry had written a story called "The Flea Who Thought He Ran Sainsbury's" all about the flea at Sainsbury's who had bitten Mr Sainsbury. And I had to say to him that, because we were a small business, any threatened litigation would wipe us out. Although I was probably being a little oversensitive, I laid my cards on the table and said: "Look, I don't think we can include this unless you change the name of the retail outlet to something that is not known." Terry, of course, said that he couldn't do that. And so that particular story did not make it into the collection. It was easier to proceed without it!'

Old Street Publishing released the story in 2007 as a slim stand-alone volume, while it was Anova Books who eventually took the chance on including the story, within Terry's *Animal Tales* in 2011. They got at least one concession from the author. The main human character was now called Mr Terry Saintsbury, and the title shortened to 'The Flea That Ran Saintsbury's', which, as the prose confirmed, was 'Yes! The one who owns all the big grocery stores and hypermarkets – that Mr Saintsbury!' No legal writs were forthcoming.

Terry was very proud of the collection as a whole. The opening story was a personal favourite. I remember the day he wrote it or, at least, started writing it. He skipped into the pub, promptly ordered himself a pint and me another of the one I was drinking, and excitedly proclaimed 'a good day of writing. I've got this new story. It's called "The Good Doctor". I've been trying to get the first line right all afternoon.' As any writer knows, that first line, while not always the hardest to come up with, is the one you know will hook in your readership. Or not, as may be. Terry recited the first line once. Then again. And once more. It was perfect. I was hooked. 'There was once a highly qualified dog, who also had a great bedside manner.'

Of all the many books by Terry that Colin Webb published: 'it's very hard to pick out a favourite, because he could write practically everything. And everything he wrote was excellent. I suppose, if I was pushed, I would say it was a delight to have published his long-form adventure novel, *The Knight and the Squire*.' A hefty tome, for children, *The Knight and the Squire* was a story very close to Terry's heart; a medieval romp that combined history with humour and bridged the past with today. The opening paragraph beautifully sets out Terry's stall: 'I suppose the things that people did six hundred years ago were just as real to them when they were doing them as the things you and I were doing two minutes ago are to us now.'

Tom, the young lad at the heart of the story, has an air of Terry himself. He has Terry's lust for life and thirst for knowledge. He's excited when he finds himself in a library stuffed to the rafters with rare volumes, with information pulsating off the page: 'As if mesmerized, Tom sat down and started to read. The here and now fell away from him.' Tired of digging ditches in the bleakness of a fourteenth-century English village, Tom dreams of fantastic adventures with the Crusades across exotic foreign lands. It is a desire for fun and freedom that leads to thrilling escapades but, as Tom explains to a pious priest: 'I'm not running away *from* anything . . . I'm running away *to* something.' Readers were engaged and enchanted, and *The Knight and the Squire* eventually begat two sequels, *The Lady and the Squire* and *The Tyrant and the Squire*.

For Colin Webb, *The Knight and the Squire* was not only an exciting story but, as chance would have it, it inadvertently had a hand in opening the door to a series that would dominate children's publishing for years to come and delight generations of readers. Colin says: 'I'm convinced that that particular novel is instrumental in the success of Harry Potter!'

Here's the theory. Pavilion, as a small company, had their titles sold and distributed by Bloomsbury. 'Bloomsbury was growing rapidly and being very successful, but they did not have a children's division. Not, that is, until we at Pavilion came along. So they sold all our children's books.' Largely thanks to the success of *The Knight and the Squire* in 1997, the company grew. As a result, Colin decided: 'We could do things better, so we gave Bloomsbury three months' notice. After that, we would sell and distribute our books ourselves.'

Bloomsbury quickly realised that they didn't have a children's book programme to replace Pavilion. Colin Webb remembers that: 'They hired a young editor called Barry Cunningham. Barry was charged with signing up as many books as he could to replace our list. The children's book market in those days was very narrow, so Barry started getting all these submissions, including one from a very doubtful agent. Frankly, it was known in the business that, if you got a submission from this particular agent, you just put it in the slush pile and ignored it.' The book was called *Harry Potter and the Philosopher's Stone* and it was published by Bloomsbury at the end of June 1997.

Bloomsbury advised young Joanne Kathleen Rowling to go with her initials in order to appeal to a wider audience and avoid the, frankly ridiculous, assumption that it would be a book just for girls. 'Imagine if that had been Terry,' says Colin. 'He would have refused point blank! Anyway, there you have it. The truth is that our departure at that time led to Harry Potter being published by Bloomsbury. So it was all down to Terry. They had to replace Terry Jones!'

So you see, dear readers, the Harry Potter reference in this chapter heading is no mere gimmick. It could well have been a case of Terry Jones and the 'Pavilion' of Secrets. Walking around Terry's Oxford today, the tourist cannot move for Harry Potter souvenirs and paraphernalia – the films having used the stunning colleges for locations. Not that Terry was ever asked to direct one, or indeed act in one. Not that he was bothered. Other people's magic wasn't for him. He had far too much of his own. Magic. And Sunshine.

# CHAPTER TEN

## CALLING THE SHOTS – TERRY
## AS A FILM DIRECTOR

*What I really like to do is write feature films. It's not
really so much about directing a film, but if I can write
myself something to direct, then I really love doing it!*

ONE Sunday afternoon, Terry was driving us back to his house
for food. Terry was never one to go to the pub after food, always
before. On this particular occasion it had been a swift pint in The
Wrestlers, a sixteenth-century pub with wood panels, stained-glass
windows, open fireplaces and very good craft beers. Partway
through the homeward bound car journey, my mobile phone –
which would usually be on silent – sparked into vocal action. In
those days, my Nokia had an array of comedy soundbites. Yes, I
was that person. These ranged from Leslie Phillips saying, 'Hello' to
Charles Hawtrey intoning, 'Drop it in the basket, I'll read it later!'
from that French Revolution Carry On film *Don't Lose Your Head*
every time an email came in. The alert for a text message was Terry,
as that outrageous ex-streetwalker Mandy and mother of Brian,
screaming: 'He's Not the Messiah, he's a very naughty boy!'

Perhaps inevitably, a text came in and Terry's unmistakable
voice rang out electronically from my pocket. Terry, with some
surprise, jerked his head and said: 'That's me!' I was slightly embarrassed, and tried to laugh it off.

Thankfully, Terry laughed. 'Isn't that really fucking annoying?'
he asked.

I swiftly turned it back on him, knowing that that most quotable of comedy film quotes had been shouted out at him, and repeated many, many times, the world over: 'Isn't *that* really fucking annoying?'

'Oh no,' chuckled Terry, 'I love it. That film has been extremely good to me!'

And so it had and continued to be. Indeed, *Monty Python's Life of Brian* is the crowning achievement of the group as a whole and of Terry as performer, writer and film-maker. It's the one that, as often as not, still tops those impossible lists of 'funniest film of all time', decades after it came out. By that rationale, Terry was the greatest comedy film director of all time. When I would cheekily point this 'fact' out to Terry he would smirk, shake his head and say: 'No, Rob. That would be Buster Keaton!'

Keaton had been his role model and idol since adolescence. Terry's eye for design had blossomed at Oxford, but the kernel of what would become his vision as a film director had been with him from childhood, through those imaginative walks in Colwyn Bay, the silly slapstick in the pages of his weekly comics and the amazing acrobatic feats of Keaton. As a young teenager, with cine-camera in hand and a limitless imagination, Terry would make those short films in and around his family home in Claygate. In these, Terry the sorcerer, using stop-motion animation, would give life to inanimate objects. He worked out how to weave his own magic spell, by positioning his mother's best dining chairs – snap – moving them forward – snap. Repeat and repeat again, with infinite patience, to create the illusion that the furniture, fed up of being sat on, was leaving through the open door, walking up the front garden path, and off, out, onto the street. And freedom. Funny freedom.

Terry's film was called 'The Chairs' and was a delight. It still is. Amusing, and sophisticated, it is the earliest extant example of a passion for making films that would never leave him. We have borne witness to the fun he gleaned from messing about with slapstick for *The Frost Report* and pulling together pastiches of arthouse cinema for *Twice a Fortnight*. His love of vintage slapstick comedy would, of course, inspire his own comedy creations. Indeed, he even played one of his heroes, Harpo Marx, for just one night only, as a super-understudy, for the double-bill comedy musical *A Day in Hollywood/A Night in Ukraine*. The voiceless Marx Brother, Keaton, Harry Langdon, Laurel and Hardy, they were all in Terry's very funny bones. Much of the humour of *Do Not Adjust Your Set* too of course relied on Terry's ability to fall over in a funny way, as well as his love of taking apart the visual tropes of television and putting them back together again – ideally in the wrong order. A style that would then make its way into Python. Everything debunked, with a loving smile.

This love of creativity – particularly on film – and Terry's need to be in control made him the natural Python to be the director. Almost by default. Throughout those film inserts on *The Frost Report* and *Twice a Fortnight* and *Monty Python's Flying Circus* Terry was very keen to vocalise his thoughts on the actual directing – as often as not to the mild chagrin of the credited director. Within the Python group, though, it was acknowledged that Terry *did* know what was best in presenting Python on screen. Michael Palin believes that Terry directing Python just felt so right. So natural. It was fun: 'Terry had this knack of keeping it fresh. There was a fluidity and spontaneity in the comedy, but the great thing about Terry was that he was very pragmatic about what he was doing.' With Terry as designated director, and actively preserving the comic integrity of the group, the others could trust him to serve Python as a concept better than anybody from outside the team.

The Pythons knew they had to produce something funny. And completely different. The joke could not be allowed to go stale. From script to screen or stage and into the audience is a long, arduous process. Terry's gift was to keep the laughter alive. To keep the group as a whole from getting complacent or, worse still, bored. Michael Palin confirms that: 'we had to still find what we were doing funny. And keep those sketches fun to perform. Even if you have done the material so often, there was still the odd moment, the odd ad lib, something very, very silly, that would set us off. Totally undetectable to the audience, one hopes, but something that would set us all off! Terry was very good at keeping Python fun for the rest of us.'

Terry's ability was to keep this sense of fun buoyant even when filming conditions were at their least enjoyable. The wet and windy wilds of Scotland for *Monty Python and the Holy Grail* could have scuppered the most seasoned of film directors. For Terry, it was his first feature film as a director, and he kept a despondent cast and crew focused on the job. His son Bill says: 'that was Dad though. He loved making movies, and he just got on with it. You know, there is that dreadful cliché that if a film is great fun to make, it's a great film. I don't buy that at all. *Holy Grail* and *Life of Brian* is the perfect example. On *Grail* everybody was miserable, the weather was awful, the two Terrys couldn't agree on anything! On *Brian* it was a wonderful time. The sun was shining, they would shoot a few scenes and be back at the hotel poolside sipping a cocktail. Both *Grail* and *Brian* are wonderful films. It's the script and the performances that matter. Always. And, to be a little bit proud of Dad here, it is his direction on both films. He was just a very good film director. Nothing fazed him. Everybody loved working with him. He just got on with the job.'

Having been an actor under the direction of other people, Terry swiftly became a real actor's director. He would maintain that: 'it's pretty easy, really. Basically, never say the actors' words. Just make suggestions. Never do it for them. As an actor, if a director says to me "Don't say it like that. Say it like this!" I would feel like saying, "Well, why don't you fucking do it then!"'

Terry's place as film director was now a given within the group as a whole. He had proved more than capable on *Holy Grail* and, with all having benefited from a complete break from Python to be energised by individual projects, another Python feature film was planned. The dynamic retained the pragmatism that had always been core to Python, while also now having a relaxed freedom. A real sense that they had all proved themselves away from the Python collective. They were all, fundamentally, writers at heart still, and the Python writing room remained very much key to the development of the film that would become *Monty Python's Life of Brian*.

Although, in fact, the *Brian* writers' room was more a writers' island. The team rented a beautiful house, Heron Bay, on a beach on the west coast of Barbados. The luxury home, designed by Ronald Tree as a Palladian Revival mansion, had been built in 1947, and made the most of the glorious Caribbean. So, in shorts and straw hats, the Pythons wrote and rewrote Python. This was a far cry from the BBC rehearsal rooms in Acton! The writing of the group was still extraordinary though. Just now in far more opulent surroundings. And Terry, as director, found himself in pole position, while relishing the sheer glee of being back within the Python group again. He had both control and support.

It was this role as an affable team captain who would fight tooth and claw for his squad, while fully appreciating that the five players around him were at the peak of their powers, that made Terry so focused and forthcoming during the pre-production stage and throughout the filming schedule. It was this creative journey that, more than the huge international success of the film, made Terry so fiercely proud of *Monty Python's Life of Brian*. And so jolly when he heard someone shout out: 'He's not the Messiah!' The very fact that people had seen the film, had loved it so much, and it had a lasting impression upon them, meant a great deal to Terry.

The very idea of *Life of Brian* sprang out of the joke suggestion that the next Monty Python film should be called 'Jesus Christ:

Lust for Glory'. Although *Life of Brian* treats Jesus as a character with huge respect, and the joke at the heart of the film is the ridiculousness of organised religion, Terry was fully aware that it was a controversial topic. But he wasn't prepared for the last-minute bombshell of financial backer Lew Grade pulling out of putting up the money. Once again, rock 'n' roll came to the rescue. George Harrison salvaged the production, remortgaging his Henley-on-Thames house, Friar Park, in order to pay for the film to be made. When asked 'Why?' by incredulous journalists, George would say: 'Because I wanted to see the film!' That 'most expensive cinema ticket ever' signalled the foundation of HandMade Films and *Monty Python's Life of Brian* was the beginning of a very lucrative and very productive decade in British film-making, with HandMade investing in many projects with various Pythons.

Somehow, throughout this production's uncertainty and location scouting and logistics balancing, Terry kept his focus on the funnies. And, as his first credited solo directorial feature film project, this was an epic. The budget was a whopping four million dollars, as opposed to the just over a quarter of a million pounds of *Holy Grail*. The storm that raged around *Life of Brian*, and the responsibility of completing the film on time and within that massive budget, never seemed to faze him at all. It may have appeared effortless but it certainly wasn't. And Terry had more than a little help from his friends.

He also had a lot of help on the domestic front. Daughter Sally was about to turn five and son Bill was a toddler. A loving father, Terry juggled this with the practicalities of his job. Whereas his own father had done his military duty during Terry's formative years, Terry had to put polishing the script and shooting the film first. Thus, following a snatched family holiday in Wales, he left the kids with Alison and jetted off to Monastir, in Tunisia, a living, breathing biblical film set whose historical fortress looked exactly like something from Ancient Rome. Terry worked to that old adage that, if the joke looks right, the audience will laugh. Besides, Franco Zeffirelli had just shot *Jesus of Nazareth* there, and if it was good enough for him it was good enough for Terry.

Monastir was also good enough for comic messiah Spike Milligan to have planned a holiday there. Some divine intervention from the Great Comedy Architect was at work here, that Spike should just happen to be there when the Python juggernaut steamed into town. The weight of Spike's achievements was great indeed though, and suddenly all the Pythons were like fidgeting schoolboys. Within the group, excited giggles erupted at the thought that maybe Spike would want to be in their film, but everybody was just too nervous to ask him. The Pythons were awestruck by this comedy god walking among them. In the end, Terry was the one to do it. He was the director, after all: 'I did think that Spike was on holiday and he might tell me to piss off! but the fan in me was so thrilled at the thought of him being in the film, I just went over to him and said: "Spike! We are making a film, do you want to be in it?"'

Spike said yes, thankfully, and Terry scuttled over to a pile of costumes, grabbed him a tunic and shouted, 'Action!' Terry felt that 'you can't really direct Spike'. He's a presence. A deity, if you will. He just wandered around in the background. He did his bit, and then he wandered off into the desert. That Spike, the godfather of alternative comedy, was on hand to endorse Terry's magnum opus meant a great deal to him. It had been Spike who had added shape and structure to the flow of his comic imagination. His Professor of Jokes, if you will.

If Spike was a talisman, a good luck charm, for Terry's first solo film as director, it certainly worked. And, while Terry was juggling budgets and locations and filming conditions and a big cast of actors, he also had to act in the film himself. Understandably, he took fewer characters, while his fellow Pythons played pretty much everybody else. Still, apart from getting completely naked

– as he does as the grey-bearded juniper-bush-obsessed hermit in the desert whose pained passion accidentally and irrevocably breaks his vow of silence – Terry was never happier than when dragging up for maximum laughs. Hence, his major acting contribution is Mandy Cohen, the mother of Brian (Graham Chapman). As Terry modestly maintained, 'playing Mandy was something like playing those shrieking women from the old television series, although she is a bit more abusive than I should have played her. She's got no redeeming features at all, and you should warm to the mum of your hero. Just a little.'

Decades before the word 'woke' got picked up, moulded, and bent out of all recognition of what it actually means, Terry was very aware that woke is a good thing; a kind thing; and an understanding thing. He certainly was the first to admit that Python could be accused of being sexist or, moreover, that the way he played women was sexist: 'It's just the background we all came from. Through school onwards. To be honest, most of the women we were writing about were grotesques. Carol [Cleveland] played the pretty ones and the sexy ones. We played the rest. We had shot the Mr Equator sketch with John [Cleese] and Fanny Carby playing his wife. It just didn't work. It wasn't funny. We reshot it, with me as Mrs Equator, and it was funnier. No matter how good the actress had been, she simply wasn't gross enough. She had to be disgusting, and I can play disgusting!' No malice or offence was ever meant. If the characters can, in actual fact, be seen to be rather feminist, then Terry's attitude certainly was – he was even selected as the very first male presenter of *Woman's Hour*, for the broadcast of April Fool's Day, 1985. And no one in the world is more qualified to comment on the representation of women in Python than Carol Cleveland: 'how could anybody be offended by Terry as a woman? It's one of the funniest, most ridiculous, most joyous things you could ever wish to see. And performed as a complete grotesque; a complete caricature. Hilarious. Not derogatory at all. Certainly no comedy director I have ever worked with understood women better than Terry. I think they all delighted in giving me very naughty things to say – Terry in particular – and I loved saying them. I was playing Dingo and Zoot, the twin sisters at Castle Anthrax, in *Monty Python and the Holy Grail* and enjoying myself so much that I even threw in an extra bit of naughtiness. When I mutter: "Oh shit!", that was an ad lib. Terry loved it and kept it in. At the premiere it got a huge reaction and I can see Terry now, turning to me and giving me the biggest smile and a thumbs-up. He was the sweetest, kindest, most encouraging of colleagues.'

Terry was also always mindful of the power of comedy. He would not be comfortable in using it to attack the persecuted or vulnerable. Terry would be delighted if his comedy offended, but only when the target of the humour was authority or an aggressor and warranted the attack. For him, comedy was always a community thing, a source of goodness, and comfort and empowerment. Even if it was a bit disgusting.

Moreover, playing disgusting, as Mandy, and directing, often while dressed as Mandy. That's a real skill set. It was a skill that super Python fan and chronicler Kim 'Howard' Johnson was there to witness. Terry, as the archivist within the group, had appreciated Johnson's passion for Python. So much so that he had welcomed him into the Python inner sanctum, given Johnson the latest film script to read and even invited him to come on location for *Life of Brian*. As an outsider looking in, Johnson was amazed that Terry just seemed to take the job of directing a major motion picture completely in his stride: 'He just couldn't be nicer to everybody. He was very busy but still had time for everybody. It was great to watch Terry in action. Although he certainly didn't seem to be the film director of a massive biblical epic. It wasn't an epic at the time. Terry just seemed to make it.' Johnson's chief memory of Terry directing the film is while the lights and cameras were being set up. Terry would spend time with the crew, pitching pennies. And, yes, he'd be directing the film, standing behind the camera, in the Mandy costume. With these great huge soccer balls for his breasts: 'Terry was so relaxed, and so well organised. He knew exactly what he was doing. He would walk the locations, the path that Michael [Palin] took as the ex-leper, everything.' As if to the manner born, Terry knew and understood every aspect of film-making: 'It was a very expensive film but Terry showed absolutely no sign of pressure at all.'

*Life of Brian* was a comedy film first and foremost, but it *was* a comic twist on a biblical epic. It was not Charlie Chaplin's ideal scenario of his tramp, a pretty girl and a park bench. This was more like something Cecil B. DeMille would have had a go at. With more laughs. Indeed, while the poster tagline for *Monty Python and the Holy Grail* had admitted that it made 'Ben Hur look like an epic', *Monty Python's Life of Brian* was a proper comedy epic. That the laughs were intrinsic to scenes such as Brian, full-frontal naked, facing a horde of obsessive followers, did not make the epic sweep of the scenes any less challenging. It was a joke, but an epic joke. Terry took these huge crowd scenes very much in his stride. Historic vistas, with five hundred people or more, were simply shading to the humour at the heart of the script. That calm strength, affability and old-fashioned charm of his successfully won over these location dilemmas that could give him – only momentary – headaches. In the BBC days of Python, he would write a sketch, with ambitious location shooting, and then hand it over to his director to figure out – with a little helpful input from himself. Now, it was Terry's responsibility. He rose to the challenge. Completely. Even when it came to that most epic of scenes when the huge crowd of people are sending up the vocal impediments of Pontius Pilate (Michael Palin). The sheer scale of the shot notwithstanding, it was only on the day of the shoot that it dawned on Terry that, of course, all of the extras who had been recruited were local Tunisians. A cast of thousands who all spoke Arabic . . . but not English. Terry thought, 'How on earth am I going to get them to say these, quite complicated, hopefully funny, lines in English?' He assumed that he would have to dub in the crowd's responses later and just hoped for the best. However, he tried shouting the lines out to them in English and, 'blow me, they just shouted them back. Perfectly. They were brilliant.'

To get the physical response he wanted from them, Terry climbed up onto a high camera platform and demonstrated, in the hope that they would imitate him as he happily rolled around on his back, laughing. And they did! 'Legs in the air, laughing uproariously at a joke they just didn't understand,' he remembered, delightedly. Modestly, Terry would say that those extras made his job easy, but it was he who, somehow, through sheer willpower, open friendliness and pure chutzpah, made that complicated shoot appear easy.

His oldest friend on location, Michael Palin, never lost sight of Terry within his all-powerful position as director: 'Because Terry was an actor, and because we had acted together for so long, we knew what each other was capable of. So he would push me in a certain way and if I resisted he would say: "Well, all right . . ." and listen and discuss and reason but generally speaking he never avoided the issue of how he wanted something done. I usually ended up doing it the way he wanted it played, but I never felt browbeaten or pressured into doing anything that I had been told to do. Rather, it was the way I wanted to do it, but, crucially, after those discussions with Terry. He had that ability to make you feel relaxed and comfortable. That's the word. Comfort. Terry could put you at ease in front of the camera.'

Terry was never one to lose his temper when directing a film. He would only lose his temper when things were not done in the way he wanted and, as director, he was in complete control of the look and feel of the production, with a skilled and dedicated cast and crew at his disposal. That cast and crew liked Terry and trusted him to do the job.

Graham Chapman, having given up drinking at the time, valued the comfort and trust of a good friend that Terry provided. Particularly in that crucial scene when Brian had to appear naked, in front of a gathering of a few British actors and a gaggle of locals, including local women. As if to seriously mirror that scene with John Cleese at the stoning: 'Are there any women here today?' – yes, there were. Lots of women. And while those British actresses, sporting beards in order to stone the heathens, were in on the joke, these local women were rather uneasy about witnessing a naked man, even in the name of a jolly good laugh. Terry's natural charm won the day again and got the shot in the can. It remains one of the shockingly funniest moments in the film. An epic laugh in fact.

Upon first seeing *Monty Python's Life of Brian*, valued Oxford chum Annabel Leventon was not only impressed but really shocked. And shocked in a good way, as she reflects: 'I still do find it quite hard to imagine my dear friend having directed such an amazing film. That sounds patronising and I don't mean it to sound patronising, but I mean, this was my mate. And it's such a big, accomplished film. It was an astonishing achievement. To control all those people and make it happen, and make such a wonderful, wonderful film. And it's Terry's! He was a brilliant film-maker.'

Michael Palin was impressed too. And he was in it. 'This was Terry proving himself as a film director. For all the Python bells and whistles, *Brian* is Terry's film. It is such a fine piece of direction. And it was the best time for Python, because everybody put their various egos to one side, for the good of the group. For this one good script. Terry was very important in getting the script together and coherent and, obviously, crucial in getting that script onto film. Without an ounce of friction. *Brian* was his finest hour – or finest hour and a half – as a director. Absolutely brilliant. Real control and focus and dedication and, yes, passion to get it right. To get everything right.'

The maelstrom of religious angst that greeted the film's release did surprise Terry, a little. He thought it would get under a lot of people's skins, but by the time they finished making it Terry felt 'it wasn't blasphemous! On the contrary – for six agnostics, it seemed remarkable that we produced a film that presupposes the existence of God and the power of Christ.' It was heretical, in that it attacked the Church, but it was not, and was never intended to be, blasphemous. Actually, they started out writing a funny life of Christ. 'We only changed it because it wasn't funny. There aren't any laughs in saying "Does God exist?" and anyway, we reread the gospels and decided that Christ is a pretty good bloke.' The comedy of *Brian* is based on human error. All comedy is people being daft or wrong in some way. As Terry explained: 'In our film we have this guy saying, "Let's all be nice to each other" and everyone goes, "Yeah, he's right!" and then they go around for two thousand years killing one another because they can't agree whether or not he was standing on a rock when he said that!' That, for Terry, was exactly where the comedy was, and, as he said, 'I'm afraid that in the end we've always gone for the comedy rather than any serious message.'

There's something reassuring in settling down to watch and rewatch *Monty Python's Life of Brian* as an alternative Christmas film. No. Scrub that. *Monty Python's Life of Brian is* a Christmas film . . . and an Easter film . . . and a film for all seasons, really . . . for people with a fabulous sense of humour. It deserves to be viewed annually. A towering, joyous achievement.

Not that, sadly, Terry could focus on either the success or notoriety that came with the film's initial release in 1979, for that Christmas saw the death of his father, Alick. It's the way of families, the circle of life, and his father had lived to see Terry and Alison be blessed with two children. Terry was, as always, philosophical about the loss of his remaining parent. It was reassuring for him to know that, in his final years, his dad had found a new lease on life and a new sense of freedom. He had treated himself to a tape deck and would merrily drive round his beloved North Wales, blaring out Scotland's finest, the Humblebums, the life-affirming folk rockers comprised of guitarist Tam Harvey, singer-songwriter Gerry Rafferty and a pre-stand-up, banjo-plucking Billy Connolly. Of an evening, Alick would sink a few pints, smoke a couple of cigarettes and play a frame or two of snooker with his mates. And so he saw out the end of his life, comfortably, with his wife, Nora, in a bungalow in St Asaph, a tiny but snug city in the shadow of its cathedral, in Denbighshire, North Wales.

Alison Telfer recalls that: 'We would see them a lot. They would spend Christmas with us – Alick loved an open fire, although it wasn't good for his chest, nor helpful for the bad smoker's cough he had developed. Even though he had only started the habit after the death of Dilys, as she hadn't approved of smoking.'

At the end of 1979, Alick was in hospital for three days in Kingston, west London. He was poorly and recuperating. Terry visited, spent an hour or so with him, and reluctantly left with his dad's reassuring words in his ears that he was fine, just fine: 'You go home, son, I'm all right.' He died that same afternoon.

Terry knew that Wales was where his dad would want to be. His ashes were scattered in the churchyard where Dilys was. It was a huge family gathering. Alick had a sister, ten years older, with a brother-in-law, Frank, who was well into his nineties. Terry and Alison had their two young children; brother Nigel had two of his own, of similar ages. The church was happy bedlam, with little ones running around, the poignancy of the occasion peppered with hope.

It was partly from Alick that Terry had inherited the steadfast integrity that he continued to pour into his work. It's the sole reason why he preferred to direct films from screenplays he himself had had a major hand in writing. That was until David Leland, the actor and theatre director friend from the Crucible, Sheffield, showed him a script for a film based on the exploits of Cynthia Payne, the celebrated Madam Cyn who had become notorious in Britain's media in 1978, when the police had raided the brothel she ran in Streatham, south London. It was a very British scandal, with vicars and politicians and solicitors handing over luncheon vouchers as proof of purchase on services rendered at saucy sex parties. David Leland's screenplay was called *Personal Services*. And although it was, from the outset, a Terry kind of a film script with its richly comic and controversial dialogue, his taking on the job of directing it was a personal favour. Several directors had been attached to the project, most notably Stephen Frears, who had even started casting the film before dropping out. David Leland had already given a copy of the script to Terry to read. He had loved it and, in desperation, Leland asked him to direct. The clincher was the fact that daughter Sally, now eleven, loved it too! Terry remembered that: 'Sally said: "Oh you must do it, Dad!" So I did!'

Not only was it the only feature film Terry directed that he claimed no writing credit for, it was also the only one he would ever direct in which he didn't even consider trying to recruit any of the Monty Python ensemble to appear. The notion of casting himself as Dolly – the cross-dressing assistant to Madam Cyn – flicked through his brain for a non-serious nanosecond before he dismissed it completely. 'I couldn't have played it. It would have been a bit of a giveaway. Straight away.' Danny Schiller is certainly wonderful in the role but auditioned with a more obvious, falsetto voice, which Terry, while immensely impressed by the gravitas of Danny himself, immediately quashed: 'I told him to just play it with his normal voice. It's not a man impersonating a woman. It's a man dressing as a woman because that is how he feels most comfortable. The big mistake we made was to screen some footage of Danny to test audiences and stupidly ask the question, "Is this a man or a woman?" They would say a man. Obviously. Simply because why would we be asking the question otherwise. If you watch the film, you don't get asked that question. You just go with it. You take what we give you on the screen, and if we had given you me in a dress you would know it was me straight away.'

The entire plot is a giveaway, of course. Although the central character is called Christine Painter, press coverage and the parallel raging interest in the controversy left it in no doubt that Christine Painter was Cynthia Payne. Even the initials are the same! Madam Cyn herself was thoroughly enjoying her celebrity status in the Britain of the 1980s, making appearances on chat shows and frequently being quoted in the tabloids. The fact that her story was being made into a feature film biopic was big news. Thus, the disclaimer at the start of *Personal Services*, which distances what follows from the real Payne, was a contractual obligation, pure and simple.

Leland's screenplay had been based on conversations he had had with Payne. However, Paul Bailey, the author of the book *An English Madam: The Life and Work of Cynthia Payne*, which had been published by Jonathan Cape in 1982, got wind of the film and put in for payment and a screen credit. Terry insisted: 'We didn't use his book at all. I hadn't even read the book!'

The script had amused Terry instantly. What had made the project so appealing were characters like Scrag-End Lil, played pitch perfectly by Victoria Hardcastle, coming out with lines such as: 'What man in his right mind wants to get his cock out in this weather?' That particular observation would tickle Terry for years to come. He would sit back in wonder at distinguished thespians like Peter Cellier, Alec McCowen, Stephen Lewis and Benjamin Whitrow in this world of blow jobs, bashed backsides and fetishes being brilliant and dedicated and true. David Leland – who plays the sleazy landlord in the film – made those characters so vividly real, carefully constructing them from Payne's first-hand descriptions and recollections.

So much so that, although Terry took control of the camera, he insisted that Leland lend a hand in the directing of the major scenes with leading lady Julie Walters: 'it would have been pointless for me to direct Julie. David knew Cynthia Payne so well, they even shared an agent, so it would have been a case of me talking Julie through the scene, and then Julie going to David to check if that was right!' Although it was no doubt true to an extent, Terry's direction certainly did contribute to a touching and hilarious performance from Walters. At the time she was cast, her standing in British film had dipped since *Educating Rita*. Both *She'll Be Wearing Pink Pyjamas* and *Car Trouble* had shaky times at the box office. So much so that Tim Bevan, producer of *Personal Services*, was not overly keen to use her. As so often in his work, Terry *was* keen *and* insistent. He had been delighted by her reading of the part. He knew she was perfect.

The only problem Julie posed for Terry was that she was too beautiful. Terry recalled that the film: 'is all set in this very old, very safe world. There's nothing very sexy about it at all. It's all very matter-of-fact. Julie's character has this disgust and fascination with sex. In equal measure.' Those early scenes of sex work had to be grubby and dispiriting, so in order to reduce Julie's attractiveness Terry had her wear a face mask in the bathtub sequence, and later, as she is putting on sexy underwear for a client: 'I had to make her look ridiculous. Pathetic. Julie just looked too good, so I told her to wear two sets of saucy underwear. The sexiness is gone. She just looks a little try-hard, a little desperate, which is what [the character] was. Even so, Julie still looks attract-ive. She ruined the shot!' he laughed.

The film was on a tight budget and the entire shoot had to be done in six weeks. Prior to this, there was a big debate about the exact era in which the film was to be set: 'Was it in the Sixties when it happened, or in the late Eighties, when we shot it? It was something that always annoyed me about films set in the past. Once an era is decided, *everything* is then geared towards that era.

The clothes, the music, everything. The era seems to be more important than the story.' In the end, Terry set the story in a contemporary reality that was also a kind of London Neverland of all eras. Simply because every era is made up of lots of eras. The now is not all modern. So the posh flat of the sex parties is something out of the 1930s; the grotty flat in the early scenes is of the late 1950s and early 1960s. It's a kind of *Steptoe and Son* poverty, set-dressed in the broadest of strokes. The little world of *Personal Services* is a secret underbelly of polite London society, full of charm and sweetness and, somehow, innocence. There is no negative creative criticism of the life choices or the lifestyle it depicts.

Terry chose to shoot the first half of the film with a handheld camera, for a cosy intimacy – almost as though his lens is eavesdropping on the scenes, peeking into this world without judgement or condemnation, merely observing. There's a sense of uncertainty, which is skilfully contrasted with the later sequences, once the character has found fame. Then the camera is on a tripod and the shots are steady. Christine has made it.

Even though he was a self-confessed hired hand on *Personal Services*, his dedication and commitment were equal to a film he had himself written. As Bill Jones asserts: 'Everyone will tell you how rewarding it was to be working on a Terry Jones film. Dad always remembered every single person's name on the set, and everyone was just so happy. He was involved in every single aspect of film-making and loved every minute of it.'

This is certainly the case with Carolyn Allen who, after wide experience in the West End, notably playing farce with the Theatre of Comedy company, was cast as one of Christine's girls, Carol: 'I was totally in awe of Terry . . . it was a thrill to be working with him. Such an open director. So warm. So lovely. Nothing showy about him at all. It was quite overwhelming on occasions when I thought about who he was and what he had achieved in his career, but he was always gentle and unassuming.'

Carolyn played the sixteenth 'birthday present' for a young lad – though the actor was actually only fourteen at the time. Terry explained the scene to the boy: 'Now, your mum is giving you a prostitute as your birthday present but you think you are going to get a bike!' And this young boy shrugged and said: 'Oh, it's no difference. You ride both of them, don't you?' Terry and Carolyn looked at each other and shrieked with laughter.

The sauce and the silliness embedded in the film adds an air of levity to the seediness of the situation. Still, the laughs are never coarse or aggressive. There is a lot of Terry's characteristic warmth and kindness on show in the way the subject matter is handled. Certainly, for Carolyn Allen, 'He seemed unruffled by anything in the script. There were these wild sex party scenes and Terry was directing them like it was nothing out of the ordinary. Mind you, he was a very sensitive man. Having got the job, I waited until being on set before saying that I didn't really want to go topless. Terry could have gone ballistic. He certainly could have recast and got somebody else. He didn't. I explained to him that I felt, although I was playing a prostitute, she was a modest prostitute. I didn't need to explain though. In the script, I was topless in this particular scene, but Terry was absolutely lovely. He gave me a teddy to wear, saying: "Don't worry. We have plenty of tits in this film. We don't need yours as well!" And that was that. It was never mentioned again.'

At the time of the film's release, in April 1987, the media were more interested in the sex than the story. Even the production's wrap party was raided by the police in the hope of, as Terry remembered it, 'finding a load of film people with their trousers down!' Carolyn Allen remembers the party vividly: 'It was wonderful. Even after the police arrived! It was just like one of Cynthia Payne's parties. I always wondered whether it had been the publicity department who had tipped them off, in order to get a few column inches. Or Cynthia Payne herself.'

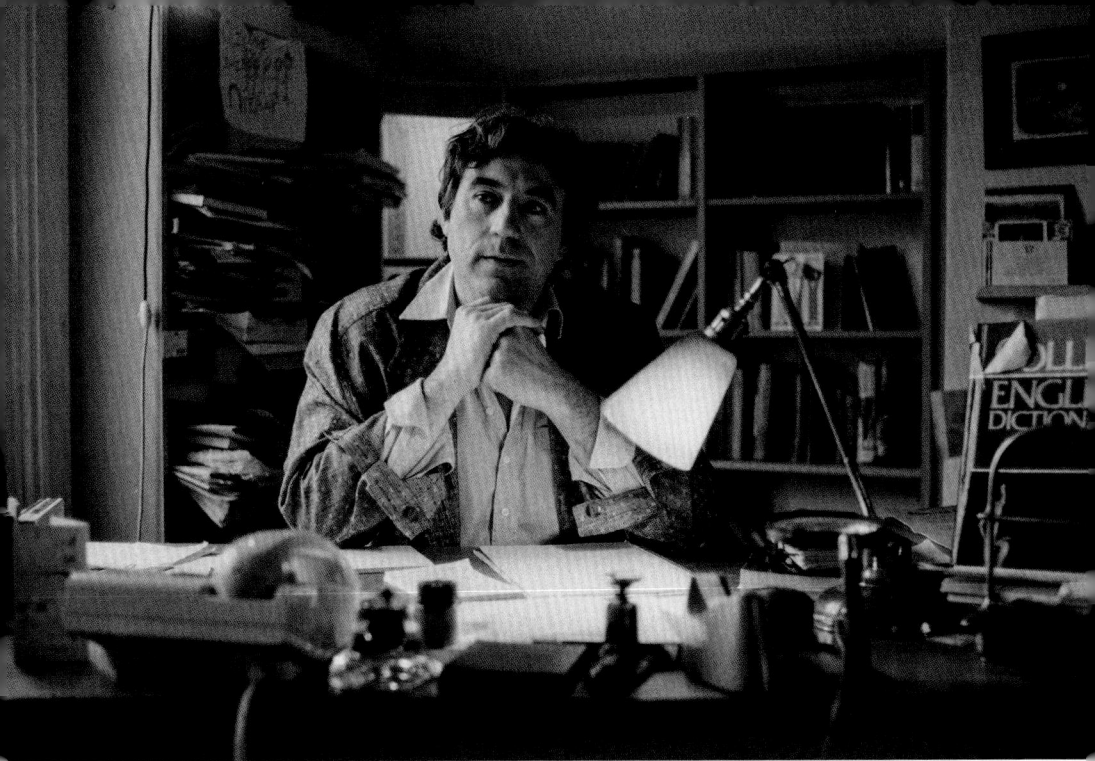

Terry's Happy Place III:
Aged 45 at home in his office of sunshine and magic at Grove Park in 1987.

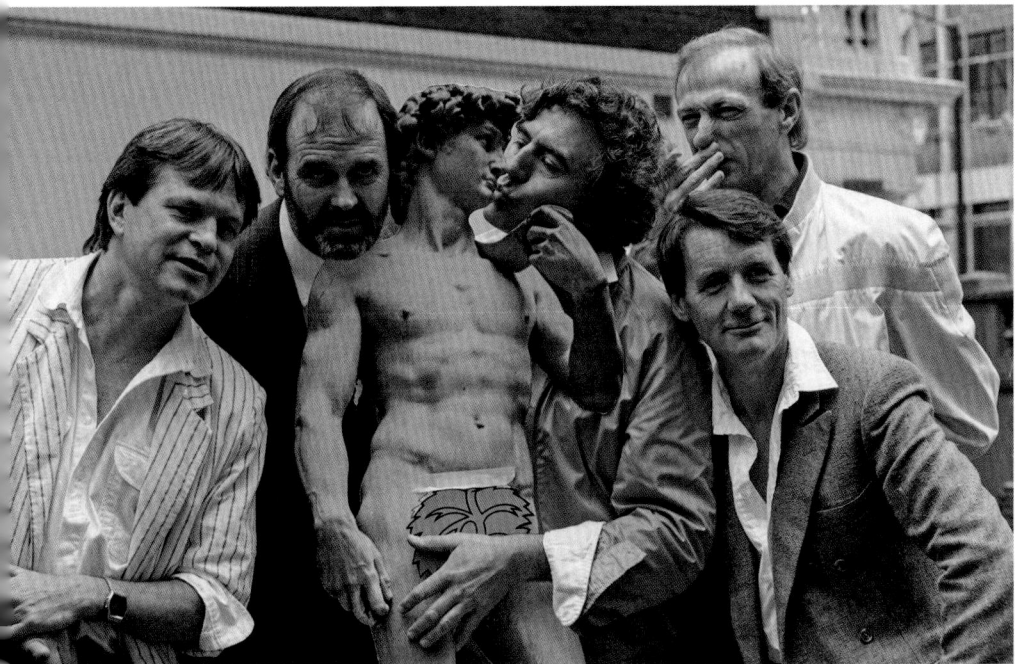

Terry, centre stage and clowning, with Terry Gilliam, John Cleese, Michael Palin and Graham Chapman to promote the BBC's first home video release of *Monty Python's Flying Circus*, on Monday, 9 September 1985.

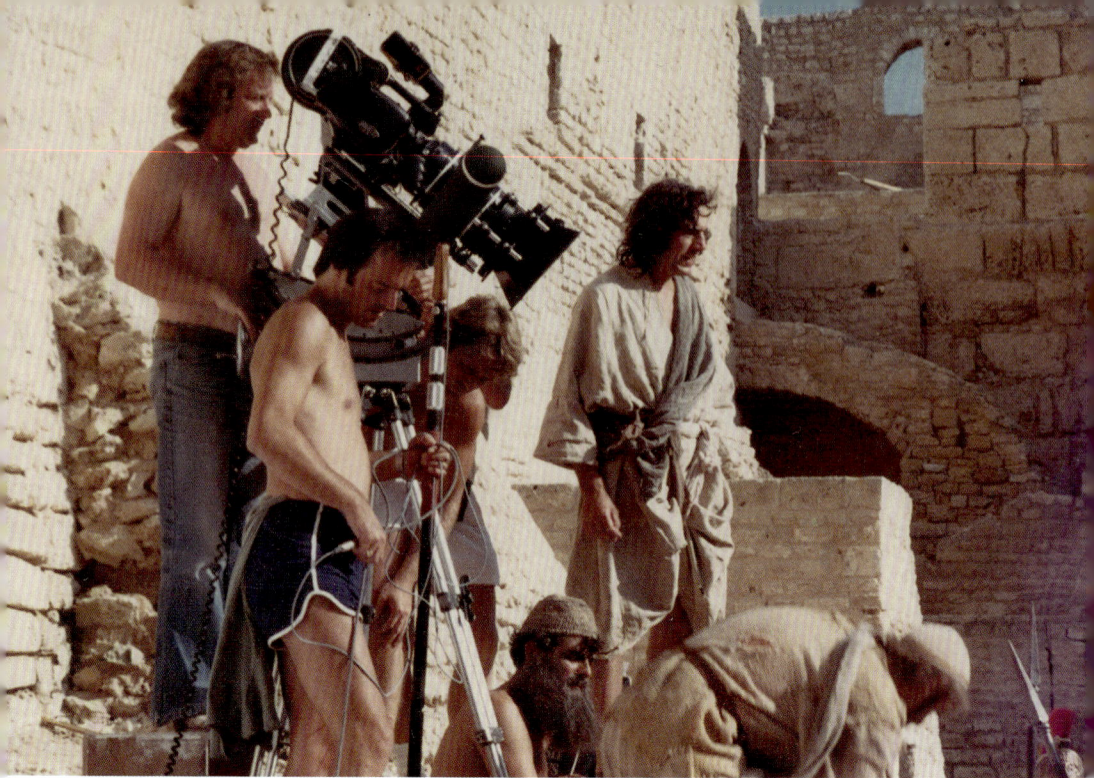

Terry, in costume and in complete control, directing *Monty Python's Life of Brian*, in Tunisia, in 1978. Actors Terence Bayler and Graham Chapman prepare.

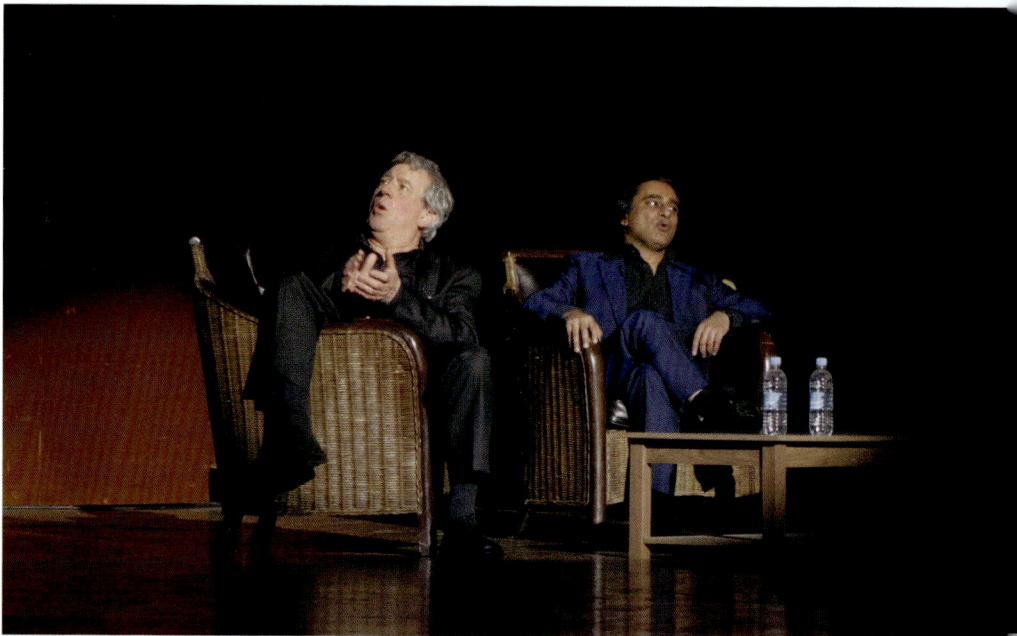

So Terry. Leg hooked over a chair as he watches his greatest achievement, *Monty Python's Life of Brian*, with *Spamalot* King Arthur Sanjeev Bhaskar at the Colston Hall, Bristol, for the Slapstick Festival, in January 2012.

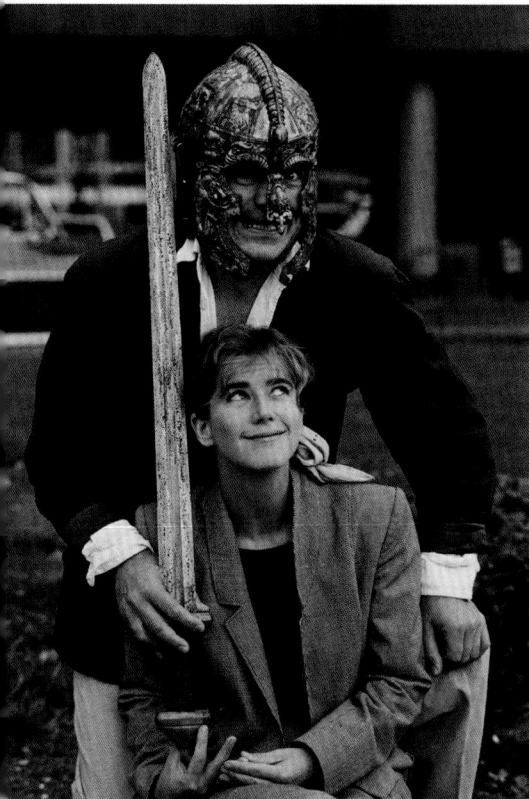

Terry as the Norseman announces his film of *Erik the Viking* at St. Katherine Docks in London's East End, on Wednesday, 12 October 1988, and introduces his leading lady Imogen Stubbs.

Posing with Julie Walters, his leading lady for *Personal Services*, in 1987, during the making of the only film Terry directed for which he receives no writing credit.

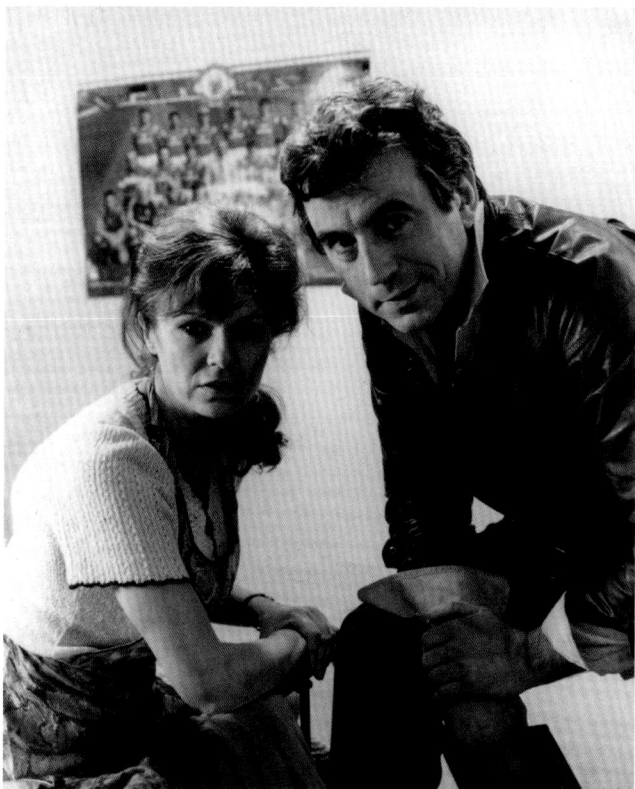

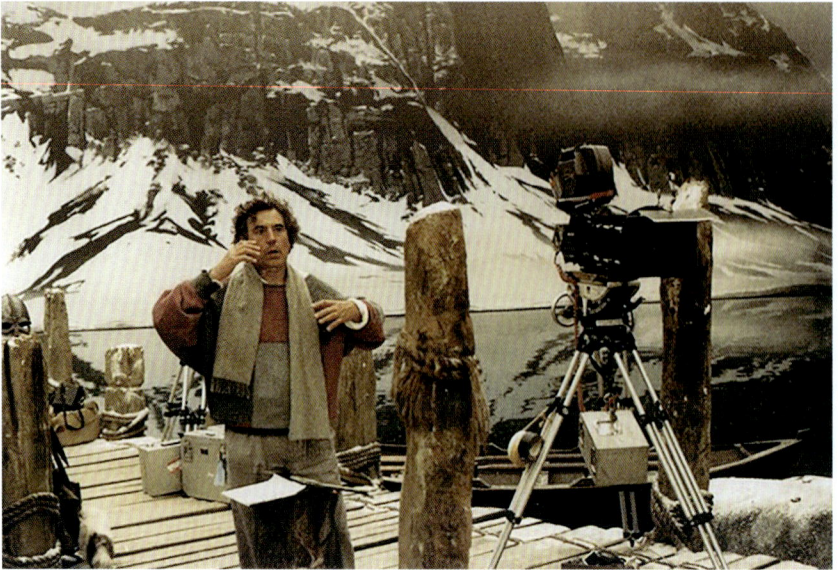

Terry Jones – Film Director, juggling every aspect of production and running a very happy ship, during location filming in Tromso, Norway, for *Erik the Viking*, in 1989.

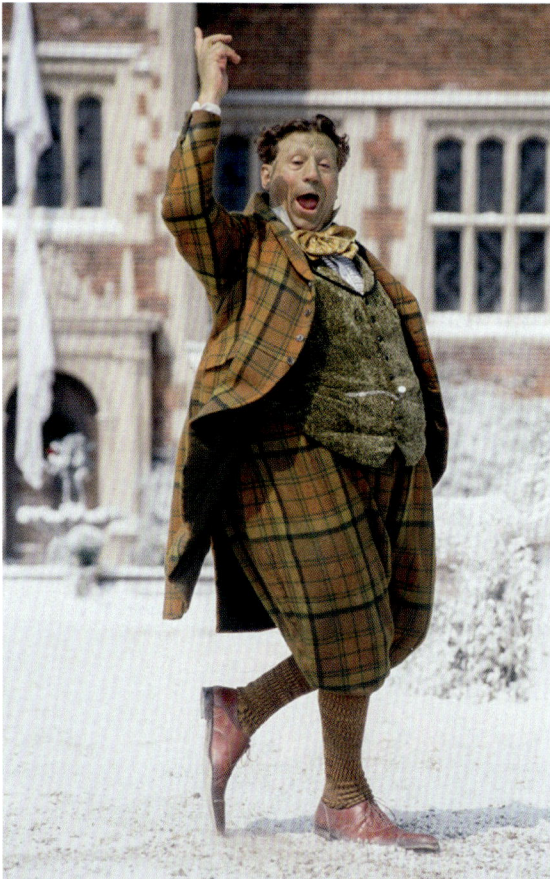

The part Terry was born to play, as Toad of Toad Hall, on location at Kentwell Hall, Long Melford, in Suffolk, for his production of *The Wind in the Willows*, 1996.

Having seen a local
Portuguese troupe
perform Python –
incomprehensibly to
him – Terry was back,
at the Sao Luis theatre
in Lisbon, in December
2007, to direct his comic
opera *Evil Machines*.

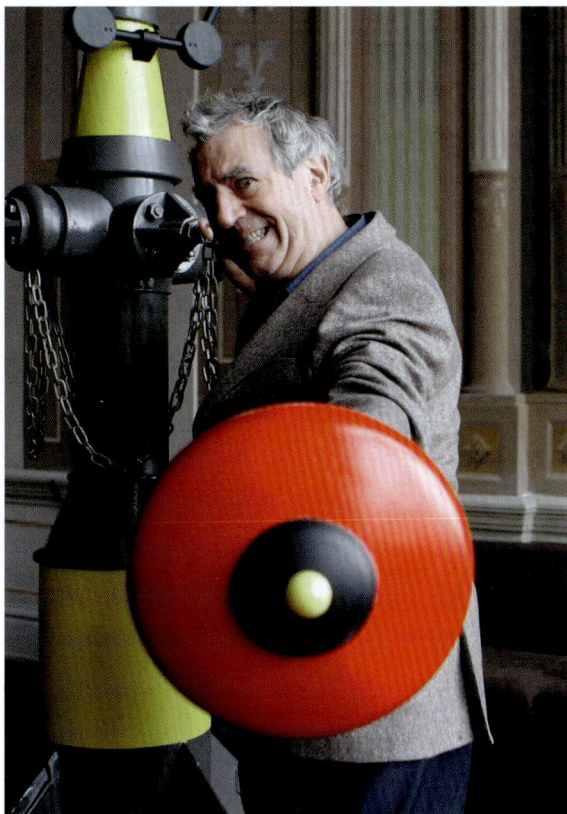

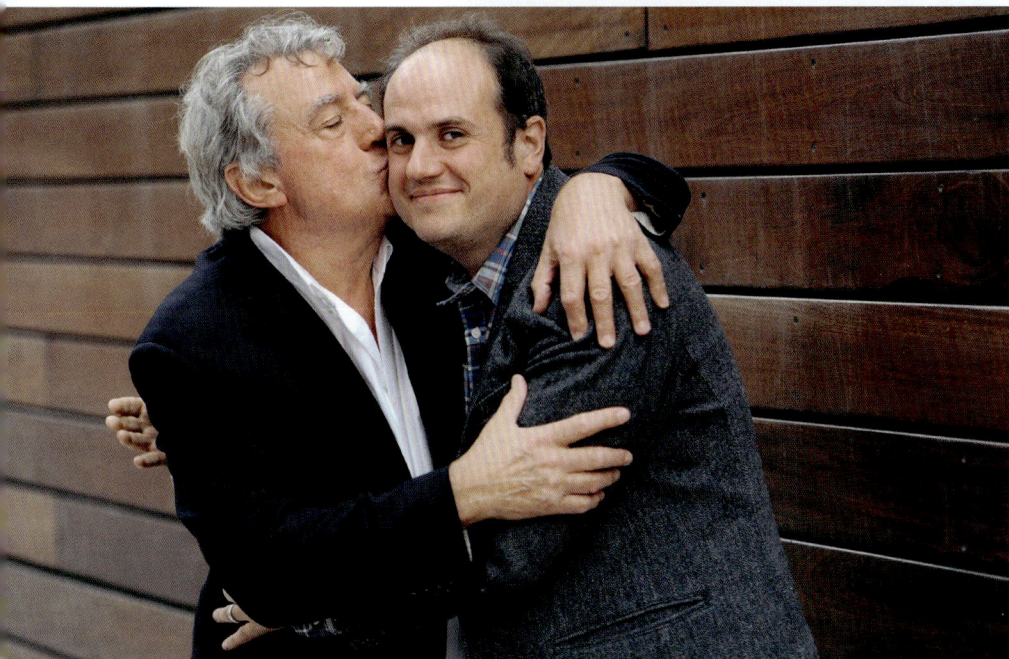

A loving moment between father and son when Terry and Bill Jones
promoted *A Liar's Autobiography: The Untrue Story of Monty Python's
Graham Chapman*, at the Toronto Film Festival, in September 2012.

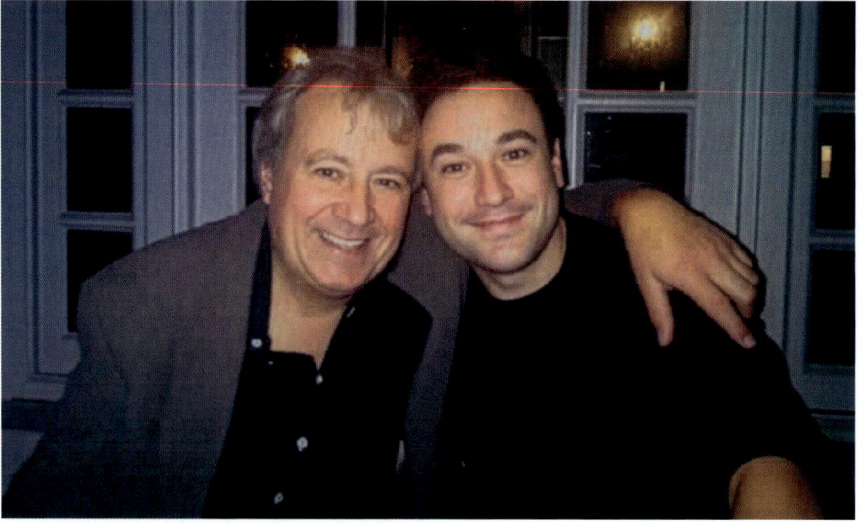

When Jones Met Jones: Terry enjoys an evening in the pub with Rufus Jones, who played him in *Holy Flying Circus*. Barry Cryer was getting them in at the bar of the Red Lion & Sun, Highgate, in 2011.

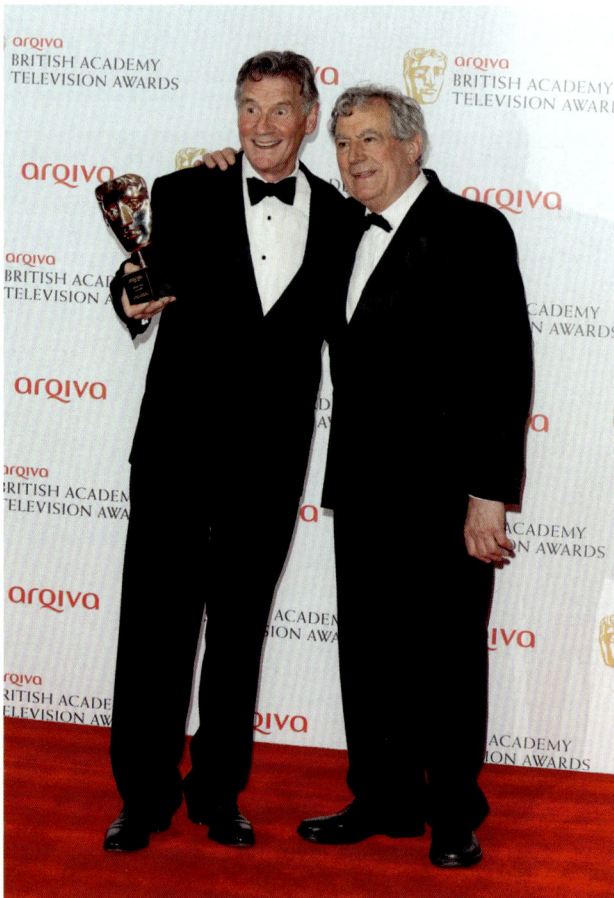

Michael Palin with his BAFTA Fellowship, presented to him by Terry at the Royal Festival Hall, on London's South Bank, on Sunday, 12 May 2013.

Still working the coconut gag after 40 years – Terry celebrates four decades of *Monty Python and the Holy Grail*, for the Tribeca Film Festival, at the Beacon Theatre, New York City, on Friday, 24 April 2015.

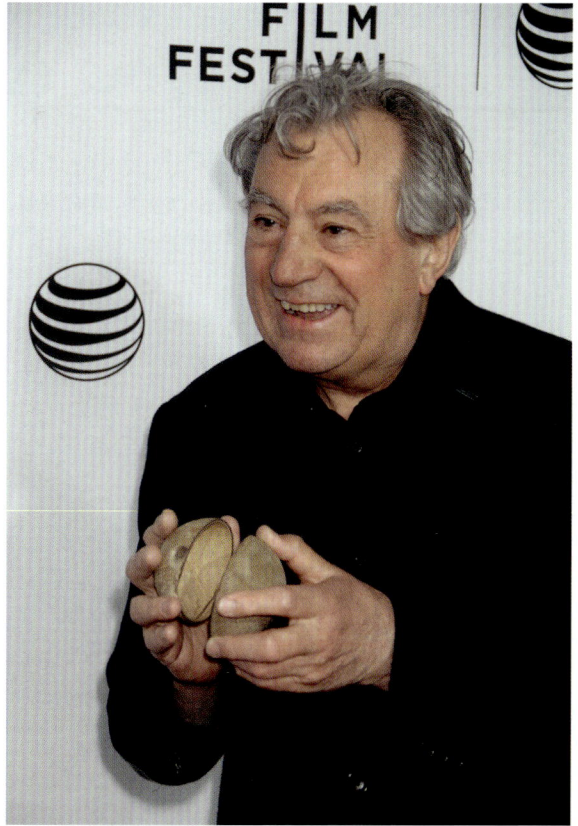

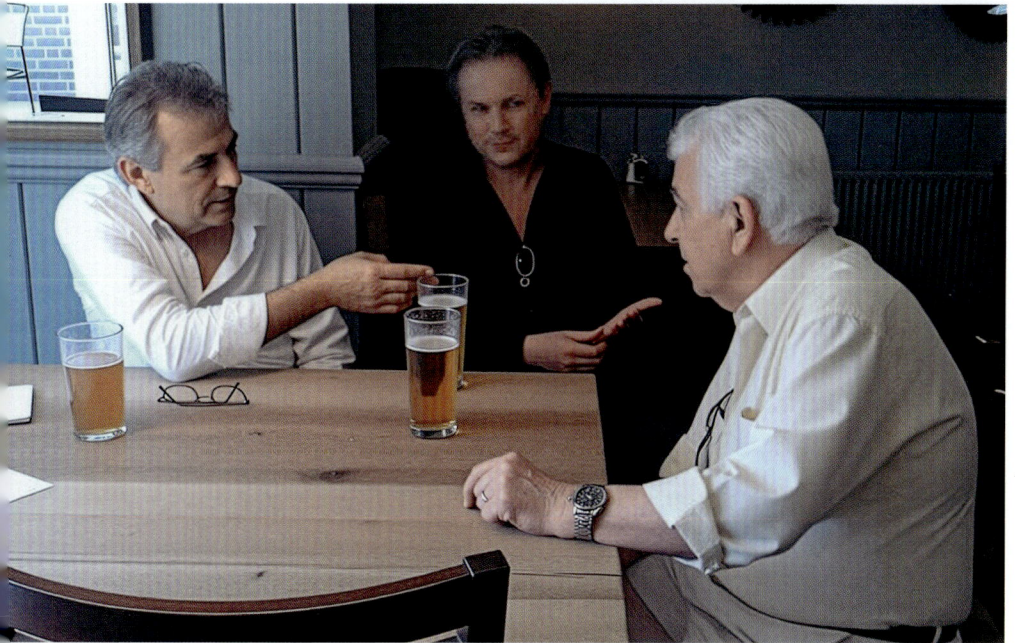

Terry and the author in deep conversation with Barry Cryer during a break in the filming of the promotional crowd-funding film for the *Forgotten Heroes of Comedy* book. Pints and puns at the Red Lion & Sun, Highgate, in July 2012.

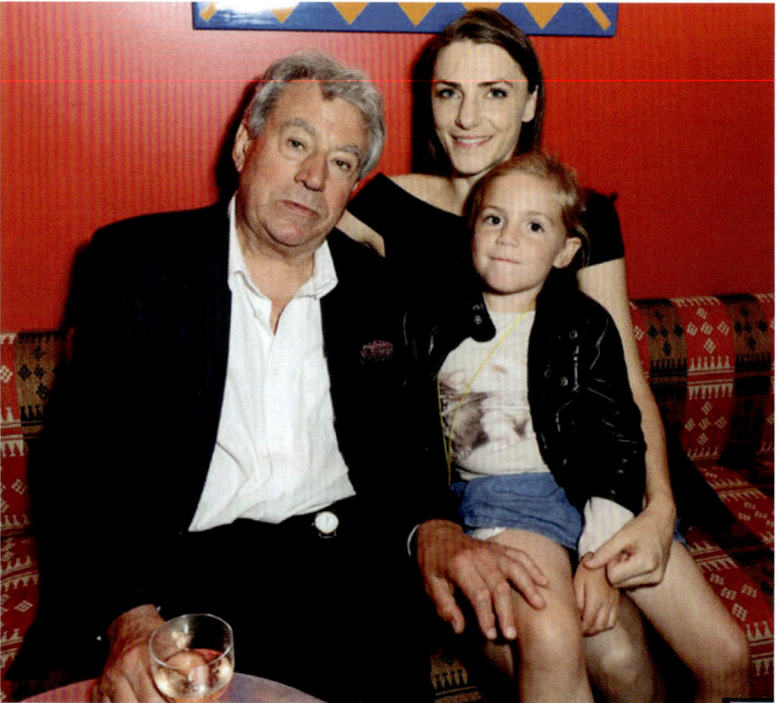

Dementia dulls Terry's expression but the twinkle remains, with wife Anna and their beloved child Siri.

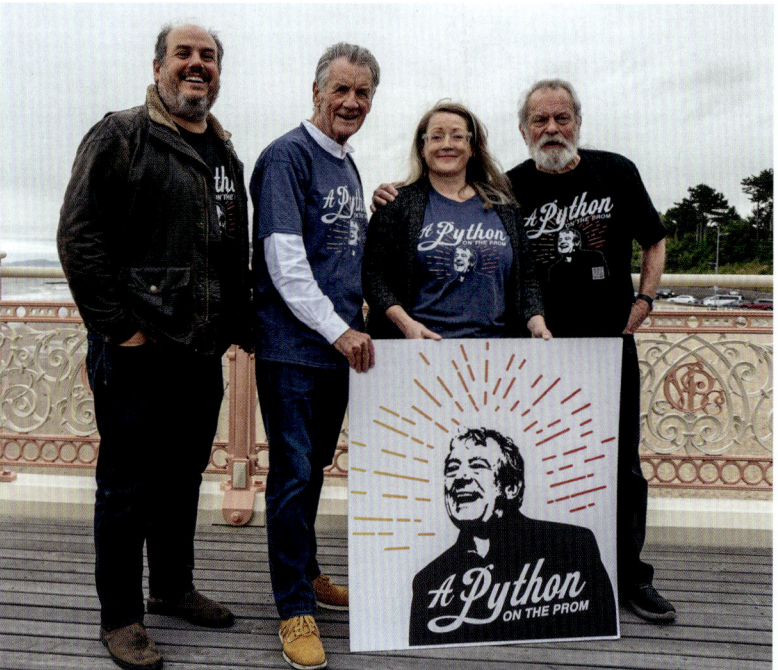

Back at Colwyn Bay. For good! Bill Jones, Sir Michael Palin, Sally Jones and Terry Gilliam launch 'A Python on the Prom', the statue appeal for Terry, on Thursday, 5 September 2024.

Cynthia had been on set and shared the most wonderful stories with Carolyn. All the crew loved her. Terry adored her. Carolyn recalls that, 'At that wrap party, Cynthia took me aside and said: "If you ever want to give up acting, come and be one of my girls. It's regular work. And honest! Unlike acting!" That was a great critique on my performance, I suppose, that she thought I looked the part so much that I could swap careers!'

There was certainly a lot of fuss made about Terry attending sex parties, which he never did, even for research, but he revelled in the controversy. One of his proudest boasts was that, of the four films banned in Northern Ireland, he had directed three of them: *Monty Python's Life of Brian*, *Monty Python's The Meaning of Life* and *Personal Services*. The other was Stanley Kubrick's *A Clockwork Orange*. Although a little apocryphal because the ban on Terry's films was ultimately lifted, and other directors' films were subsequently banned even though he continued to say it, it was a lovely, oft-repeated soundbite that proved Terry's sheer, child-like delight in his comic talent to shock. He would continue to battle censorship, adding his name to a petition in 1996 to support the cinema release of David Cronenberg's controversial thriller *Crash*.

For Carolyn Allen, it was Terry being 'amiable, friendly, and funny' that made *Personal Services* a favourite job: 'It's lovely. I'm very proud to be part of it.' And it was Graham Chapman's favourite Terry Jones film too. No flippant recommendation, considering it was Terry's direction that had brought out Graham's finest film performances. One can see what appealed to Graham in *Personal Services* though. This was his post-war London of illicit pleasures and loveable misfits.

For Terry's daughter, Sally, who had clinched Terry's decision to direct the film in the first place, there are: 'fond memories of Dad taking us into town on days when he was editing in Soho. He knew Soho so well. He would drive over to do some shopping. All these wonderfully exotic places like Algerian Coffee Stores, and the old

Italian businesses there. He wouldn't suffer fools though. I would see him getting cross with the street traders on the market, trying to palm him off with something that wasn't ripe!'

These Soho field trips would translate to packed lunches for Sally: 'when Mum was off to exotic places for conferences in July and August, and Dad was directing a film, it would fall to him to prepare my lunch for secondary school. I would open my plastic box and find fifteen sandwiches in it! I could feed the whole class. Dad did know how to cook and was domestic, he just didn't grasp the economy of scale!'

A dab hand in the kitchen, if not with a lunchbox, Terry was always at his happiest when he was working. Even if he was a hired hand on somebody else's film.

One such assignment was an episode of *The Young Indiana Jones Chronicles*, a TV series dreamt up by George Lucas off the back of the opening scene of *Indiana Jones and the Last Crusade* (1989), which had seen River Phoenix as the young archaeologist in a flashback scene before series star Harrison Ford takes over. The television series was conceived as 'edutainment' for ABC, with two series airing from March 1992. The instalment Terry worked on, 'Barcelona, May 1917', also gave him a nice little acting job, as the rather duplicitous Marcello. Gavin Scott wrote the episode, as well as playing a German spy, George Lucas was executive producer, and the dashing Sean Patrick Flanery was our heroic archaeologist. Despite the feature film-level locations and budgets, and the educational bit of 'edutainment' coming from Indy's encounters with historical figures, the series was only a muted success, and by 1994 the episodes had been sold to the Family Channel, who spliced together separate programmes to produce a makeshift feature. *The Adventures of Young Indiana Jones: Espionage Escapades*, coupled Terry's episode with a Robert Young-directed segment set in the Prague of 1917. Terry was blunt about the experience: 'it was a fun one, and a nice script by a friend. And a lovely location. It was an easy job between two films I really wanted to do.'

The first of those two films Terry really wanted to do had been *Erik the Viking*, released in September 1989, and very much inspired by his children's book *The Saga of Erik the Viking*. In fact, his old Oxford friend David Wood had originally been approached with the idea of turning the book into a stage play. Colin Webb, at Pavilion, invited David to lunch. They went to a nice restaurant and Colin said, 'I want to ask you if you would be interested in adapting Terry Jones's *Erik the Viking* as a Christmas show for the Lyric Hammersmith.' Colin was rather surprised when David said, 'No!' David loved the book but he explained 'that you either need to do it with great imagination, in a black box with just nothing – the studio at the Lyric, not the Main House – or you need to do it very, very big – a spectacular – which the Lyric Main House would be too small for.'

*Erik the Viking* certainly needed something spectacular, and if the stage couldn't do it justice then a feature film might. Certainly the book's illustrator, Michael Foreman, believed 'Terry wrote cinematically. During the course of a single sentence, Terry's viewing angle can change, zoom in, out, up, down, swing round to the rear and disappear into the far horizon. This makes his books great to read and difficult to illustrate!' Michael used to show Terry his single image for a whole section of his story and Terry would stare at it with a look that said disappointment, despair and disillusionment: 'He would always be kind, but deep down I know he wanted to turn all his stories into movies.'

And so it was with *The Saga of Erik the Viking*. In the film, as in the book, Erik would set sail in the *Golden Dragon* and discover the Edge of the World. Terry's cinematic retelling of the original tale – which, at one early point in pre-production, he considered making with the Muppets of Jim Henson's workshop – would retain all the visual epic sweep and adventure of the novel, although the tone of the film would be very different. With that wide canvas that the big screen gave Terry, these bullet points in the book became a much more realistic feature film with a galaxy of special effects, practical effects, artistic backdrops and international locations, allowing him to bring his story to vivid, visual life. The setting was more gritty; more realistic. It was the darkest of Dark Ages, centred on Erik's quest to use the Horn Resounding to awaken the gods and welcome a new era of peace and light. The comedy was told in much broader strokes, and the plot ventured into much more adult territory, allowing the Viking invaders to live up to their historical reputations and do all that raping and pillaging that struck terror into the hearts of all. Terry would have thought about all of this seriously, and indeed producer John Goldstone flagged up the problem. He also produced *Life of Brian*, and he assured Terry that such violence and death would work in a Python comedy but could detract from a film aimed at a family audience. Even while writing *The Saga of Erik the Viking*, Terry had remembered that the Monty Python series three sketch of Njorl's Saga had been rather dull. As were the Icelandic stories that had inspired it. Terry recalled that: 'they were all about families moving into different valleys and the murderous results of this relocation. I was much more interested in the monsters and the magic.' For the film of *Erik the Viking* he wanted to include both; his reasoning was that after all that raping and pillaging, any Viking at the heart of his film had to feel some sense of remorse and guilt at his murderous ways. Terry had written something similar for the last series of Python on television, but the idea had been dropped. Now, with the film, he could develop this interesting idea. A Viking who was sorry for his actions would be the ideal starting point for the plot of his film. The magic and monsters would all be part of the redemptive journey too, but that redemption needed an opening act of violence. That opening scene in *Erik the Viking* is harrowing indeed, and features Samantha Bond as

Helga the peasant girl, who is raped and dies. Her chilling fate is discussed with desperation and poignancy, while the script counterbalances the tragedy with sitcom-style dialogue. The confusion and regret was the catalyst to reveal the humanity of Erik the Viking, and spark off his need for an adventure of self-discovery. Terry would not compromise on this idea. And it would divide opinion on the film.

Some audiences wanted *Erik the Viking* to be a bit Python; others wanted it to be a bit historical, or a children's film in the spirit of the book that almost shared its name . . . and with that wonderful sweetness and innocence of his, Terry wanted it to be all of those things at once. A near-impossible juggling act with perhaps just too much ambition, just too many disparate ideas working against each other. Terry wanted it to have the spirit of the book, but with some cold, hard historical truths in it too. He wanted the film to be authentic, up to a point, and so these Vikings don't wear helmets with horns on. Still, it's a fantasy, and a comedy. As the poster screamed, it's 'a fun trip through the Dark Ages'. The darkness sits within the light. Uncomfortably, maybe, but that's life for you. Still, it is fact and fiction all sealed together with loads of jolly moonshine sprinkled all over it. *Erik the Viking* may jar at times, but there is plenty of Terry's trademark magic and sunshine.

This *is* a family adventure, with need for parental guidance. The 12 certificate from the British Board of Film Classification put it just about in its place. Even so, at the heart of it, the film represents the boundless enthusiasm and off-the-wall humour and playfulness of the man who made it.

Imogen Stubbs, sweet and sexy in equal measure as the sun-kissed Princess Aud, remembers Terry as someone who: 'just seemed to love you from the word go. He made you feel very special. He was a very wooing man in any case, but this amazing, surging, child-like energy just won me over. I had been offered something else, which was really quite serious, but doing a children's film appealed to me. In the end, I suppose it fell between two stools, because Terry seemed a little vulnerable, and a little naive in what he was doing. And excited to be doing it. Just this lovely, friendly quality. Terry made you feel like you were part of his family.'

An eight-week location shoot in Malta appealed to Imogen too: 'I had been doing wonderful ensemble television plays of Ayckbourn and Rattigan. It was very much like theatre. Then along came *Erik the Viking*. A fun, silly film. In Malta. I had been used to the rehearsal room in Acton!'

Not that Malta was at its best at the time: 'we were staying in the nicest hotel in the area but everything used salty water. You would have salty coffee at breakfast; awful food; and when we were falling off the edge of the world into the pit of hell, or whatever it was, these huge water jets were spraying us with sea water, full of sewage! Despite all that, it was absolutely great. Terry made it great. He was like a kid in a toy shop. And we felt the same. I had a Viking ship to play with! For Terry, directing a film just seemed to be party time. There was a great restaurant near the hotel, and Terry was a lovely host. He was such a brilliant and funny anecdote-teller. And brilliantly bonkers. The hotel had this round swimming pool. One evening, when nobody was in it, someone challenged Terry to try to run on the water! He did try to do this mad thing. He took a run at the pool and tried to run across it. Obviously, not being Jesus, it wasn't going to happen! Then everyone started trying to do it. It was that mad kind of fun we had. It is such a happy memory. Hysterically funny, and utterly wonderful.'

This crazy affection shines through the film, particularly in Imogen's innocently seductive performance: 'I felt quite young and intimidated. I too had been to Oxford, but I certainly didn't share that information with Terry. I pitifully kept quiet about that to everybody. I had played Sally Bowles on stage and done a few nice theatre things, but I don't think Terry had ever seen me in anything. And there I was. In Malta. With lots of very experienced people in the cast. I was playing the granddaughter of Eartha Kitt and Mickey Rooney. I'm also playing Terry's daughter, and Terry is kind of my father and my mother. It's all gloriously modern. And gloriously silly.'

While Imogen is naturalistic and coy and truthful, Terry allows himself to go gloriously camp, foppish and chew-the-scenery large at every opportunity. It works. His performance as the King of Hy-Brasil, the Celtic version of Atlantis, pulsates with hedonistic pleasure and a winning inability to see his flawed musical talents. Wallowing in Norse myth and injecting a Nero-like disregard for the inevitable collapse of his empire, Terry vanishes beneath the waves with an enthused and effervescent song bubbling on his lips. It was all very Pythonesque.

Certainly Tim Robbins, starring as Erik the Viking, came to the project with the intention of having fun in a Python film and being a serious method actor too. The silliness is at a peak in the scene when it's decided that all the beard-wearers should be sat on the opposite side of the boat to all the moustache-wearers. Tim's frustrated yell of: 'That doesn't matter!' is pure Python indeed. And it's funny, thanks to an early note from Terry: 'Tim came to the set with this English accent that was just odd. Not odd enough to be hilarious. Just odd. I told him just to play it with his own accent. It was an anachronistic film in any case, so an American Viking would fit in. And be funny!' It was similar to the advice that Terry had given on *Personal Services* to Danny Schiller, an actor employed again in *Erik the Viking*, as Snorri the Miserable.

It was quite the cast: Charles McKeown. Tim McInnerny. Jim Broadbent. 'John Gordon Sinclair was so funny,' remembers Imogen Stubbs, 'and lovely. Freddie Jones. All in silly beards and lots of hair, and being better paid than they had ever been. Freddie Jones did get a little naughty, when we were back in England, in the studio filming all the freezing cold land of ice. Freddie was a wonderful actor and he liked a drink. By four o'clock he was getting a little sleepy and a little thirsty so, in that booming, sensuous voice of his, he would shout out "It's a wrap!" so convincingly that all the crew would start packing up, and Terry would be wailing: "No, it's not! Stop it, Freddie . . . we've got another three scenes to shoot . . ." but even then, Terry would always keep his cool and never lose his temper. He was always good natured. I don't remember him being anything other than ebullient and delightful and fun. And did he wear the responsibility lightly. God, nobody was less authoritarian or presumptuous about the position he held. Terry was a man of such generosity of spirit. He appeared totally uncomplicated. A bubbling effervescence.'

It's this spirit of fun and adventure that radiates throughout *Erik the Viking*. Terry's totally free hand on the tiller is clear to see. As writer and director and actor it is his absolute prerogative to make the film he wanted to make. That light and shade, his sense of wonderment and adventure, and his understanding of dramatic tension and spinning tomfoolery is all in *Erik the Viking*. However, he was a little miffed, to put it mildly, that a rough cut of the film was released before his final, approved edit; that some later releases upped the certificate to viewers of the age of fifteen and over; and that some territories insisted on billing it as 'from the Monty Python team'. It's true, though, that the embodiment of both the lovely and the threatening essence of Python is there. Neil Innes, a source of eternal sunshine in any case, prances through the film with a wistful smile and a musical score of pure joy. While John Cleese, as Halfdan the Black, is the symbol of death and destruction at the blackest heart of the film.

For Imogen Stubbs: 'Neil Innes was an absolute delight. And John Cleese couldn't have been more supportive or nicer. People were always leaning out of cars driving round Malta and saying "Hey, you're John Cleese!" and John would go: "I know!"'

He was still John Cleese nearly a full decade later when Terry was dream-casting his own adaptation of Kenneth Grahame's 1908 publication *The Wind in the Willows*. This really would be very much more a family film, from a children's book lovingly channelled through Terry's playful but, yes, still dark imagination. The call to adapt *The Wind in the Willows* came in 1994. Terry was in Syria, filming *Crusades*, his history documentary for BBC Television. The caller had miscalculated the time difference and, for Terry, it was three o'clock in the morning. What's more, he was suffering from a severe case of the flu. Those unmitigated circumstances, along with the fact that Terry had never read the book, made him blurt out: 'Get lost!'

Anyway, having returned to Greenwich Mean Time, and actually now read the book, he realised that *The Wind in the Willows* was a brilliant allegory for the potential destruction of the countryside through human intervention, from the dawn of the Industrial Revolution and on through until the invention of the motor car. Within the magical pages of Grahame's writing, Terry found a kindred spirit. The passion of nature and a hint at a love letter to environmental issues, all wrapped up in a story for children, appealed to him greatly. This was the key to his interpretation of *The Wind in the Willows*. Terry's version would address Kenneth Grahame's fear, as expressed in his book written in the first decade of the twentieth century. Terry's film, coming at the very end of the twentieth century, had a satisfying sense of closure.

Typically of the British film industry, no sooner had Terry's interest in the project reached fever pitch than the original production company withdrew. Terry recalled that: 'because it was fifty years after the death of Kenneth Grahame the book was out of copyright. That meant there were up to six different film versions of *The Wind in the Willows* in pre-production at the time, including an adaptation of Alan Bennett's brilliant play, over at Paramount Pictures. There was something of a race on, and I seemed to have fallen at the first hurdle.' Enter the Canadian film producer Jake Eberts, who had heard Terry was interested in making the film. Eberts shared Terry's concern for the environment – at Goldcrest Films he had commissioned the animated feature of *Watership Down*. With Eberts behind this production of *The Wind in the Willows*, Terry was assured to be the first past the finishing post. With freedom to take the beloved characters of Mr Toad and Ratty and Mole and the rest, and do what he would with them with his usual glee, it was one of Terry's easiest and most rewarding writing processes.

Terry even wrote some of the original songs: '*Oh, the clever men at Oxford, Knows all there is to be knowed, But nobody knows as half as much as clever old Mr Toad!*'

Terry's screenplay and direction heightens the threat and danger presented in the book by the weasels, chief protagonists in the attack on the natural beauty of the countryside. In his mid-Nineties reworking, the weasels are very much 'Thatcher's children', so money-obsessed that they are keen to destroy even their own green and pleasant land in order to build a dog food factory. This is the environmental consciousness of Terry's short-lived *Vole* magazine within a children's film narrative, with the threatening, munching and crunching machinery a symbol for the greed of the age.

Cast as the Chief Weasel was that fine classical actor of immense presence Antony Sher, who had whispered and sneaked his way through *Erik the Viking*, as Loki. In *The Wind in the Willows* he gives a darkly witty, sarcastic and gloriously slapstick performance. He plays his villainy with richly broad strokes, and enjoys the film's blackest comic moment, with a grotesque musical number of dismembered limbs and ever-rising profits.

As the chief initiator and protector of the Monty Python group, Terry also wanted the best of his comedy colleagues in the cast. John Cleese gives a memorable cameo performance as a supercilious solicitor in court; while Michael Palin beams in a lovely burst of fun as the sun: 'Very nice. Lovely. I was done by nine a.m. Brilliant. Over the Moon, I was. Well, over the sun at least.' Terry Gilliam was to have given an equally powerful, force-of-nature performance, as the babbling voice of the river, but Terry Jones cut the scenes down to a gurgle before filming began. Eric Idle, however, was offered and grabbed one of the jolliest leading roles, as Ratty. It is the Water Rat, of course, who in Kenneth Grahame's story memorably says that: 'Believe me, my young friend, there is nothing – absolutely nothing – half so much worth doing as simply messing about in boats.'

There was an awful lot of Toad in Terry, and an awful lot of Terry in Toad. So it was obvious that Terry would have to, once again, cast himself, and direct himself, in the role. And, as befits the writer and the director, Terry gives himself an unforgettable entrance. The excited conversation between Ratty (Eric Idle) and Mole (Steve Coogan) builds up the importance of Mr Toad as a character long before we, the audience, meet him. When he does appear, it is at the very end of a long, sweeping panning shot across the luxurious grounds of Toad Hall. As the camera settles on an extreme close-up of a huge pile of newspapers, Terry's directorial reveal of his own Mr Toad character proves him to be perfectly pompous but playful: that long, sticky tongue darts out to entrap a snack-sized fly. In Terry's screenplay too there is a weighty and worthy comic battle between Toad and Ratty. Fought with sharpened tools of false modesty and false promises, this war of words between the two Pythons is the comic centre of the film.

There wasn't very much method in Terry's acting, just sheer, undiluted glee. Really just playing an extended version of himself, Terry indeed behaved very like Toad and had once owned an old steamer, which had been docked at Canary Wharf. He would mess about in his own boat, play his accordion, and encourage his dog Mitch to howl along to the tune. In the end, the boat sank. Very Terry; very Toad. All that was needed to turn Terry into Toad for the film was a skilful make-up job and let him rip. 'Actually, we had the devil's own job in getting the green of my skin right. It just didn't look green enough on camera. We got through two or three make-up ladies who had nervous breakdowns trying to get it right!' Terry told me.

They got it right. And Terry's performance is so magical, so much fun. His enthusiasm was palpable as he bounded around the location – Kentwell Hall in Suffolk – every inch the amphibious landed gentry. To the manor born. The role also allowed Terry to deploy his slapstick skill. Toad is a clown. A loveable fool. At one point he is in drag, disguised in order to escape from prison.

After fifty years those gymnasts' muscles were still supple, and Terry was very much up for doing his own stunts. At one point he does a backflip, while wearing a voluminous dress, over a wall at Dover Castle; and later into a vat of water. So good was he that Marc Boyle, the stunt coordinator on the film, gifted him the same cap and a jacket that his stunt team all wore, in recognition of having done so many of his own stunts. Boyle considered him to be deserving of the honour. As far as Terry's son, Bill Jones, is concerned: 'Dad was the English version of Tom Cruise!'

Terry's action-packed performance in *The Wind in the Willows* was complemented by a cast of quality thespians and comedy heavy hitters: Nicol Williamson brought a gentle authority to Badger, his Scottish brogue adding gravitas to his pearls of wisdom. While that youthful Steve Coogan – in between begging Terry and Eric to recreate Python sketches – gave a perfectly judged, fidgety and self-doubting quality to Mole. Terry would tell everyone that Steve was a great comedy actor, and would often compare him to his favourite screen comedy actors: Peter Sellers and Michael Palin. Praise indeed. Victoria Wood playing the prison Tea Lady who Mr Toad ties up and disguises himself as during his escape plan, Stephen Fry as the Judge and greasy car salesman Nigel Planer all gave their comic clout to the film. One that everybody involved loved making and was extremely proud of. None more so than Terry, who felt it was his most complete family film. One he hoped every subsequent generation would discover and enjoy.

The film received wide distribution in British cinemas from October 1996 but, already, unscrupulous film people were set to get their hands on it. The outcome for *The Wind in the Willows* in America would prove demoralising and annoying for Terry.

Although the book had previously been protected by copyright, Kenneth Grahame's cuddly characters had been the property of Walt Disney Productions since the 1949 animated feature *The Adventures of Ichabod and Mr Toad*, narrated in part by arch Hollywood baddie and definitive Sherlock Holmes Basil Rathbone. The characters had also inspired a favourite attraction at Disneyland: Mr Toad's Wild Ride. In order that Terry's film of *The Wind in the Willows* would not cause confusion, and in order to make a bit of money too, the – now rebranded – Walt Disney Company bought up the American distribution rights and released it straight to video, under the Disney-friendly title of *Mr Toad's Wild Ride*, as if it was nothing more than the movie of the theme park amusement ride. Terry didn't have a say in the matter. He threw a Toad-sized tantrum though. He also loathed the marketing of his film: 'I hated the poster Disney used. It was like a cartoon. Like that bloody Disneyland ride. My film was a classy piece of film-making. It really deserved a classy feel to the publicity. The people in charge clearly didn't know, or care, what they were doing.'

Columbia Pictures, who were handling the film in every other territory in the world, got wind, through the willows, of what Disney was planning. As a result, a court case decided that Disney had to give Columbia the right to screen the film in American theatres. By this stage, though, the home video of Terry's film had been released and few, on either side of the court case, were bothered. Apart from Terry, that is: 'Columbia did hurriedly release my film to a few cinemas in Los Angeles and a couple in New York. I was actually in New York, filming, at the time, and my producer rang me and excitedly said: "Hey, Terry. *The Wind in the Willows* is showing just round the block from where you are staying!" I couldn't quite believe it.'

The film was getting terrific reviews too, with a whole page in the *New York Times*. But it was all too little, too late, sadly. Terry rushed round to this tiny cinema in Times Square – the kind of place that showed sex films! But, sure enough, there was this little marquee, with funny, handwritten lettering. It just said: *Wind in the Willows*. No cast. Nothing. But it was Terry's film. Terry didn't have a camera with him, so he went off to buy an instant camera and take a photograph. However, by the time he got back to the cinema they'd taken the film off. He'd only been gone ten minutes!

Disappointed and beaten, Terry did get a little satisfaction at the fact that when audiences did see *The Wind in the Willows* they loved it. And it won a fair few awards at children's film festivals, in Chicago and Wisconsin. And Terry got a little misty-eyed when I told him that I saw the film at my local Odeon cinema, as part of a packed house, all of whom were clearly enjoying the film as much as I was. That time, I paid for a ticket, unlike the time I had sneaked in to see my first Terry Jones film at the cinema. At least I could see *The Wind in the Willows* legally at that point! That made Terry laugh. As he often said: 'I thought it was a really nice movie.' It still is, Terry. A rollicking film for all the family. A treasure for generations. Just like you wanted.

The battle-scars of fighting on behalf of *The Wind in the Willows* took a long time to heal, however. It would be nearly twenty years before Terry would direct another feature film. Which is something of a crying shame, for, like those other wonderful auteurs Michael Powell, Orson Welles and Ken Russell, Terry should have been given a government grant every two or three years to make whatever film he damned well chose to make.

Regardless, all those films that he did make will live on, imbued as they are with his utter joy in making them – a joy he seems, as the man in charge, the captain of the ship, to have been able to always communicate on set, no matter what the creative, time or budgetary challenges he was up against at various points.

Imogen Stubbs describes Terry's open-hearted enthusiasm as being unusual at the time. 'Everybody else in this business tried to be terribly cool and seemed to have this attitude that you should be so lucky to work with them. You got the impression you were being judged. The film world is full of dictators and narcissists. Terry was the complete opposite. He just rushed forward and gave me a big hug. He was delightful, and genuinely happy to be working with his actors. And he was fully aware that film is an absolute privilege. To be paid to have lots of fun and make something that, hopefully, an audience will glean a lot of fun from too. Simply put, being directed by Terry Jones spoiled me for every other film I have done since!'

While I was putting the finishing touches to the first draft of this affectionate memoir, on the Comedy Historian Facebook page I marked the anniversary of the birthday of George Harrison, beloved Beatle and without whom no *Life of Brian*. The photograph pictured George, standing with, to his right, Graham Chapman. To George's left, standing on his head, is Terry. A couple of much-missed Python pals larking about. One lovely comment, from social media follower David Farmbrough, celebrated 'three unique men': a great writer/actor (Graham); a great songwriter/guitarist (George, of course) and for Terry something beautiful: a 'great film director'. I can imagine his dreamy and appreciative smile now, as to be considered a great film director was one of his most treasured ambitions. That he achieved it, at least seven, well, six and a half, maybe six and three-quarter times over, in the forever bewildering and belligerent British film industry, is something to be amazed at and, yes, proud of.

# CHAPTER ELEVEN

## ALBATROSS? PYTHON REUNITED

*The one thing we all agreed on was that our chief aim was to be totally unpredictable and never to repeat ourselves. We wanted to be unquantifiable. The very fact that 'Pythonesque' is now an adjective in the* Oxford English Dictionary *means we failed utterly!*

So is *The Wind in the Willows* a Monty Python film? Well, no, obviously not. But is it a Python reunion film? Well, yes, kind of. And this was the blessing and the curse for Terry. The albatross round his neck, if you will. Terry valued and understood the lasting legacy of Python. He could somehow detach himself from the Pythons, look at it as an abstract entity; as a very good unit. The whole group together had a natural comedy chemistry. So, as director and instigator, it was Terry who worked hardest to get them all back together again – whether for the Python films proper or by casting his fellow Pythons in his own films.

In a practical sense, such was their comedy bond and working relationship of long standing and international appeal, that, when Terry wrote lines of dialogue for Michael or John or any of them, he not only knew exactly how they would deliver them but also that he could trust them, completely, to understand them. The Python sense of humour was Terry's sense of humour and, sometimes, it was only another Python who could fully grasp the idea that Terry had in his head. Moreover, not only would the integrity of Terry's screenplay be preserved, but the film set would be a fun one, of shared memories, shared jokes and shared comradeship. You only have to watch ten seconds of a scene with Terry and Eric in *The Wind in the Willows* to see that. Terry admired and respected his fellow Pythons, yes, but the verve and energy and sheer electricity that sparked to life when the Pythons assembled often gave him a much-needed fillip.

It seemed the public also needed the feel-good lift that the comedy of Monty Python provided. That initial burst of television episodes ignited a seemingly insatiable need for more Python, in whatever form that might take. Python had always had a very serious business head on its silly shoulders and the demand was lucrative to say the least. However far the six members might wish to drift or move on, reunions, reissues and recycling kept the brand potent; while funerals, feuds and financial meetings kept them in the papers. Every so often, with a sense of inevitability, they would be dragged back together again – yet another fascinating clash of the Python planets, rather like amicably separated parents meeting up once in a while to see how their grown-up children are getting on.

Few writers and performers would eschew the chance of success in order not to occasionally feel like a victim of it. Although, without getting out any small violins, it is possible to see how public demand to make more of something you know has realistically run its course could be frustrating, if everything you do subsequently is liable to be compared unfavourably with it. For example, every lazy journalist would bemoan the fact that *Erik the Viking* wasn't as funny as the Python films. Well, it wasn't a Python film. Terry Gilliam's *Brazil* had a chillingly nice Michael Palin; while *The Adventures of Baron Munchausen* had a bald-pate, speedy Eric Idle. Neither of those were Python films either.

Throughout the late Seventies, even as Terry and Mike were concocting *Ripping Yarns*, John Cleese and Connie Booth were running *Fawlty Towers*, Eric was playing with the Rutles, Terry G.

was making *Jabberwocky* and Graham was writing good film roles for himself to play, the Python nostalgia juggernaut continued. Classic sketches were repackaged for *The Monty Python Instant Record Collection* for Christmas 1977. With this, the Python branding embraced, even encouraged, its naysayers by blatantly admitting that this lavish greatest hits package was nothing more than a complete and utter rip-off. The fact was, of course, that the biggest rock acts, the Beatles and the Rolling Stones, had already issued several such greatest hits packages; and that the Python audience wanted a similar such handy compendium of their favourite group. However, the group mentality had been set in stone. The Pythons would always send up the regurgitation of old material; and the audience would laugh at the joke, and laugh as they re-bought. Brilliant comedy as bare-faced commerce.

As a group, since the early days they had taken on commercial ventures. For Michael Palin: 'it was always fun, and it was going to be paid work. We took on most things. We did a few ads, although neither Terry nor myself were particularly interested in commercials. It paid a lot of money. Politically we didn't feel right about doing it. It was exploitation of the workers.' As an antidote for directing adverts for Guinness, and Gibs Shampoo, and Harmony hairspray, and Bird's Eye frozen food, Terry also delivered *Who's There?*, an instructional short film about canvassing for the general election of 1970, on behalf of Harold Wilson's Labour Party. Deploying his talents to amuse to sell products or help the party was always a means to an end to support Terry's entrepreneurial ventures and his community spirit, embodied in *Vole* and the Penrhos Brewery. Terry would also counterbalance the corporate pound by readily performing vintage comedy sketches for Amnesty International concerts and other charitable events.

Resurrecting old Python material was also a means to an end. It brought in money, yes, but it also galvanised the audiences. It kept old fans happy and, it was hoped, attracted new fans. Although, following the success of *Monty Python's Life of Brian*, Terry was predictably keen to build on the repackaged legend and generate new Python material. Ideally, another feature film. However, films take a long time to put together and, first and foremost, there was the minor matter of recording one more album outstanding from the contract the group had signed with Charisma Records. Still, Python being Python, they managed to make a benefit out of a beholden promise. *Monty Python's Contractual Obligation Album* was recorded over lengthy sessions throughout January, February, March and April of 1980 and, while, as the title suggests, a lot of the material was rehashed sketches from previous comedies, dating back to the *I'm Sorry, I'll Read That Again* days, there was fresh material too, including a silly songbook of brand new numbers written by Terry.

Python sound engineer André Jacquemin remembers: 'everybody was very good and relaxed in the studio. It was fun, as always. And they all worked very hard on it. Terry more than most. Despite that very funny title, there was never a feeling that they were doing the record to get it done. Absolutely no feeling that they were just throwing it together. We recorded far too much material, actually. They all came with their individual bits. That was the only difference. It was less of a team effort, more individuals all working on the same album.'

This more individual approach, along with the vast number of sketches and songs recorded, gives the album a slight sense of the Beatles' mammoth 1968 release commonly known today as the *White Album*. The world awaits the full, double record, concept album from the Pythons. *The Shite Album*, perhaps.

The orchestral version of Terry's 'I'm So Worried' – a song listing things he purported to be concerned about, particularly the baggage retrieval system at Heathrow – was even recorded at Abbey Road. In his wisdom, Terry decided to actually sing it live 'with this bloody huge orchestra'. So they built a sound booth in the studio and Terry went in and started singing. They did a few takes but the time was running out and it was André who was getting worried. Then Terry wanted to do one more take. André explained to him: 'Terry, it's going to be a bit expensive . . .' But Terry was adamant: 'No, no, no, don't worry. We've got time to do it'. So they did. 'That cost us ten grand extra! Just because Terry was being passionate about wanting to do another take!' recalls André. 'Terry was really good to work with. And a lot of fun. And very appreciative. Although, at times, he would go off on a tangent because he had his typical Terry feeling that I have to do it this way . . . even if it would get him into trouble and cost us even more money!'

Terry was so enamoured of the 'I'm So Worried' song that he asked André to record several different versions of it. One was the country and western version: 'This was after we had blown a load of money at Abbey Road! Anyway, we did that version back at Redwood Studios [the studio André ran, largely funded by Terry, Michael Palin and various Python-related projects]. But Terry couldn't quite get it working properly. We had a few attempts at it and Terry stopped and said: "I just don't know what's wrong!" Then he had a lightbulb moment. Terry said: "Let me take my trousers down to see if that makes a difference!" So he undid his belt, and dropped his trousers down round his ankles. I had a load of my muso mates, and Terry Jones, in the studio, stood there in his underpants, singing his heart out on "I'm So Worried". And that's the version we used!'

So, dear reader, the next time you hear 'I'm So Worried', just imagine Terry singing in his underpants, with a studio full of musicians, fit to burst with laughter. Or why not ask your device to play it now. As André remembers: 'Terry was so chuffed with that. He finished the song, looked at me and said: "I knew that would work!"'

Any songs that required a certain kind of doom-laden weight would generally fall to Terry, with his semi-operatic kind of

Welsh booming voice, memorably on the deliberately dull 'Here Comes Another One'. He would often ad-lib in a recording session, changing lines as he went and wrong-footing the engineers. 'Here Comes Another One' just goes on and on and on, hilariously so, until he comes to a halt and then, after a moment's pause, goes on a bit longer.

There was an energetic relentlessness about Terry at all times. Particularly when the creative juices were flowing. André remembers him just making up the song 'Traffic Lights' on the spot. 'Terry said: "I've got an idea. Hang on . . ." I would be recording everything, all the time, anyway, just in case, but Terry just went into "I Like Traffic Lights . . ." and wouldn't stop! He wandered over to the piano and started plinking and plonking out this tune. Just making up this really funny, annoyingly unforgettable little song. Totally spontaneous. Organic. That's why I think there's this magic affection for what the Pythons did. Just off the cuff. It's a kind of magic comic genius.'

*Monty Python's Contractual Obligation Album* may have been made because it was just that – something they were obligated to do. And yet, perhaps because it forced the team to both delve into their back catalogue and focus their minds on new material, the sessions for the album seem to have energised the Pythons. They certainly energised Terry.

Over in America, a cult Python fandom had been growing since *Flying Circus* had first aired on PBS in 1972, particularly among students. This grew hugely in the slipstream of *Holy Grail* and *Life of Brian*, presenting the Pythons with the opportunity to put on a live show on a scale unimaginable in Britain at the time, and make rather a lot of cash doing it.

*Monty Python Live at the Hollywood Bowl* galvanised the student hysteria for the now-classic silly sketches and songs and indulged the group in rehashing and re-performing the tried and tested favourites they had been doing on stage since the early Seventies. Only this time the audience capacity was seventeen and a half thousand people. And at the four Python gigs, performed at the end of September 1980, the majority of that capacity audience were stoned. They still chanted along to all the familiar routines, though. Yet again, Terry did 'Nudge, Nudge' and 'The Lumberjack Song', not to mention the blueprint for Python, the Slapstick Lecture from his Oxford days. Terry, as the bashed, bruised and battered victim of the wooden plank, threw himself into this pivotal, pioneering sketch. It was placed right before the intermission, in order for him to shower and compose himself for the second half of the performance.

Despite the huge audiences and love for Python among a certain demographic, the rest of America were not always entirely clear on who or what this 'Monty Python' might be. The booker of one television chat show in Philadelphia thought that 'Monty Python' was one person. Various lopsided seats had to be dragged onto the set in order to get them all in shot. Terry ended up perching himself upon the knee of fellow guest, singer and *Starsky and Hutch* action hero David Soul.

Despite the success in America, Terry was never, not for one second, tempted to greedily embrace the strong dollar, even when they were getting amazing offers and the super-tax at home – at a peak of 90 pence in the pound – was less than super for those earning the big money: 'I love England too much to become a tax exile,' he explained. Terry supposed it all depended on just how interested you were in money. If he had gone off to Los Angeles and become a tax exile, he'd be cutting himself off from his roots. And Terry could never have done that. He was never particularly motivated by money and fame, for a start. And the beer was rubbish! His ambitions had always been centred around making things.

Safely back in England, Terry couldn't resist an opportunity to make something with his beloved old writing partner – though strictly speaking it was a filming of a thing from their past. *The Box* was a television adaptation, directed by Monkee Micky Dolenz, of the 'Buchanan's Finest Hour' play from *Their Finest Hours*, which Terry had written, with Michael Palin, for the stage and performed at the Sheffield Crucible five years earlier. This version was edited to a commercial television half-hour, with a large packing crate in shot and three dismembered voices: Charles McKeown, as disgraced Member of Parliament Sir Clive Buchanan, Terry as his assistant Harrington and Michael as a French escapologist, complete with dead and decomposing girlfriend.

The tongue-in-cheek commentary has Britishness at its heart – a parody of an advertising campaign on behalf of the strength and durability of British manufacturing. Terry would have revelled in this product of the old Jones and Palin writing partnership. It was further fuel on the fire that Python, and the separate Python factions, were still operational – another example of that inescapable law of comedy physics that would always bring the Pythons back together at some point or another. Although, the next full-fat Python project would see shifts in the writing dynamic.

Again it was Terry, the terrier, who went about chasing up the group to work together again. As with the previous film, *Life of Brian*, he reasoned that lovely weather might invigorate ideas. A writers' retreat to Jamaica was decided upon and Terry desperately tried to inspire a film project. Scraps of unconnected sketches – brilliant but incoherent – was the result. Michael Palin suggested that they all go home to England and write a fifth television series. Terry reflected, 'the old style of writing Python – me and Mike; John and Graham; Eric alone and Terry G. doing his animations in isolation and then just unleashing them upon us – was irretrievably gone.'

However, Terry persisted. Early one morning, he emerged into the sunshine with the revelation that all they needed was another twenty minutes of good material and they would have the film he so wanted to make. In length, at the very least. Terry thought that all the really good sketches could be linked together as a passage of time, someone's life story: 'we should have focused it all on just one person, to give the film that central narrative flow, but that is with the benefit of hindsight.' In the event, the sketches could and should relate to all of us. It was *Monty Python's The Meaning of Life*.

*The Meaning of Life* is a Python sketch film. There's no denying that. In many ways, it is a fitting closing bookend with *And Now for Something Completely Different*, the film that started their collective big screen career. By that rationale, in that they went back to a sketch format, many considered it a retrograde step, but, with Terry as the film's director and overseer of the final cut, *The Meaning of Life* is undoubtedly very much something completely different. It is all new material, for one thing. A collection of sketches with the confidence and freedom of comic expression that the BBC would never have allowed, together with the controversial and commercial clout that the success of *Life of Brian* had brought. *The Meaning of Life* is the most assured and mature of Terry's directorial work for Python. As a result, Terry was not only proud and protective of *Monty Python's The Meaning of Life* but genuinely believed that the film contained the very greatest of Python comedy: 'when I'm asked to pick out the sketches I consider as the best we ever did, I do tend to select one, two, three or four segments from *The Meaning of Life*.'

It's easy to understand why. There is such epic sweep and style to every foot of that film, from the startling Zulu battle scenes to its gloriously open and frank discussion of sex and its knowing and self-mocking pokes at religion and university education. The 'Every Sperm Is Sacred' sequence is an outstanding musical number that, because of the increased budget for the film, funded by Universal Studios, could be given the full film musical treatment. Terry was delighted that his vision could be achieved: 'we had the money. At last. I could really go for that Dickensian London feel, with loads of really talented singers and dancers, all choreographed by the brilliant Arlene Phillips.' Although Terry insisted that: 'it was never intended to be a parody of Lionel Bart and *Oliver!* It *is* Lionel Bart and *Oliver!* It's done with great affection. To compliment that musical, not take the piss out of it!'

With such a child-like understanding, Terry certainly found directing the young children easy. With the parents having read the script and the kids even knowing what the song was all about or, better still, not knowing what the song was all about, Terry just shot it: 'they weren't embarrassed at all. They were all brilliant. The only concession we made, to appease the parents and the nannies, was when Mike [Palin] had to talk about wearing a little rubber thing on the end of his cock. On the studio floor, I asked Mike to say, "on the end of my sock"! We dubbed in the cock later!'

Terry's masterstroke in the 'Sperm' musical number was in persuading Michael that the role of his wife should not be played by an actress but by Terry himself. As always, Terry knew the comedic power of him playing drag: 'Mike was convinced it would detract from the song! I twisted his arm. Probably the only time I ever insisted on any casting. I just knew I would be funnier. That's why I played the woman in Eric's "Galaxy Song" bit too. *That's* another favourite scene.'

The trust within the group mentality of Python was at play when Terry Gilliam baulked at the idea of playing Mr Creosote. Terry G. was convinced that Terry J. would be better at it. The arduous make-up job may have had something to do with it, as Terry J. remembered: 'I was in the make-up chair for three and a half days!' That scene was very much a team effort though. And that was very Terry: 'We were still working as a group. We would still chip in on other people's material. Mr Creosote was my idea, but it was John and Graham who came up with the wafer-thin mint and the scene's motivation for his exploding at the end.

When the Python team worked, it worked amazingly well. Far better than anything one of us as an individual could ever have done.' That explosive finale to the scene certainly remains the most unforgettable and certainly most gross-out, disgusting moment in the film, although Terry, as the director, had a problem to overcome: 'My main concern was making the vomit look authentic!'

In order to give the illusion that the sprays of sick were coming out of Terry's mouth, an elaborate tube was erected to the side of him. Although obscured from the camera, this tube cast a shadow on his face. Terry as director was not happy. So Terry as an actor had to suffer the discomfort of having the end of the tube actually in his mouth: 'I was covered in this stuff. A sort of mixture of vegetable soup and Russian salad dressing. It looked great! Then we catapulted thirty gallons of the stuff over the extras playing the other restaurant diners. We dressed them all up in cheap costumes!'

Terry was proud when audiences and critics would walk out of the cinema in disgust at the scene. Nearly a third of the 300-strong preview audience did just that. Terry and Universal saw it as a brilliant tagline. The blurb asked: 'Have you been grossed out yet?' That was the whole point. That image of Terry, vital organs exposed, dripping with blood and vomit, and still chewing, was *the* image of the film. For Michael Palin it is 'one of the best things Python and Terry in particular ever did. He takes this little idea and makes it into a Gothic extravaganza. It's the very essence of what Python should be.'

And, typically, a throwaway comment from Michael Palin was Terry's very favourite moment in the entire film: 'we were shooting the dinner party scene with the deadly salmon mousse and the Grim Reaper claiming his victims. Just as the ghosts were going out of the door, Mike's character suddenly says, "Hey, I didn't even eat the mousse!" He just threw it in on that take.'

Fitting then, that it is Michael Palin, still in drag, who ends the film. The Meaning of Life is revealed. It's all pretty simple really.

Just be nice to each other. Still, after an impassioned rant about the violent state of modern cinema, the revelation is the nostalgic embracing of the old television series. With a petulant 'oh well, here's the theme tune' those grainy old Gilliam animations flicker away on a tiny television screen as it drifts off and into the 'Galaxy Song' once more. It is such a final, knowing crystallising of a comedy collective's legacy that it's easy to overlook the fact that *Monty Python's The Meaning of Life* was in cinemas only a little over thirteen years since *Monty Python's Flying Circus* had first been broadcast. A comedy heartbeat, in the great scheme of things.

British reviews did tend to harp on the film being a tad old hat, just another load of Python sketches. Certainly, Terry got very aggrieved about it; for many years afterwards he would berate critics who have written that the Pythons were just trying to be too clever by being deliberately unoriginal. For Terry, though, *The Meaning of Life* was the perfect Python sketch film: 'That's what we set out to make. It was a challenge to make the film like the old sketch shows, but now we were totally in control. We were good at sketches and some of the best sketches we ever did are in that film, and still we got these niggly comments. I rose above it. Sort of! That's exactly why I put in the reference to the original series at the end.'

European and American responses were very much better. Indeed, Hollywood's very own Mr Creosote, Orson Welles, loved it. I'm sure Welles himself was absolutely stuffed when he sat on the panel of the 36th Cannes Film Festival when *Monty Python's The Meaning of Life* was awarded the Special Jury Prize.

The positive reactions were more than enough to keep Terry's nose to the Python grindstone. He was bubbling over with ways and means and cunning plans to get the Pythons back together again. For him, the sheer joy of doing Python again was irresistible.

To celebrate, Terry had bought himself a big fluffy coat for a fiver. It was like his student days again. This particular coat was a dark brown job, made entirely of nylon. It was voluminous, original and utterly cheerful. Alison Telfer remembers it well: 'Terry loved it and wore it often. One day we had been to the theatre, in the West End, with Sally and Bill. We came out and we were trying to cross at the Aldwych, which is always nightmarish. This particular day the cars just weren't stopping. Terry suddenly curled himself up into a ball and rolled across the zebra crossing. In this furry coat! The cars stopped. Well you would, wouldn't you!'

However, others within the Python collective were simply and exclusively interested in their individual pursuits. A return to a somewhat fractured and fragmented team did not appeal to them. They were all very keen to take the Python pound though, and Terry was at the forefront of this as well. He had always been a kind of Indiana Terry Jones, Raider of the Lost Archives, in any case, instrumental in salvaging and curating and promoting the Python vault. It had been Terry who, eager to catalogue exactly what the BBC held in the way of Python episodes, had located a pile of film cans, sat on a shelf destined to be demagnetised – in other words, wiped clean to be used to record other programmes. Without Terry's efforts to find and preserve these tapes, great swathes of original Python on television would have been lost for ever.

With *Monty Python's The Meaning of Life* in cinemas, the BBC were being asked left, right and centre for vintage clips of the group. Even at that stage, no one at the corporation seemed to know, or indeed care, which Python had written which Python sketch. Through legal battles with everybody from American television channels to unscrupulous film producers, the Pythons, by and large, stood shoulder to shoulder to protect their legacy. And their financial interests.

Certainly, as the twentieth anniversary was fast approaching, all the Pythons were eager to capitalise on the landmark. And, as ever, very amused and happy to be depicted as greedy bastards while doing it! Virgin Records released *The Final Rip Off* compilation album in 1987. *Monty Python Sings*, which would quickly become the team's best-selling album, had been planned as the spearhead for twenty years of Python in 1989. It was released that December, a little over a month since the bitterest of blows to the group.

Graham Chapman had been diagnosed with throat cancer in 1988. As a qualified doctor, he was well aware that the outlook was not good but, for the group, and for his own joy of living, he reassured everybody that he was absolutely fine. None more so than his fellow Pythons, all set to celebrate the twentieth anniversary. And for the television compilation show *Parrot Sketch Not Included*, introduced by American comic Steve Martin, it was decided that the occasion warranted something very special indeed. On 3 September 1989 they filmed a brand new sketch with the Pythons dressed as schoolboys – all except Terry, of course, who was a schoolgirl. It was not written by any of the Pythons and Graham – visibly very ill by this point – was noticeably under par in his performance. In the end, as was in their powers, the Pythons vetoed the sketch. Terry was relieved that the group, as a whole, had decided not to include it: 'Poor Graham really didn't look well at all, and it was the first time Python had performed a sketch that none of us had written. Hardly the best way to celebrate something that meant a lot to all of us.' Instead, the show concluded with the six Pythons crouched within a large cupboard. Steve Martin poses the question, 'Where are they now?', opens the cupboard and shuts it with a 'Sad, isn't it?' The lone voice of Michael Palin nicely calls out, begging for the cupboard door to be reopened, so the fans can see them together again. This goes unheeded. The single, bitter word: 'Bastard!' caps the most perfect final moment any of them could have written.

Graham died, at the age of just forty-eight, on 4 October 1989, a month after the filming day and just one day before the official twentieth anniversary of Monty Python. In a comment to the press Terry called it 'the worst case of party-pooping ever'. In private reflection, of course, he was devastated: 'You never felt you got to know Graham. Not completely. He was always brilliantly in a world of his own, but he had been part of my world for a very long time. I had gone to visit him in the hospital in Maidstone, but arrived just after Graham had died. I missed saying a proper "goodbye" to him. We all still miss him terribly.'

Terry had always thought another Python film was a possibility, even though, 'if it was to have happened, it would have been in a different way in any case. I might have written something and said to Mike and the others, "This would be really good for the whole team, wouldn't it?"' In the aftermath of Graham's death, the idea of a brand new Python project was redundant. Python was a team of six. Without one element, the comedy equation would simply not add up. Terry 'certainly wouldn't have sat down in a Python group meeting and said: "Right, let's write something especially tailor-made for the Pythons. Let's initiate a new Python film."'

But even as the remaining five mourned the loss of their comrade, the Python franchise continued. From the BBC *Omnibus* documentary *Life of Python*, broadcast to mark the show's twenty-first anniversary, in 1990, to the nearly six-hour miniseries *Monty Python: Almost the Truth (The Lawyer's Cut)*, for the fortieth, chatting with director Alan G. Parker over a two-day Python reminisce, in 2009, Terry remained serenely benevolent about the history of Python and the Python legacy. He would repeat and remould familiar anecdotes for every interviewer. Never complacent though, but always with that twinkle of glee. Always with a sense of pride in a comedy bag of tricks that still held the world bewitched. Terry would be actively funny too. Hands-on funny. Danny Scheinmann, as frantic lawyer Abe Appenheimer, was on hand to absolutely make sure that the film-makers would have no legal come-back on the contents of the documentary. The legal eagle would be bombarded and blown up but he would go through anything in order to cover the show by branding the film with a 'The Lawyer's Cut' stamp. That 'get-out-of-jail' card had been Terry's idea. He insisted upon it. And it cost an absolute fortune. Terry, eagerly claiming the right to record the introductory voice-over himself, was happy to be funny with other people's money until the very end.

While allowing for such flashes of brand new Python comedy, these retrospectives could also include Graham in archival contributions. They were still a six-man-strong team. And, of course, every Python anniversary also had to resurrect Graham's finest performance, in *Monty Python's Life of Brian*. As Terry was the director, he was invariably asked to introduce screenings and put the film in context. He did this all over the world. Including at the Bristol Slapstick Festival. And in Aberystwyth. Sue Jones-Davies, who played Judith in the film and subsequently became mayor of the Welsh town, personally lifted the ban on *Brian* just ahead of the film's thirtieth anniversary. Terry was on hand for that very first showing. Colin Webb, too, called on his friend to support the Little Theatre, a small independent cinema, in Bath: 'Terry was delighted to come along and talk to the audience. Understandably, once the film started running he and I went out for some dinner. He had seen it so many times!'

The Python parade just kept on going. There had been *The Ultimate Monty Python Rip Off*, on CD, and video games based upon *The Holy Grail* and *The Meaning of Life*. When the first, double-disc DVD release for *The Meaning of Life* was issued in 2003, it generated a reunion of the Pythons. Of sorts. All five of them were dropped into a virtual chat room, sharing anecdotes, as they were beamed in from video links from different parts of the world. That Special Edition release of *Monty Python's The Meaning of Life* was even promoted by a small, in-store, cut-out Mr Creosote, on a bouncy spring. Terry, in all his gross-out glory, was still symbolising the film for this advertising gimmick. Three years later, in 2006, Terry would even recreate his role of Mr Creosote for an uncredited cameo in the film *Stranger Than Fiction*, directed by Marc Forster, written by Zach Helm, and starring Will Ferrell as Internal Revenue Service auditor Harold Crick, whose bland reality is invaded by fictional characters.

Thoughts ahead of the thirtieth anniversary of Python in 1999 had seen the group get together in 1997 for a meeting that engendered all sorts of possible ways in which to mark the event: from a new feature film to an international stage tour. In the end, on 7 March 1998 the five surviving Pythons were interviewed on stage at the Wheeler Opera House, Colorado, by American stand-up comedian Robert Klein, as part of the US Comedy Arts Festival. Broadcast as *Monty Python Live at Aspen*, it reiterated the impact that Python had had and was still having on comedy. Eddie Izzard was invited to 'gatecrash' the proceedings before being swiftly evicted from the stage. This was real, living comedy history. It was the first time the troupe had performed live on stage since the Hollywood Bowl shows in 1980. And Graham was at Aspen too. Well, an urn supposedly containing his ashes was on stage throughout, before the lid was removed and Graham's mortal remains spilled forth! They would do the ashes gag once more for a funeral-based reunion photo shoot, with Terry in a skirt and slippers once more, and in a coffin, decidedly cheerful about facing the aftermath, thanks to a bikini-clad Cameron Diaz being interred alongside him.

In October 1999, the actual thirtieth anniversary was marked by *Python Night* on BBC Television, a whole evening of Python-related programming: documentaries and travelogues and retrospectives but with the added bonus of brand new sketches interwoven throughout. Graham, once again, was represented in vintage material, while the two Terrys, Michael, John, Carol Cleveland and a little bit of Eric Idle, linked in from his home in

America, did Python, thirty years on. For Terry, this involved everything from donning a knotted handkerchief to play one of the moronic Gumbies (alongside Eddie Izzard again as a guest Python) to wearing sensible female clothing of tweed and brogues as a shrieking pepper-pot. Terry opened *Python Night* with an outrageous resurrection of tasteless variety theatre turn Ken Ewing, with his Musical Mice – those poor music hall rodents who squeak, in tune, every time Terry whacks them with mallets!

The year saw the closure of the Museum of the Moving Image, the British Film Institute cinema collection, which had Python all over it. That giant foot was with you every step of the way, gradually getting more and more calloused as you made your way through. As one door closes another opens, though, and Terry had directed John Cleese in a seven-minute film to introduce and explain the BFI London Imax Cinema. Also in 1999 Terry, along with the other survivors, had been asked by Python publisher Methuen to pick his favourite Python sketches for the first volume of *A Pocketful of Python*. There were, unsurprisingly, five to collect, with Terry's featuring him on the front cover as the Nude Organist. Terry also wrote the cheeky preface for the selection made by Eric Idle. It certainly put paid to Terry's thought, due to Eric's necessarily limited input into *Python Night*, 'that we have all pissed Eric off!'

With *Spamalot* still doing big business in London and New York, Eric also wrote and presented *Not the Messiah (He's a Very Naughty Boy)*, a comic oratorio based upon *Monty Python's Life of Brian*. Described by Eric as 'baroque 'n' roll', the show premiered in Toronto, before playing in New York, Brisbane and in London at the Royal Albert Hall. The London gig was recorded and attracted an almost full cast of Pythons on stage, with Michael Palin resurrecting his speech-impaired Pontius Pilate; Terry Gilliam as the individual who says 'I'm not!' when assured that everyone is an individual; and Terry as a hard-hatted, choral-singing Welsh miner. No less wonderful was Terry's vocal performance as Graham's mum in the abstract and absurdist animated biopic *A Liar's Autobiography: The Untrue Story of Monty Python's Graham Chapman*. Terry couldn't help getting into drag – even if it was audio only. Based on previously unreleased tapes of Graham reading his memoirs, this was the new Monty Python film that Terry had wished for. Michael Palin added his vocal talent to the mix, as Graham's father, while Terry G. was the psychiatrist and John was David Frost. How very meta. Eric dropped in a little something limited too. And Cameron Diaz was back with the team, as Sigmund Freud!

For, you see, for all the aborted attempts at reuniting Python the group, in one permutation or other they were forever getting up and giving the people a little bit of joyful irreverence. George Harrison, who had long maintained that 'the only thing worth getting out of bed for is Monty Python', saw his devotion to the team and his entrepreneurial saving of *Life of Brian* commemorated in the *Concert for George*, staged in 2002, a year after his death. The Pythons performed 'The Lumberjack Song', beside guest Python Tom Hanks. The team of Neil Innes, Eric Idle and the two Terrys also sang the barber shop quartet rendition of 'Sit On My Face': all, dutifully, exposed their naked bottoms at the end. For George.

The major Python reunion would come in 2014 though, when the full team – complete with Graham on screen – would take the O2 in London. The nightly guest list of contemporary comedy greats was incredible, each eagerly lining up to pay homage to the Pythons. Having guested with them twice already, Eddie Izzard was one, and he also saw the majority of the ten shows as an audience member.

The O2 reunion shows were a monumental comedy event. For all the pomp and circumstance and sheer excitement, it was a financial necessity too. After all those years of sending up the reissues and repackaging as a commercial rip-off, this time they really did need the money.

With the huge box office success of *Spamalot*, a legal case was instigated by Mark Forstater, who had been one of the producers on *Monty Python and the Holy Grail*, the film on which the stage spectacular had been based. Terry joined Michael and Eric to testify in the five-day-long High Court reading in which Forstater was claiming £250,000 in lost earnings as 'the seventh Python'. The six Pythons lost the case in July 2013.

As a practical and swift way to replace the coins in the Python coffers, the group agreed to the reunion show. Eric would direct this full Python reunion, with Graham on film.

The Python residency at the O2 was split into two chunks of five performances each, with the ten sold-out gigs attracting a total crowd of nearly a quarter of a million people. You can buy an awful lot of Spam with that kind of takings. Plus there was the worldwide audience who paid to see the final show – the absolutely planned, last of Python – relayed, live, in cinemas, on 20 July 2014. *Monty Python's Total Rubbish*, a vinyl and CD box set of all the albums, was released ahead of the O2 shows too. Along with a glut of collectibles, too humorous to mention!

For Terry, resurrecting the classic Python sketches in between West End-sized musical numbers allowed him to perform – one final time – 'Nudge, Nudge' and 'The Lumberjack Song'. The O2 shows ended with a clear farewell: Monty Python 1969–2014 writ large on big screens, but even that wasn't the end. Despite the reluctance of some members of the team to tour the live show around the globe – including, ironically, that master globetrotter Michael Palin – the renewed interest and unquestioned love for Python had inspired Terry to return to film directing. It was the first time since *The Wind in the Willows* . . . and it would be the last time.

Terry had had the idea on his desk for years. *Absolutely Anything,* a modern reworking of the late-Victorian short story by H.G. Wells, 'The Man Who Could Work Miracles'. It also had more than a tinge of *The Good Person of Setzuan* in which Terry had played one of the gods, in Oxford. *Absolutely Anything* was written with his *Blazing Dragons* chum Gavin Scott. The Wells story concerns pub bore George McWhirter Fotheringay, who continually denies the possibility of miracles. As if to prove how wrong he is, a group of celestial beings single him out to give him the gift. He becomes the man who can work miracles. In Terry's version it is school-teacher Neil Clarke who is given all the power.

Like most feature films, *Absolutely Anything* had a torturous pre-production history. Terry was always quite candid about the battles for funding and the shifting sands in casting. Bill and Ben Productions – that's Terry's son, Bill, and his business partner, Ben Timlett – were the producers. Having been behind the *Almost the Truth* documentary and the Graham Chapman animation, Bill and Ben Productions secured the money for Terry to shoot the film in six weeks across April and May 2014.

In the preceding years, Terry had discussed and dissected the screenplay, of which he was very proud. American financing was set to be secured with the central casting of John Oliver, from *The Daily Show*. His attachment had been hinted at in the autumn of 2010, but, by the time the production was set to roll, he had become unavailable. Hugh Laurie, a hit in the States at the time as grumpy medic House, was in the frame too. Finally, and winningly, it was the man who could work miracles for Generation X, Simon Pegg, who secured the role. Pegg, the Nerd who did very Well, was at the time concurrently chalking up roles in the *Star Trek* and *Mission Impossible* series.

The object of Pegg's character's impossible mission in *Absolutely Anything* is Kate Beckinsale, playing his hot and happy next-door neighbour Catherine West (Kate's equally glamorous mother, Judy Loe, had played the dashed attractive Chief Petty Officer

Russell in the *Ripping Yarns* episode 'The Curse of the Claw'). Terry peppered the supporting cast of *Absolutely Anything* with the cream of comedy. His friend of long standing, Sanjeev Bhaskar, who had been a guest Mountie for 'The Lumberjack Song' at the *Concert for George*, and one of the many King Arthurs in the West End run of *Spamalot*, was cast as Ray, the best friend, while long-time Python aficionado Eddie Izzard played the no-nonsense headmaster Mr Robinson. Terry was most delighted with the stoic and straight-faced performance of Rob Riggle, real-life US marine and stand-up comedian, playing the bullish Colonel Grant Kotchev.

*Absolutely Anything* would mark the final screen credit of Robin Williams. Terry had renewed his friendship with Robin as far back as 2009, when the *Almost the Truth* documentary was nominated for two 'Outstanding Nonfiction' Emmy awards. Terry found himself sitting behind Robin in the auditorium of the NOKIA Theatre in Los Angeles, for the ceremony. Terry, as enthused and forthright as ever, explained the premise of his new film, *Absolutely Anything*, and offered Robin the voice-over role of Dennis the Dog, our hapless hero's hound who gets the power of speech. Robin agreed on the spot. Terry followed up by sending over the script, to which Robin emailed back immediately: 'Let's get this film made now!' Of course, the film industry being the way the film industry is, the mill grinds slowly . . .

By the time the cameras were rolling in 2014, Terry had the real dog, Mojo, performing visual wonders before his very eyes, but still hoped against hope that Robin would be willing and, most importantly, available to provide the vocal talent. Of course he was. He was dedicated to the project and Terry was thrilled that Robin was still keen to do it. He later told me about Robin's intricate perfectionism: 'The first time we tried to voice Dennis, it was a Skype call with an interminable delay. Robin was not satisfied with the result. He kept on saying: "I don't mind if you get someone else to voice it." But we couldn't do that. Eventually Bill and I went over to San Francisco to re-record Robin. And he still wasn't satisfied. A couple of hours after the recording, he rang me on my mobile and said: "I just had an inspiration! Dennis is a 16-year-old boy!"' It was third time lucky, with Terry back in London, and Robin, at home, channelling his overeager, oversexed teenage self into the canine star of the film. It was his hilarious, inspired and joyful cinematic swansong. For Terry, 'what I remember about Robin was his humility. He could be funny as no one else could be funny – like he had another monumental voice telling him to be funny – let it rip!' And he certainly let it rip for *Absolutely Anything*. Terry even gave Robin the killer last line, although it was a line consciously and unapologetically borrowed from another comedy film. One of the greatest comedy films of all time.

Terry and I were sitting in the pub one evening, discussing the script and the latest obstacle in a seemingly endless course of obstacles in the way of the production. Terry suddenly blurted out that he was so keen to make the film. Desperate, in fact. 'We have the greatest closing line,' he said. I, having not read the script but knowing my comedy film history, gasped: 'Great! Just like "Nobody's perfect!"' Terry stopped in his tracks and put down his pint:

'I've not sent you the script yet, have I?'

'No, why?'

'Well, that's it. That's the last line!'

'What, Nobody's perfect?'

'Yes!'

'Nobody's perfect? from Billy Wilder's *Some Like It Hot*? As said by Joe E. Brown? That Nobody's perfect?'

'Yes. Nobody's perfect is the last line of our film too!'

'Oh, right! OK!'

It was one of those moments that, if it had been almost anybody else in this cockamamie business, I would have turned a fetching shade of bright pink and clammed up. Terry, being the lovely bloke he was, just put his hand over mine, smiled and said: 'That's good, Rob. That's good. It's a line they'll remember. You've remembered it already!'

This innocence at incorporating such a very famous film quote was an indication of the playful joy Terry was taking in the pre-production of the film. Still frustrating, but fun. It may well have been his final feature film as a director, but he was as eager and hands-on as ever he had been. Bill Jones recalls that: 'we were looking for a bus for the scene when the Simon Pegg character gets zapped into the engine compartment of a double decker. Dad went on the recce to look over this bus and they opened it up and pondered whether anyone could fit in there. Without a moment's hesitation Dad said: "Well, let's find out!" and he climbed up and got in. It seems you *can* fit a person in with a bus engine. Our friend Ken Tuohy, who was a co-producer, said: "I've never seen a film director do that before!"'

Terry was also very happy to be physically manhandled while casting for the film's heavies. In one scene, a policeman has to hoist Simon Pegg up off his feet. As a test to see if the actors in line for the role had the strength for the scene, Terry happily asked each and every one of them to lift him up. Bill remembers: 'It was James Kermack who got the job and, to this day, delights in telling everybody about his unusual audition but, in fact, Dad spent all morning being roughly lifted up, in order to get the right actor. He was happy to be lifted here, there and everywhere for the good of the film!'

Not only is *Absolutely Anything* a fabulous comedy film, but it has Terry's final directorial flourish. Unsurprisingly, he gave himself an Alfred Hitchcock-style cameo – as a sour-faced cab driver forced to have an orgasm while driving. Our man with the miracles tells him to go fuck himself – and he does! But, you see, in this twenty-first century twist on H.G. Wells it isn't playful gods that bestow the power, it's aliens, and who better to provide the voices for the aliens but Monty Python.

With rehearsals for the O2 reunion shows hotting up, *Absolutely Anything* proved to be the first film since *Monty Python's The Meaning of Life* to feature every surviving member of the team. And, under the direction of Terry Jones, *Absolutely Anything* can, just, be cited as the last Monty Python film. Certainly the casting of Terry as the Scientist; John as the Chief Alien; Terry G. as the Nasty Alien; Eric as Salubrious Gat; and, naturally enough, Michael as the Kindly Alien, warranted the inclusion of Monty Python on the film poster. So it is a Monty Python film. Just.

Released in the summer of 2015, with the tagline: 'Great Power. Total Irresponsibility', *Absolutely Anything* did fair business in British cinemas. Although the American release didn't come until May 2017. And it was Terry's way to prove, if nothing else, that the O2 claim that Python was dead, done and dusted in 2014 was a fallacy. Of course Python wasn't bereft of life. It still isn't.

That the Pythons would always rally and always make each other laugh was very important to Terry. He wasn't sentimental though, just philosophical: 'We never really stopped being friends; but I'm not sure we ever *started* being friends. We've always liked each other in a work situation. I will have dinner with Eric on rare occasions and it is always smashing. Great fun. I will throw the occasional chair at John. Nothing malicious. Just for old times' sake. Mike and I are friends, but we have always been friends. Whenever any of us get together, there are lots of memories and lots of laughter. Then we go home to our separate lives. You don't have to play golf every alternate weekend in order to make good comedy. Although I did play squash with Mike.' Regardless, for Terry, 'Python was a heavily guarded group of six. Even after one of us was bereft of life, it was the six of us.' That strong foundation has been rocked over the years, but it is as firm as ever it was.

# CHAPTER TWELVE

## IS NO ONE INTERESTED IN HISTORY?!
## PRESENTED BY TERRY JONES

*Every age has its own history. History is really the stories that
we retell to ourselves to make them relevant to every age.*

TERRY, ankle deep in the snowy tundra of Antarctica, trudges
through a forbidding landscape, his lips tinged somewhat blue
with the cold, his well-padded red coat, tightly furled scarf and
massive fur hat keeping out the icy blasts. All at once, this enthused
commentator happens upon a waddle of penguins. As Terry told
astonished journalists ahead of releasing the footage: 'we'd been
watching the penguins and filming them for days, without a hint
of what was to come. But then the weather took a turn for the
worse. It was quite amazing. Rather than getting together in a
huddle to protect themselves from the cold, they did something
quite unexpected that no other penguins can do.' That something
quite unexpected was that these famously flightless birds took to
the air. Terry gushed that he had been witness to the penguins
hot-winging it to far-off sunnier climes, to hobnob with toucans
in the leafy rainforests of South America, thousands of miles
across the ocean.

The 'trailer' for a series apparently called *Miracles of Evolution*,
Terry's film was in fact a beautifully coordinated 90-second spoof
made by the BBC for April Fool's Day 2008. It was a glorious joke
with a serious purpose – to promote the still new streaming service
the BBC iPlayer. Terry, of course, was thousands of miles away

from the Antarctic when he filmed his presentation of this extraordinary film: on a soundstage at BBC Elstree. The choice of a Python as the presenter could be seen as a signal to the viewer that there was something silly going on, though, equally, by this point in his career, TV audiences had become used to Terry as a relaxed and fearless presenter of documentaries – although there were a few stumbling blocks to get over first.

Terry had dabbled with presenting television shows, notably book review *Paperbacks*, in the early Eighties, but he had felt uncomfortable and uneasy in the position. The key worry for him was that he felt there was nothing to protect him. There was no barrier between Terry Jones the presenter and the subject he was talking about. His frequent documentary collaborator Professor Alan Ereira found this initial nervousness on Terry's part surprising: 'He felt very self-conscious about it. He had always had a comedy character to hide behind, now it was his own personality that was being pushed to the fore.'

However, when Terry was offered more and more opportunities to present television documentaries, there was an even bigger concern. Added to his great reluctance to be himself on screen, there was a genuine fear of encroaching upon the territory of and stepping upon the toes of his dearest friend. *Around the World in 80 Days with Michael Palin* had aired on the BBC in 1989, and Michael's natural, likeable and affable presenting style, along with the impressive challenge of completing a similar journey to that of Phileas Fogg in Jules Verne's book, had proved a hit with audiences. It led to further TV adventures and Terry's Python pal becoming the nation's ideal travelling companion.

Terry had appeared in 'The Challenge', episode one of Michael's *Around the World in 80 Days*. Both Terrys, in fact, are at the railway station of London Victoria to see Mike off, with our Terry summing up his friend's journey as a quest to 'celebrate travel'. But, upon Michael's breathless return, Gilliam is there to greet him, but no

Jones. There is a lovely moment, in the seventh and final episode 'Dateline to Deadline', when, having completed the journey successfully in under eighty days, Michael arrives back at the Reform Club, as Phileas Fogg did in Verne's novel. Michael looks round and the first thing he says is: 'Where's Terry?' Where was Terry? I asked Michael. 'I don't know!' he replied. 'I hadn't even realised I'd said that. I obviously missed Terry. He was probably in the pub! Or watching a Harry Langdon film at home! Something far more interesting than congratulating me,' he chuckled.

In the early 1990s, possibly in part motivated by the huge success of Palin's travel programmes, the BBC were very interested in securing Terry as another celebrity presenter. As Alan Ereira explains: 'People in telly were sniffing around Terry with the idea of using him as a documentary presenter. At the time that was very much the fashion of television, to take somebody who had an established television identity for something else and draw in an audience, an audience that might not have previously been interested in watching a documentary.'

Professor Ereira was then a staff producer at the BBC. He thought Terry would be a wonderful presenter and he decided to take on the challenge of convincing him. Alan had been told internally at the corporation that Terry was scared and, while that was putting it a bit strongly, he was certainly reticent. Sure enough, when he got in touch with Terry, Terry promptly explained exactly why he didn't want to do it. Skilfully, Alan countered with the perfect persuading argument: 'I told him, "You shouldn't be worried. I *know* it's something you want to do and I *know* you will be good at it. All you have to do is still see yourself as a performer. You have to invent an identity that is not you but is 'Terry Jones. The Documentary Maker'. And you inhabit it, and you perform it. It's not you. It's just another character you are playing." Once he took that little note on board, which he did fully, he recognised that hook as something he could work with.'

It's easy to see why Terry was seen as the perfect person to present a documentary series with a history angle. In the wake of Monty Python's twentieth anniversary, and with the public affection for the team still high, the surviving Pythons were now turning fifty. Whether they liked it or not, they had evolved from countercultural figures sending up the British Establishment to being much-loved Establishment figures themselves. Terry might have seen himself as a 'pseudo-historian', but his knowledge of and passion for history was deep and authentic, which is an important ingredient for good TV. Plus, Terry cared about many topics and, despite his initial reluctance to present a TV show as himself, he was more aware than most that television was the perfect platform from which to share those things closest to his heart with the widest possible audience.

Understanding all of this too, Alan Ereira proposed a project that he knew would very much appeal to Terry. The programme was called *And God Blew* and was one section of a BBC2 themed evening on the weather. The programme set out to take a look at how the weather or, possibly, 'God's master plan', had shaped and changed history. As Ereira explains: 'it all started with the one everybody sort of knows, the Spanish Armada of 1588, when the Spaniards of King Philip II tried to restore Catholicism to the England of Queen Elizabeth I. The crux of the documentary was whether we could unpick the weather events that add up to some kind of coherent plan on the part of the Almighty! Is the weather all down to God's intervention?' History and religion had been pretty central to all the Monty Python films Terry had directed and, for Alan: 'Quite honestly, I couldn't think of a better presenter for it.' Having read Terry's book *Chaucer's Knight*, Alan felt he was coming from a similar point of view: 'I genuinely thought the subject would interest Terry.'

Although the historical arguments were sound, Terry would not have to try to defend a stubborn academic viewpoint. The approach of the documentary was serious, but the tone encouraged Terry to be a little bit silly. Indeed, the style of presentation is unashamedly Pythonesque. With Terry on board, the history and accredited historians could speak for themselves. The character that Ereira gave Terry was a heightened version of himself. An inquisitive but rather sceptical presenter who would look for the joke within the history, pull incredulous faces at unusual facts, and fundamentally lighten the weight of the information. It was this slightly whimsical angle that meant they had a certain amount of creative freedom in how they could approach the topic. All of which, as Alan Ereira had predicted, appealed to Terry, and his reluctance to present quickly began to fall away.

Knowing Terry, I doubt that he thought much about how a heightened profile on television would give him extra sway in getting pet publishing and feature film projects commissioned, and how, in turn, this increased celebrity would grant him further opportunities to promote this work. For Terry, it was all about the project and subject matter. If something grabbed his interest, then that is what he wanted to do. If this meant that he had to emerge from behind his writing desk and actually present his interesting findings on television, then that was all part of the process. He had long proved himself an engaging orator on the lecture circuit, his enthused voice getting more and more excited, more and more high-pitched, stumbling over his Rs, giggling as his arms flailed about with almost uncontrollable passion for what he was saying. All of those elements would inform his on-screen persona too. Unconsciously or otherwise, the television appearances were all adding to the Terry Jones brand. This was Terry saying, 'Here I am. This is what I do. Join me . . .'

So, eventually, Alan Ereira's conviction prevailed and Terry wholeheartedly bought into it. Alan's job then was to convert the idea for *And God Blew* into something Terry could work with. To that end, he scripted the documentary, provided Terry with all the material and then, as Alan remembers: 'allowed him to do what he would call "Terry-ify it!"' – giving him the opportunity to completely put his individual stamp on it, to turn Ereira's script into something uniquely his. Terry accepted the challenge.

Terry, as the ever-questioning, comedically blinkered host, was faced with a conveyor belt of proper historians who undermined his misguided authority with accurate facts and figures as he, increasingly desperate and flustered, still attempted to be proved right at every turn. It was an approach to comedy-meets-history that would be used brilliantly some decades later by Philomena Cunk, Charlie Brooker's wonderfully deluded creation as played by Diane Morgan. Although with the difference being that Philomena bamboozles the experts she meets while remaining steadfast in her ridiculously misinformed views. By contrast, the historians who appeared in *And God Blew* had a great sense of humour and completely engaged with this freewheeling approach to history. And Terry Jones played the perfect fall guy.

The programme begins with the tinkling piano and intertitle text cards of a silent movie, then Terry, as host, deploys a different historical artefact and a different style of storytelling for each one, with a weather forecaster's map to bed it within recognised television convention. And in a budget-squeezing coup that no doubt pleased the BBC hugely, all these links were filmed in and around the Travellers Club, in London's Pall Mall. In fact the whole programme was shot, on two cameras, in just one single day: 'Yes!' confirms Ereira. 'One day. It was an utter joy. And I had a little reason for doing that. Not just to save money. Terry was a natural on camera. He found this extra, hidden talent on that day's filming and, honestly, we never looked back, but I had thought it sensible to get everything shot in one fell swoop.' Essentially, Alan didn't want Terry reflecting too much on what was going on and what he was doing. He wanted him to just go with it and, the faster they could get through it all, the more fun it would be for Terry and the audience.

This trick to avoid Terry overthinking what he was doing proved successful. *And God Blew* zips along at a cracking pace, with Terry as jolly presenter constructing a tongue-in-cheek argument that God must have been on the side of the British aristocracy as all these historical weather interventions had worked out very well for the established order. That is until we get to the very last example. The actual former Japanese Ambassador to the United Kingdom, Professor Kazuo Chiba, creeps up behind Terry, to the hilarious comic shock reaction of our host. Chiba then proceeds to explain that the Japanese too had had the gods on their side. Quite brilliantly, he relates the two attempts of the Mongols to take over Japan in the thirteenth century, both times defeated by the 'divine wind' – a storm that destroyed the invasion fleet. So clearly the divine purpose here was the protection of Japan and not the glory of Britain. Much to Terry's well-honed mock chagrin at having his presenting skills usurped. That's history for you. Ereira was delighted: 'As was Terry. It was a complete takeover of the show and made for a great ending. The end credits then ran in Japanese, with Terry trying to stop them, saying: "This wasn't what I wanted to say at all!" It became history as a comedy.'

The *Radio Times* billed the programme as 'Monty Python team member Terry Jones explains how Britain has been saved from invasion and insurrection by the elements.' Just as he always wanted to, Terry succeeded in making history funny and accessible while keeping the historical facts totally accurate.

The BBC certainly recognised Terry's ability to come across as your favourite eccentric history teacher who would make study fun, with his endearing style and comic knowledge of how to deliver a joke as well as a truth. They were more than eager to engage this Professor of Popular History for more of the same. And, Terry having discovered another new talent, happily concluded that presenting programmes may well be something worth doing.

Of course, these projects take time to discuss, plan and achieve, but the BBC pretty much immediately commissioned a very ambitious series for Terry to present and Alan Ereira to produce, simply called *Crusades*.

Just as with his passion project, *Chaucer's Knight*, over a decade previously, Terry would relish the opportunity to shine a spotlight on history that had become mythologised and misunderstood, and search for the truth. Terry's *Crusades* would, by and large, reveal the Arab perspective of the eleventh- and twelfth-century invasions of the Middle East by Christian Europeans. This approach sat perfectly with Terry's multiculturalism and refusal to simply accept the Europe-centric view of the past. The starting point was that Richard the Lionheart was not the great hero he had been portrayed as. Very much akin to Terry's interpretation of Chaucer's Knight as a mercenary, this was an exposé of the Crusaders as the villains of history. Through Terry's presentation, it would be made clear that the Arabs were every bit as convinced as the Christians that God was on their side. Not only this, but that they were a much more sophisticated, well-organised and intellectually worthwhile society, and the crusaders were basically a bunch of travelling, badly organised thugs, nothing better than football hooligans on the razzle.

*Crusades* was shot in 1994, when the aftermath of the first Gulf War was still being felt and – despite various peace treaties between Israel and the Arab states being signed or in the process of being negotiated – the situation in the Middle East remained unstable, to put it mildly. The intention was that, as a TV programme, *Crusades* would be fun and interesting, but important in terms of redressing the historical balance too. The original idea, before Terry was brought on board as the presenter, had been inspired by a 1983 book, *The Crusades Through Arab Eyes* by Amin Maalouf. As Alan Ereira explains: 'Once I had told Terry about that book, and he had fully absorbed it, he knew that was the way our show had to go. I knew Terry was now in the mindset to do it, and he would be excellent.'

In the early stages, perhaps because of all he had read and the intended scope of the show, Alan thinks that Terry was more deferential than he should have been to his producer's view. Ereira remembers sitting down with him and saying: 'OK, I am driving this and shaping it, but you are the face. And nobody is going to blame me for what they see on the television. They are going to blame you. So take possession of it. Be conscious that what you are saying – whether it has come from you or from me – is going to be on your shoulders.' Despite the fact that the series would of course be looking at events nearly a thousand years in the past, the nature of the region is such that it would be possible to wander into areas of controversy. Ereira did not want to put Terry 'in a position where he might be doing something that could attract a press response. This could be something that the BBC would not know how to deal with. I couldn't have Terry carrying the can for that.' Terry had to be willing and able to stand behind what he said, in other words. 'That's where the trust came in.'

Michael Palin was just about to circumnavigate the globe for *Full Circle* and, again, Terry was concerned about stepping on the toes of his good chum. But Terry was reassured that what Michael's project amounted to was that celebration of travel that Terry himself had perceived as his unique gift, whereas Terry's was travel in the name of history.

And Terry would cover an awful lot of ground in the name of *Crusades*. Location filming took place in Asia Minor, the Mediterranean and Tel Aviv. Effortlessly shifting from clown to serious scholar, often in a single shot, Terry, seemingly with confident ease, used his skills to sugarcoat cold, hard historic facts with laughter, while never once undermining the power of what he was imparting. He recreated the Fourth Crusade for the Venice Carnival, displaying his still-sharp mime and pratfalling elegance as he demonstrated the trickiness of stepping off a boat in full armour. He explained the 1,000-mile trek from the Bosphorus to the Holy City, driving home the point that four out of five died on the journey. What's more, Terry didn't pull back from discussing the cannibal-ism of the survivors, the slaughter of the innocent, the impaling and then consuming of children. This was a gory, unpleasant history dished up with honesty, glee and enthusiasm. Terry crossed Syria and Jordan, detailing the Arabs' counter-crusade to win back Jerusalem. He told of the rise of the young Kurd, Saladin, and his destruction of the Christian Kingdom in the space of a day; the murderous ideals of King Philip II of France and the unscrupulous thirst for victory of Richard the Lionheart – who, at one point, with funds running out, had vowed to sell London to the highest bidder in order that he could continue fighting.

The locations where they filmed were not dangerous, but there were various factors that had to be considered for the safety and comfort of Terry and the crew. Ereira's main difficulty was to make sure that Terry didn't inadvertently get into trouble: 'We were working in Syria. The Syrians had a peculiar notion about what needs to be represented to the world as part of Syria. It's a surpris-ingly large area . . . and you can be imprisoned if you are carrying a map that shows something different. I had to keep going through Terry's luggage removing maps!' They also filmed in the West Bank, in Palestine, but, despite his natural ebullience, Terry was fully aware of how to behave and what not to say. It no doubt helped that his affability and charm were always to the fore.

As ever, when Terry developed a trusting working relationship with someone, he was loyal. When he and Alan came to produce a book of the television series, despite it being obvious that it was primarily his name that would attract readers and sell copies, the money earned was split equally between them. 'I never asked for that, I didn't have to. That was Terry. We never negotiated on anything,' says Ereira.

When it came to the writing, Terry and Alan had a system: 'We would write alternate chapters. Terry would send me his chapter, I would make my alterations, make a few cuts, and send it back to Terry. And Terry would, sometimes, put it all back in again and send it back to me! I would then take it all out again, and put back all the stuff he had taken out of my chapters, and we would keep on like this . . . but we never had an argument! We always found a middle ground. Eventually.'

An unexpected outcome of the series' success – though no doubt one that delighted Terry – was that, after the show had aired, universities saw an uptick in students applying for places on medieval history courses: four times the usual number. The BBC was very satisfied with its new history presenter and his evident ability to connect with audiences from different age groups. Further series, *Medieval Lives* and *Barbarians*, were commissioned, both of which saw Terry again giving the BBC history programme a fresh twist, asking questions about the misinterpretation of history and pointing out the ridiculousness of accepting established narratives as truth without asking any questions.

The driving force that underpinned these programmes was always this flipping of perceived knowledge. Initially, *Medieval Lives* was made by an independent production company for the BBC without Alan Ereira's direct involvement. But when the project hit difficulties, as Alan remembers, Terry insisted he come in to salvage it: 'That was the loyalty and trust that Terry had with me. Terry said: "This doesn't work. You have to get Alan in!" And so they did. I used to joke with the makers that you have got the producer, you have got the executive producers – if you are looking for a job description for me you can just bill me as "Terry's Friend".'

Ereira admits that he was not popular at the BBC, but Terry's loyalty and the popularity of the excellent series essentially removed any potential problems that his involvement could have raised. 'I did have one of those notorious BBC Christmas trees on my file. I was a troublemaker, but Terry wanted me around. We shared the same vision.' And Terry was someone you would also want on your team if things got tricky: 'he was marvellous company and the personification of extreme generosity'. On one occasion, they were filming in the United States and the budget was low. They were all put up in a hotel that Terry was not at all comfortable with, so, 'off his own bat, he moved everybody into a hotel that he did feel comfortable with. All of the crew. At his own expense. It wasn't a conversation, he just did it.'

The one-off documentary *Gladiators: The Brutal Truth*, hosted by Terry and produced and directed by Alan, was shown as part of BBC2's Roman Day in 2000, the year of the release of the smash-hit Russell Crowe film *Gladiator*. It uncovered the 'natural history meets showbiz' of the arena, and the sex appeal of the gladiator. Terry (now aged nearly sixty) even did some basic weapons train-ing – and was often on camera in not much clothing. Just the way he liked it – hilarious history with a serious purpose.

The BBC continued to be happy with the films Terry was making for them – but with one important caveat: that the history Terry wanted to present in his own, now trademark style was at a suit-ably long-distance arm's length. Once Terry started making noises about looking at the nineteenth century and later, the powers that be at the BBC got a little more hot under the collar. As far as Michael Palin was concerned, Terry could, on occasions, be his own worst enemy:

'Terry would take up causes that would make him very cross if anybody tried to dissuade him. Rather than trying to understand other people's points of view and make a situation work, Terry could be very confrontational. You can only push your pole position so far. He could be very stubborn, and that attitude created a slight frisson around Terry, which was a real shame. Terry was such a lovely, funny, easy-going, loveable, trusting, wonderful man and yet he always seemed to manage to get himself into this cycle of irritation with the BBC and the way they were doing things. And they, of course, as the broadcaster, would tell him: "No. We are doing it this way!" Terry wouldn't take kindly to that.'

Terry trusted his own judgement, emphatically. And he continued to trust Alan Ereira, who wrote and directed the 2008 series *Terry Jones' Great Map Mystery*. Initially broadcast on BBC Two Wales, the four-part series followed Terry's journey through the world's first road atlas. This was John Ogilby's *Britannia*, which had been published in 1675. This pilgrimage took Terry from Aberystwyth, on to St David's, Holywell, Chester and Holyhead. The last leg of the journey, along a route in severe disrepair, was the most hazardous of all. Indeed, Terry was the first person in 180 years to successfully navigate the road. The programme was political, historical and full of intrigue. Just up Terry's street.

If Terry's passion projects were blocked by the BBC – which they often were – he would take them away from the corporation to independent film-makers. For *Ancient Inventions*, originally broadcast on the Discovery Channel, Terry tackled three separate threads: war, sex and city life. Based upon the 1994 book by historians and archaeologists Peter James and Nick Thorpe, the series debunked popular myths of history with odd facts and curious revelations. Terry would stop at nothing to prove that our modern way of life was pretty much dependent on ideas from history. He was still as fit as a butcher's dog, and the series saw him leaping over cannons and whizzing round such favourite haunts as New York, Rome and Venice. He would do *really* silly things too, like sitting in a bath fully clothed. Our favourite history teacher is clearly enjoying himself hugely, usually with a glass of wine and a plate of good food in front of him.

But the best teachers never think they know it all, and Terry loved that he got to learn about historical periods completely new to him. This was certainly the case with *The Hidden History of Rome* and *The Hidden History of Egypt*, both for the Discovery Channel. 'It's an absolute pleasure and a rare privilege to host shows like those,' he said. 'The producers line up loads of experts in their field, who share their latest research with you, and bring all this history up to date. It's wonderful. I feel like I'm getting a crash university course.'

Terry brought his relaxed and unorthodox style to other subjects that fascinated him. He had so many different and diverse interests, and, with his history presenter stripes now fully earned and worn with comfortable ease, he would jump at the chance to explore them on telly. Terry readily dressed up and played the slapstick fool for the Wild Pictures documentary *In Charlie Chaplin's Footsteps*, investigating the comic genius who took physical comedy to new heights, from abject poverty in south London to becoming the highest-paid star in Hollywood. Although Chaplin was not one of his long-standing silent comedy heroes, Terry had become bewitched by him. He rewatched his films, he re-addressed his politics and he tracked down members of Chaplin's family. There was no doubt that Terry was still in possession of those very funny bones that had been getting audiences laughing as he did backflips and pratfalls for over sixty years, and it was a talent that engendered a renewed respect for Chaplin's comedy legacy.

Terry's interest in the history of love and sex went way back to *The Love Show*, the trouble-struck theatrical project from 1965. Terry had returned to the subject for an episode in the *Ancient Inventions* series; and his lengthy research into the ins and outs of copulation was now to be extended for a further programme, *The Surprising History of Sex and Love*. 'Terry's Friend' Alan Ereira was involved too and remembers it as 'the best documentary Terry had ever worked on.'

However, it proved a tricky subject and yet another example of how Terry's single-minded vision could come into conflict with the organisations commissioning his work. The rough cut worried the Discovery Channel people because, as Alan recalls, 'the American sensibility over sexual imagery was far more touchy than Britain's but, more importantly than that, Terry wasn't prepared for the reaction to the central theme of his film. That was the argument that sex had been turned from a sacrament to a sin. In the ancient world sex was sacramental. Indeed, there was such a thing as sacred prostitution, and all that quickly became unacceptable to the powers that be at Discovery. Sex being something to be repressed and controlled is a relatively new phenomenon. An entire industry was built on this: when something that was open and free was forced to become secret and expensive! And this concerned the core values of Discovery.'

Although a truncated version of *The Surprising History of Sex and Love* was broadcast, to award-winning praise, it had been re-edited outside of Terry's jurisdiction. Terry was livid, of course, but, in the end, philosophical, reasoning that what remained was still powerful and historical, just a little sanitised. Which was not his style at all.

Terry's final documentary film was *Boom Bust Boom*, released to cinemas in 2016. Produced by Bill and Ben Productions, with Terry directing, narrating and presenting, alongside some adorable, financially savvy puppets, the film ripped off the lid of economics to reveal that word is pretty much devoid of meaning. Or common sense. It is another history lesson, of course. This time at the expense of mankind's thirst for wealth and power through the speculation of ideas and opportunities.

From his initial position of reluctant presenter, worried about appearing as himself on camera and being seen to tread on the well-travelled toes of a friend, Terry had gone on to develop his own typically unique sensibility as a documentary film-maker: as a friendly but forceful face of truth and understanding. This is largely thanks to the healthy respect that he had for the past and the people of the past, and his imaginative powers, which let him see the world as it would have looked from their point of view. They were, he thought, when all was said and done, just like us. It was that idea of living history which was at Terry's very core. Using his modern sensibilities, he could think his way into a non-modern world, a world where Christianity wasn't the full story; the European way wasn't the only way; where civilisations from centuries ago could tell you more about the here and now than national newspapers, and where the past, for all its terrors, was fundamentally a foolish and funny place.

'Of course the past is funny!' Terry would explode. You are missing *everything* if you don't see the ridiculousness of what went on. That arrogance of not learning from anybody else – this was the joke of history. People don't like being told; they like being let in. And if he changed just one viewer; made just one person question their perception of the past, then his job had been done. If that story wasn't worth telling, wasn't worth delving into and explaining, then why do it? And a rhetorical question is just how Terry would have left it.

# CHAPTER THIRTEEN

## FANTASY AND REALITY

*I think fame is great. It makes it easier to do things, and much harder to pay for things. People keep buying you dinner!*

TERRY always was something of a brilliant butterfly brain. He could spin many creative plates all at once, juggling a film in the can; a film in the camera; and a film in those early stages of getting funding. He'd be playing the fool as an active Python for the latest documentary or revival; presenting a show and pitching the next one. And there would always be a book in the offing, on the table or in his mental notepad. He wouldn't know for a while that that unique mind of his would one day let him down, but, even so, he certainly wrung out every drop of inspiration that he possibly could.

Terry was a writer, first and foremost. He was a talented actor and a brilliant comic, of course, and a lauded director, much respected by the performers with whom he worked. But crucially, writing was something that he had pretty much complete control over. He didn't have to hassle for the budget or toe the line with a hard-bitten producer. Hours spent on the telephone trying to secure the money for production were hours of creativity wasted, as far as Terry was concerned. He would get very vocal about the state of the film industry, holding up both America and France as countries where film attendance was on the increase while his home market was being hit by a steady stream of cinema closures. But when Terry could just write the words, he was in his element. It was the perfect immediate outlet for his restlessly inspired mind and avalanche of ideas.

The other thing that lay at his core, his very essence, was that Terry was a collaborator. Though almost everyone who worked with him has a wry story to tell about him digging his heels in, refusing to compromise on his creative vision, he always sought out people to work with. Perhaps – as a naturally gregarious man who loved people – it was a way to offset the typically lonely, solitary life of a writer. Maybe it goes all the way back to his natural affinity for team sports at school. Or was irrevocably cemented in his mind through the process of putting on plays and productions with his gang at Oxford and then in writers' rooms in the early days at the BBC. And for all his occasional irascibility, there was never a shortage of people who wanted to work with him. Many of his collaborators became friends, and he was always looking for ways to work with his friends, usually on ideas cooked up over famously long lunches or dinner parties at his house.

Not all of the very many projects that Terry was at some point involved with got off the ground, of course. Any creative, multi-talented firebrand has many ideas and scripts that will never sell – and Terry had more ideas than most. As is often the way with the film business, he would sometimes be called to work for a time on something that then morphed into something else to be finished by another writer. But from the 1980s all the way through to the early part of the new millennium, he was called up by a roster of famous names who all wanted to tap into the Terry Jones wellspring of creativity and gloriously silly ideas. His fingerprints – even if at times only faintly – can be found all over the place if you know where to look.

For example, in the mid-Eighties, executive producer Steven Spielberg was on the lookout for a swift sequel to the 1984 horror-comedy smash hit *Gremlins*, which he had executive produced. Terry delivered an ambitious script that saw the frantic, destructive goblins take on Manhattan and ultimately do what King Kong couldn't and completely destroy the Empire State Building. It was deemed a little too nutty, and certainly too expensive, and was abandoned. In the eventual sequel – *Gremlins 2: The New Batch*, written by Charles S. Haas – the furry creatures who you shouldn't get wet do indeed get to Manhattan, though generally stick to the more budget-friendly confines of a department store. Still, for those in the know, there remains an essence of Terry in the project.

Conversely, Terry did receive the sole writing credit for another film made by a Hollywood big-hitter, Jim Henson, despite the fact that much of the plot he came up with was written out of existence. What would become the enduring cult hit *Labyrinth* certainly feels like it has emerged from the darkest comic recesses of Terry's imagination, if not being completely the project he had envisaged. It had all come about as an act of defiance on Terry's part. He had seen Jim Henson's *The Dark Crystal* in a cinema in New York, and thoroughly enjoyed it. Typically of Terry, who had an enduringly cavalier attitude to time-keeping, he had missed the first five minutes of the screening. At the end, he left the cinema with the sense of having been thoroughly entertained and engaged by the film. Then he read review after review that ripped *The Dark Crystal* to smithereens, in the main complaining that the plot was far too obvious. Terry didn't think the plot was obvious at all. Not until he saw the film again. From the beginning. Then he discovered that they had put a voice-over narration in the first couple of minutes that gave the entire plot away and ruined any sense of wonder or adventure that the rest of the film would have had. Terry commiserated with Henson, and eagerly accepted the offer to write the screenplay for his next film. This was *Labyrinth*, which was always intended to be far, far funnier than *The Dark Crystal*. Terry saw Henson's idea for something stranger and more grown-up than his output with the Muppets sitting comfortably within the tradition of Lewis Carroll's *Alice's Adventures in Wonderland* and the dark, symbolic thrills of magical manipulation. Terry's version of the film – written well before David Bowie was cast as Jareth, the King of the Goblins – also had a little girl as the central character; and as the representative of the audience in a weird and wonderful world. However, Terry's notion was that the real star of the story is the labyrinth itself. And with Terry on board the story inevitably had plenty of silly situations and jolly japes. Not least of which are the guards on duty. A two-hander scene between a general and a foot soldier, who just happens to be a skeleton, has all the hallmarks of wacky and off-the-wall comedy that had been Terry's style for decades. Typically of Terry, this darkly comic scene had a soft centre. The discussion was all about an attempt to launch a massive jelly bomb. Destructive things that come across as rather nice had been in his armoury since that explosive gift box in *The Oxford Revue* and would become a recurring theme in the fantasy fiction of Terry Jones.

Although Terry's first draft of *Labyrinth* forms the basis for the film, Jim Henson felt the screenplay needed a re-buff and re-polish, and employed a glut of established writers to take over, including children's poet Dennis Lee and pioneering comedy performer, writer and director Elaine May. Along the way was added to the mix the thrilling and disgusting 'Bog of Eternal Stench', which, for Terry: 'sounds very much like something I would have come up with but, honestly, it wasn't in my original screenplay'. Maybe an old idea and a new, off-the-cuff joke, lingering in the labyrinth that he had come up with and others developed. Anyway: 'I'm very happy if people enjoy it and think I wrote it.' Although, for Terry, in the end, *Labyrinth* didn't quite work, didn't quite come together. Though he was more critical of his own contribution than that of anybody else. Indeed, he claimed his favourite bits of the film were those scenes where he couldn't recognise a single line or idea of his own. He reflected at the time: 'I've got the film there, but it doesn't work. It needs an injection of meaning. I shouldn't say that, but you can inject meaning into things. And I do feel that comedy or fantasy needs to contain a *reflection* of reality to work.'

Perhaps the first audiences felt the same way. *Labyrinth* was famously met with a somewhat bemused reception on release, and enjoyed only modest success in the US. It took some years for it to become the cult favourite and fantasy classic that it's seen as now – the memory of seeing it for the first time is seared into the minds of many who watched it as children, up past their bedtimes.

Terry was at least able to get a book out of his work on *Labyrinth* – and a new collaborator. *Goblins of the Labyrinth* was very much inspired by the Jim Henson film – or, more accurately, inspired by the largely aborted ideas that Terry had conjured up for *Labyrinth*, here refreshed and energised by the illustrations of Brian Froud. It was Brian's intricate concept designs that had created the visual feel of the *Labyrinth* film, and his beautiful but creepy and occasionally disturbing imagery matched Terry's writing style perfectly. Brian and Terry forged a firm friendship almost immediately, helped by a mutual appreciation for the finer things in life, and much wine was stopped from going sour.

Steven Spielberg had remained a Hollywood big-hitter who flirted with Terry with regards to possible film projects. Having been brought in by Disney, Spielberg and his Amblin Entertainment had turned the live-action meets Toontown *Who Framed Roger Rabbit* into a blockbuster. One of that film's animation directors, Rob Minkoff, befriended Terry. Minkoff had ambitions to move into directing live-action films and commissioned a fantasy screenplay from Terry, which went unmade. By the end of the Nineties, heartily fed up with these film ideas that went nowhere, Terry followed the British film trend of the time and decided to start his own production company. So, inspired by his greatest directorial achievement, *Monty Python's Life of Brian*, he launched Messiah Pictures in 2000. The first slated release was to have been *Das Cowboy*, a five-million-dollar comedy about the making of a

Western. Julian Doyle, who had edited both *Life of Brian* and *The Meaning of Life*, as well as Terry's *The Wind in the Willows*, was to direct, on location in Spain. Robert Carlyle was signed up to play the B-movie horror writer assigned a spaghetti Western. Stacy Keach was to be the washed-up Hollywood actor who would star in the film within the film. Terry himself was set to give a cameo performance as a manic preacher. Alas, it turns out that even when you are Terry Jones and you have your own production company, films are very difficult things to get made. It never happened. Also on that initial Messiah Pictures schedule was *Mirror Man*, a collaboration with French screenwriter Philippe Le Guay, which Terry was set to direct. The plot revolved around a man's mirror image, which emerges from the glass and, quite understandably, disrupts his entire life. Later drafts of the screenplay would include contributions from Gavin Scott and Kim 'Howard' Johnson, but Terry never did make the film.

Indeed, Terry would have so many projects on the go and up in the air at any one time that it was often a relentless conveyor belt of serious propositions and silly ideas. Some of those serious propositions did come about. Some of the silly ideas did too. But all of them were by-products of Terry's excessive creative energy and an excuse for those long lingering lunches with people whose company he enjoyed.

Terry's involvement with an early version of a musical based on the pop songs of the Kinks certainly seems like it was a serious proposition, though in the end it didn't come to anything for him. His group of friends had always included rock music royalty and, by the dawn of the twenty-first century, Ray Davies was a close neighbour in Highgate. Terry was to write the book for the musical but, despite several drafts and much hard work, the production didn't happen. *Sunny Afternoon*, as it would eventually be called, would be written by playwright Joe Penhall, and opened at Hampstead Theatre in 2014 before transferring to the West End, where it won four Laurence Olivier Awards. There was to have been another jukebox musical project, in collaboration with Meat Loaf's favourite songwriter, Jim Steinman. Terry wrote the book for a rock 'n' rap retelling of Tchaikovsky's *The Nutcracker*, which he called *Nutcracked*. It was set for a West End premiere in early 2013, but escalating budgets saw the production abandoned.

Singer-songwriter Kate Bush and Terry often discussed the possibility of collaborating on a stage or film project together. In Tim Walker's portfolio of photographs for Kate's 2011 album, *Director's Cut*, Terry is seen sitting on a train, next to Python costume designer Hazel Pethig, gazing with wide-mouthed wonder at an active laptop. He is credited as 'Professor Need'. A mad and eccentric and delightful character indeed. Terry attended a couple of Kate's *Before the Dawn* concerts, in September 2014, and again the notion was raised about his directing Kate in something. Although this never happened, this friendship remained undimmed. Ever modest and ever encouraging of others to try something outside of their comfort zone, Terry reflected: 'I told Kate that she should direct it herself!'

Of course, what many fans and opportunistic producers wanted to know was whether there was ever going to be another Python film. The Pythons themselves would often ponder this, even after the loss of Graham. Although, of course, the enthusiasm of the different members waxed and waned over the years. And even if it ever felt like there was some momentum building, they could never agree on what exactly to do. As late as the end of the 1990s, the team rallied round to discuss an intriguing project that was close to Terry's heart, 'Monty Python and the Last Crusade'. However, staging a direct sequel to *Monty Python and the Holy Grail*, only with the Pythons as aged knights and archive recordings of Graham as the voice of King Arthur's ashes, proved impossible to agree upon. Eric went off to write *Spamalot* instead. Another idea, an ingenious one indeed with a central idea of cancel culture that was very much ahead of its time, was about Python facing a lengthy court case over copyright infringement and offence caused to over-sensitive viewers. This film never got off the ground either. Yet another aborted project was 'Monty Python's Third World War', which was to have been a clever indictment of the business of mass murder, and a comedic exposure of the scandal and commercialism of modern warfare. In the end, despite his enthusiasm, Terry would have to accept that the days of new Python were well and truly over. We will never know if these projects could have blossomed into a wonderful Python renaissance. The big risk was of course that they could have proved a last-gasp attempt at holding on to something that should have been left in the past.

For Michael Palin, though their friendship endured, the days of him and Terry regularly writing together were also over. Terry was often asked whether he would work with his old sparring partner again. It was something he was always very keen on but, as Michael remembers, 'To be honest, after *Ripping Yarns* Terry and I went our own ways. We still remained the very closest of friends but we had our own projects. We grew up and grew apart in terms of writing together, but we enjoyed our dinners and our pints and our chats.' Then, one enterprising publisher suggested more *Ripping Yarns*. In book form, for the twenty-first century. Michael recalls that: 'Terry and I discussed it and we came to the conclusion that we were both a bit past it by then. What would we write? Biggles in the retirement home?' Resurrections of past glories were often mentioned though, including doing something with Bert Fegg. A radio series was mooted; even a West End stage musical. Eventually Aardman Animations in Bristol approached them with regards to a Bert Fegg feature film. Several fun project meetings resulted, but alas no film.

Then there were the history documentaries that Terry could never make. As his long-time collaborator Alan Ereira reflects:

'Those are the ones you really remember. The ones you can't do! It was our main aim. To get people to recognise new ways of seeing the past. The kind of stories that would interest Terry were, for example, a series we pitched a lot: "Heroes and Villains", in which Terry would have reversed perceived knowledge.' Another pet project that never happened was 'Lies My Father Told Me', which Terry would make copious notes about. This idea was concerned with upending some of the incorrect received ideas that many of us have from how our parents want us to see the past and see our futures. The reason for the lack of a green light on these ideas was, as Alan believes, because 'all the broadcasting finance was dominated by America, and a lot of our ideas were considered unAmerican'. There was one about the American Civil War and another about the appropriation of the prairies from the Native Americans – both subjects with long-reaching consequences in the States. As Alan remembers, ruefully, 'lots of shaking heads at the Discovery Channel met that suggestion. How dare these two Limeys tell us about our own history!'

Although Terry became frustrated at not being able to make all the things he wanted to, there's no doubt that he loved the process of meeting potential collaborators and working together on ideas. Monty Python – but also his successful books and documentaries – served as a passport that took him to all sorts of interesting places where he got to talk to interesting people about interesting things. This highly sociable curiosity and his gleeful determination to find fun and enlightenment would always start with companionship and invariably lead to projects, both unachieved and achieved.

One of the most intriguing was 'The Two Terries', a touring show that allowed Terry Jones and Terry Pratchett a free hand to talk about absolutely anything. The publicity promised that 'whatever else comes to mind!' would be the subject of the show, though the crux was, inevitably, comedy writing. For Terry, it always came back to writing.

Terry loved to get up in front of a live audience and discuss his past; our collective past; his latest project – or anything, really – and was always totally happy when the audience questions turned back, time and time again, to Monty Python. Colin Webb explains how Terry was a dream author in the sense that, unlike many high-profile writers, he absolutely loved to attend book festivals, and would happily accept any invitation that his packed schedule would allow. Colin remembers: 'Terry wasn't the kind of writer who would deliver the manuscript and move on to the next project. He was very proud of what he had written.' This garrulous passion for discussing his work, meeting groups of readers and signing books made Terry both likeable and bankable. A publisher knew his name would carry weight; and that he would beat the drum when the time came to sell the book.

Sometimes Terry's determination to have fun would try the patience of those around him. Though such was the loyalty he inspired that he would usually get away with it. Colin Webb tells of one unexpected, unscheduled pitch meeting late on a Friday afternoon. 'Pavilion Books had offices at the top of Covent Garden, and the receptionist said, "I've got Terry Jones and Brian Froud to see you." This was at four o'clock in the afternoon. And they were both absolutely smashed. They came up to my office and would only speak to me if I first opened a bottle of white wine. This I did. Then Terry started explaining this book between mouthfuls of wine. It was an idea they had had over lunch all about this old Edwardian lady who sat around in her garden, catching fairies by snapping shut her book on them! I really had to get home that Friday evening so, just to get Terry and Brian out of the office, I said: "Fine. OK. You're on. Here's a contract. We'll do it!" That's what happened. That's how publishing worked back then.'

*Lady Cottington's Pressed Fairy Book* was a strange fantasy publication, somewhat inspired by *The Country Diary of an Edwardian Lady*, a surprise best-seller when it was published in

1977. Terry's book was all about another Edwardian lady, who collected the psychic impressions of the mysterious fairies who lived in her garden. Her name was a reference to the Cottingley Fairies – a series of photos, purportedly of fairies, taken by two young girls, Elsie Wright and Frances Griffiths, in 1917. Sir Arthur Conan Doyle believed them to be genuine and, although the subject matter of Terry's book may suggest it was aimed at children, *Lady Cottington's Pressed Fairy Book* was very much for adults. Brian Froud's lavish, rather saucy illustrations gave the publication a unique, mystical look and Terry's off-kilter and just plain bizarre comic brain did the rest.

Terry being Terry, he was very keen to dress up as Lady Cottington for a shaky, monochrome film to promote the book, supposedly shot just before the Great War – the conceit being that, when this lady had died in 1990 in comparative obscurity, an investigation of the loft at her home had revealed this extraordinary volume. The merry promotional campaign that Terry revelled in certainly worked. *Lady Cottington's Pressed Fairy Book* sold all round the world and Terry joined forces once more with illustrator Brian Froud for a sequel, *Strange Stains and Mysterious Smells*, published by Simon & Schuster in 1996. This was apparently the previously unknown protoplasmic research into the psychic images and psychic odours of fairies undertaken by Lady Cottington's twin brother, Quentin Cottington. Uncannily, he looked the spitting image of Terry too. Froud's sketches and oil paintings endlessly inspired Terry's weird and wonderful imagination, and this was a fantasy world of grotesque comedy and outlandish, vivid images.

Another skilled collaborator and partner in drink was Douglas Adams. A product of the Cambridge Footlights – he had graduated from St John's college a decade after the Pythons' Cambridge contingent – Adams had joined the Python party, having briefly teamed up to write with Graham for the very last episode of the television series, the *Holy Grail* album and *Out of the Trees*. Adams even made a couple of appearances in the last series of Python, memorably in the 'Mr Neutron' episode, where he loaded a missile onto the scrap metal cart driven by Terry. As a result, Adams had become a chum of the team, and the British Pythons had endorsed – after a fashion – his breakthrough science fiction comedy novel *The Hitchhiker's Guide to the Galaxy*. In fact the comic, semicircular words of praise were as follows:

'Really entertaining and fun.' John Cleese.

'Much funnier than anything John Cleese has ever written.' Terry Jones.

'I know for a fact that John Cleese hasn't read it.' Graham Chapman.

'Who is John Cleese?' Eric Idle.

'Really entertaining and fun.' Michael Palin.

That Terry's tongue-in-cheek dig doesn't really reference Douglas Adams at all is perhaps significant, as when he first heard the radio series – the first episode of which was broadcast in March 1978 – he was only mildly impressed. He found it amusing enough but it wasn't really his kind of thing. Through friendship and collaboration, though, Terry would later get it, and, in turn, write an introduction to the Folio Society edition of *The Hitchhiker's Guide*. It was a novel in which, Terry enthused, Douglas Adams 'brilliantly combines science fiction with the finest tradition of English humour.'

There had even been talk of Douglas and Terry collaborating on a screenplay for a feature film of *The Hitchhiker's Guide*. As Terry remembered, however: 'Douglas loved ideas but hated writing' and, as a result, he swiftly fell out of love with the idea of revisiting *Hitchhiker's* for cinema. Other, fresh film ideas were discussed though, and the two did join forces to write 'A Christmas Story', a very silly seasonal saga for the 1986 charity publication *The Utterly Utterly Merry Comic Relief Christmas Book*. For Terry and Douglas always got on well. As well as obvious mutual interests in absurdist humour, science and history, they both liked a drink. Douglas was someone very much cut from the same good-time cloth as Terry himself. Kim 'Howard' Johnson and his wife Laurie can testify to the gloriously boozy clash that usually occurred when Terry and Douglas got together, including one (hazy) memory of a more-than-convivial time at the Four Seasons hotel in Chicago: 'Oh, my Lord. I have never drunk so much in my life. And they drank more than I did. We are all amateurs compared to Terry and Douglas. We were politely asked to move on from the restaurant and were given a private room to continue drinking, such was the hilarious, disruptive ruckus we caused. Well, *they* caused!'

Having created his very own, hugely, internationally successful universe, Douglas Adams always had his finger on the now and, more potently, a bright eye on the future. To that end, in the late 1990s Douglas turned his attention to a CD-ROM comedy-adventure game. *Starship Titanic* would allow the player to journey on a stellar-galactic version of the ill-fated ship that, allegedly, couldn't sink, meeting a typical Douglas Adams collection of oddball aliens along the way.

As Douglas Adams wrote in his introduction to the novelisation: 'about this time, Terry Jones came into the production office. One of the characters in the game is a semi-deranged workman's parrot that had been left on board the ship, and Terry had agreed to play the voice part.' Terry's reaction to the vivid graphics and exciting character animations was so enthusiastic that, again to quote Adams, he 'uttered the fateful words, "Is there anything else you need doing?" I said, "You wanna write a novel?" and Terry said, "Yeah, all right. Provided," he said, "I can write it in the nude." Terry is one of the most famous people in the known universe, and his bottom is only slightly less well known than his face.'

And so the deal was struck. Terry wrote the tie-in novel to the game that Douglas didn't have time to write himself – although whether Terry actually did write every single word without a single item of clothing is debatable. The novel is called *Douglas Adams's Starship Titanic*. The publicity department of the American publisher, Ballantine, billed it as 'Arguably the Greatest Collaboration in the Whole History of Comedy!' The glowing reviews did seem to agree that it was a successful blend. *Publishers Weekly* called it 'absurd' and 'rollicking', while *The Washington Post* bandied around words like 'zany' and 'irreverent'.

Though the book was clearly aimed at the American market, Terry's earth-bound points of reference are all very British; he zings his characters through the sleepy countryside of Oxfordshire. The most endearing alien character is a rather bumbling and naive and easily distracted bomb, voiced on the CD-ROM game by John Cleese. Douglas Adams was thrilled with it, delighting in his friend's unique project credit: 'Parrot and novel by Terry Jones.' In the novel, the parrot is very much the catalyst for the adventure.

It was a winning combination but never to happen again. Douglas Adams collapsed and died after his regular gymnastic workout in Montecito, California, in May 2001. He was just forty-nine. Terry, ever the dutiful friend, jumped on the next plane out of London to comfort and console Douglas's distressed family. Terry's eulogy would be included in the American paperback edition of *The Salmon of Doubt*, a collection of tributes and unpublished material, released exactly a year after Douglas's untimely death.

The shocking news had come when Terry was losing a lot of those closest to him, with George Harrison's death that November. The previous year, his Oxford friend and colleague Doug Fisher had died at the age of fifty-eight. A memorial concert was organised at the Soho Theatre, part of which reunited a group of contemporaries performing the 'Slapstick' routine from nearly forty years earlier. David Wood remembered: 'Annabel Leventon was the lecturer on that occasion, I was playing the chap in the middle, between Mike Palin and Terry. I had to swing right, banging Terry on the head with this plank of wood! It was a prop but it was still pretty heavy, and I didn't want to hurt them. They were my friends. It was the only time I ever saw Terry get angry. He said: "Look! If you can't do it properly I'll get somebody else!" So I did it properly! It went down beautifully but, my God, it must have hurt him. He was delighted. Anything in the name of comedy. Anything for a laugh. And especially anything for a good friend like Dougie Fisher, who we all greatly loved and admired.'

Even though these occasions were an upbeat way to remember his happy days at Oxford and those people who had made them so happy, Terry would always have this sense of comic perfectionism too. John Gould, the musical director of *The Oxford Revue* and those pantos that Terry and Michael had written, was also so honoured with a memorial concert, in 2013. Terry sang 'Forgive Me'; and joined in on the communal, counter-melody number 'Last One Home's A Custard (or, Six Characters In Search of a Song)'. There was another piece from *The Oxford Revue* that was also performed at the John Gould tribute. 'Sotto Voice (Piano Thoughts)' had always been accredited to Gould, with a little help from Chopin. There was, it seems, also a little help from Terry. David Wood had never realised Terry had been involved, until: 'he received the copy of the CD of the show I sent him. Terry noticed that he was uncredited! He was very good about it. He just wanted to let me know. Ever the historian!'

Undoubtedly, the most shocking loss for Terry had been the sudden death of his elder brother, Nigel, in 1993. He had been ever supportive of his sibling, and Terry was ever conscious of the potential jealousy over his fame. The brotherly relationship had certainly had its moments over the years, but Terry found solace in the beautiful funeral service, and his precious memories of their playful childhood together; a sense of always looking up to Nigel, of being happy when he impressed his older brother and keen to embrace the mutual love of jazz that always brought them closer together. Jazz played an important part in the funeral service, as well as that of old school friend Geoffrey Burgon. It was music that brought Geoff back into Terry's inner circle; he had written the biblical score for *Monty Python's Life of Brian*. Typically, soon after, Terry and Geoffrey had planned to collaborate on a musical based on the writings of William Shakespeare, which never happened. At the funeral of Terry's brother, Geoff 'realised just how much Nige had meant to Terry'. It was a shared passion for creating things that was at Terry's core. As Geoff confirmed: 'it's our primary interest in life.'

It sometimes seemed that Terry's social energy was as limitless as his capacity for creativity. His wide circle of friends and acquaintances included many whom he had known for decades, as well as people who he had picked up from various places along the way. There was little separation between life and work – collaborators often became friends, and friends invariably became collaborators. Terry would jump at the chance to work on anything with those whose company he enjoyed. Alongside writing, food was his great passion, as a comfort or a reward, but particularly as a way to get people together.

David Wood recalls Terry always being a very good cook and very welcoming, while fellow Oxford friend Nigel Pegram dined with Terry many, many times, often with his distinguished ballerina wife April Olrich. 'It was Terry's goodness of spirit that always struck me,' he recalls. 'On the wall of his home, Terry had an amazing telephone. April said: "My golly, that's lovely!" and Terry, ever generous, said: "You can have it!" She said, "Oh no, I couldn't . . ." Anyway, Terry got a screwdriver, unhooked it and gave it to April, saying: "I want you to have it!" A few months later he came to have dinner with us and saw the telephone hanging on our wall and said: "I've got one of those!" And I said: "No you haven't! Not any more!" He just laughed. He was affectionate. He was a hugging, giving, wonderful guy.'

Terry's regime while writing was fairly strict. Work would always come first, but in the middle of the day he would factor in a brief break during which he would go for a brisk walk to get himself a sandwich. Or he would head to the local shops and markets to pick up exotic ingredients for the evening meal. He was a brilliant self-taught cook, forever trying adventurous new things in the kitchen. Daughter Sally recalls that: 'he would bring back these wonders from around the world. He had visited Syria while he was making the *Crusades* series and had discovered sumac, this gorgeous spice, made from berries. Dad would start smearing it on everything!'

Michael Palin – of course a very regular guest of Terry's – agrees: 'Terry was a really, really good cook. And he would try absolutely anything! He was always on the lookout for the most obscure, outrageous items to prepare. He would ask me: "Ooh Mike, could you get me some Afghan sheep's eyes!" I'd say: "Sounds horrible, Terry!", but he would enthuse: "No, no. They are really lovely. Really nice!"'

When Sally and Bill were young, they would be bathed and put to bed, and then often six or eight people would arrive for dinner. Or Terry would arrange to meet friends in the pub before trooping back to eat. Terry's lovingly prepared meal would of course be accompanied by copious amounts of alcohol to wash it all down with. I was privileged to be invited to one or two of these gatherings at Camberwell and many more after he had moved to Highgate. For those lucky enough to be in that amazing inner sanctum, the dinner parties have become the stuff of legend. The guest list was eclectic and electric. Terry's circle of friends was wide and various. One evening, you could find yourself in conversation with *Blood on Satan's Claw* writer Robert Wynne-Simmons, film-maker Sara Sugarman, broadcaster Zeb Soanes, *Viz* comic founder Simon Donald and yachtswoman Clare Francis. All at the same table. In the early days of our acquaintance in particular, Terry would be excited to share his friends and introduce me to people who he thought I'd like to meet. He also knew that I would be tickled pink at certain attendees at these relaxed and elephantine gatherings. Often, when another Python was going to be in the house, Terry would phone me in the morning:

'Rob, are you still coming tonight?'

'Absolutely. Can't wait.'

'Fantastic,' Terry would gush. 'Terry G. has just confirmed. See you in the Red Lion and Sun at five . . .'

Alternatively, Terry would be crestfallen when he phoned one morning: 'Rob. Sorry, but Mike's just called. He can't make tonight. Do you still want to come?'

'Of course, Terry!'

He would brighten: 'Oh, brilliant. See you in the Gatehouse at five thirty . . .'

In the *Ancient Inventions* series of documentaries Terry says: 'Who invented cooking? I don't know, but thank God for them!' Never were truer words spoken. Terry was passionate about, borderline obsessed with food. To the extent that, be it at home or, more often than not, out at a restaurant, he would always, but always want to try the food that you were eating. Michael Palin remembers that: 'Terry just couldn't be satisfied with what he was eating. He always needed to eat some of your food too. It used to make my wife Helen really cross. She would just have been served a nice plate of food and Terry would say: "Ooh, that looks good!" and just dive in. Protests would do no good. They were always too late in any case. Terry would want to share everything, even if the other person didn't want to!'

I can testify to this. And I can see Terry now, like a hungry hamster, cheeks stuffed with his food, and the food of his friends and their partners. Sat there, happy and content, making yummy food noises as he reached for someone else's plateful. At least up to a certain point. Late in our friendship, I became a vegan and the food I was enjoying was very much not to Terry's taste. In fact, he couldn't stand it. There was now nothing he wanted to pinch off my plate. Michael Palin is delighted at the thought: 'That's hilarious. And brilliant. What a wonderful way to avoid Terry nicking stuff off your plate. We should have all gone vegan!' I was never one of those evangelistic vegans, I was simply into kind cuisine. Although I did try to tempt Terry with vegan-friendly ales. We also had some very serious conversations about the health benefits of a vegan diet.

Throughout 1999 Terry suffered chronic hip pain – which was strangely alleviated when John Cleese went into hospital for a hip replacement operation! Terry's problem didn't go away completely, though – as wonderfully silly as it would have been had John's treatment provided the solution. Terry would gleefully show you his X-rays displaying the damaged cartilage in his hip, and he eventually had his own hip replacement operation. Terry was also always mindful of his cholesterol levels rocketing. He had serious concerns about his heart and he was not blind to the fact that his food and alcohol intake were inadvisable, to put it mildly. There were warning signs that, when he got them checked, led to him being diagnosed in October 2006 with colon cancer. He rather took the verdict on the chin, and seized on the medical fact that a man in his early sixties, with a Terry-sized appetite for booze and rich food, was more than prone to the ailment. Treatment and care and thought saw him through the cancer. A distressing tumour was cut out, and a course of chemotherapy stopped the cancer spreading. The only side effect he suffered was a slight freezing sensation in the feet.

As I got to know Terry, I experienced first-hand how his sociability coupled with his love of collaboration could lead to all sorts of comedy adventures that you might not have seen coming but which were a joy to embark on. All fuelled by the force of his will and personality. From our first meeting, Terry caught on to my deep interest in vintage comedy, and was immediately fascinated by this young lad whose knowledge and passion both surprised and delighted him. Terry wanted to bask in it and cultivate it, and was quick to pull out his vast collection of 78rpm comedy recordings.

One day, we began talking about veteran comedian Ronald Frankau, a chap with a plummy voice who invariably dressed in a swanky dinner jacket. He would often tell anybody who cared to listen that 'I went to Oxford, you know!', for the comic effect, of course. Frankau's songs were also often enriched by utter smut. Terry loved him, though he was flabbergasted that I had even heard of him, never mind knew his work: 'But he's been dead fifty years!' he said in disbelief. My acquaintance with Frankau's comedy had been via an LP in my dad's collection called *Listen to the Banned* – a collection of 1930s recordings so filthy that the BBC had refused to broadcast them. Typically of Terry, his amazement at my knowledge of Frankau swiftly turned to admiration, and that quickly became determination to channel this knowledge and appreciation into something. A project! 'He's a Forgotten Hero of Comedy,' Terry shouted. 'That would make a fabulous book. You write it, and I'll do the foreword!'

And so it was. For our next meeting Terry and I had a notebook each and, over a couple of pints, we chatted and joked and reminisced and jotted down literally hundreds of names for possible inclusion in the *Forgotten Heroes of Comedy* book. Terry's limited viewing of television throughout the 1950s and early 1960s gave him brilliant blind spots. Arthur Haynes, for one. He was a towering character comedian who, with scripts by Alf Garnett creator Johnny Speight, became as big a star as Tony Hancock and who, following his untimely death in 1966, aged fifty-two, was promptly confined to the archives. Although Terry had lived throughout Arthur's heyday he had never heard of him. He trusted me, though, and the name went into both our pads. Terry was determined to include Roy Kinnear, the roly-poly, sweating actor who could steal a scene with a perfectly timed glance. For me, Kinnear was anything but forgotten, but Terry reasoned that while he may not be forgotten he was misremembered. Kinnear was, he insisted, more than the one-trick pony the public thought he was. So he went on the list. There was Leslie Sarony too – another outrageous purveyor of glorious comic filth both as a solo turn and, with Leslie Holmes, as The Two Leslies. Terry's delight in once meeting Leslie Sarony was palpable. Sarony had been one of the very, very old commercial pirates in Terry Gilliam's *The Crimson Permanent Assurance* and, on set, Terry J. went into full fanboy mode. 'Sarony was so humble and nice and lovely,' he remembered. 'I don't think he could quite get over how thrilled I was to meet him. I had been listening to his records since I was a boy. And they were old even then!' So Leslie Sarony's name went on the list. And so it went on.

When it came to trying to find a publisher, none we approached cared very much for the title *Forgotten Heroes of Comedy* – 'if they are forgotten, who cares?', they would say. With that old, often-deployed bravado of Terry behind me, we stuck in our heels and refused to compromise. That was the title Terry wanted so that was the title the book would have. The pioneering publishing company Unbound came to the rescue. Terry was a champion of the firm, with one of his own books being the very first Unbound publication. That was *Evil Machines*, a typically sophisticated collection of young adult short stories featuring villainous motor-bikes, a truthful telephone, a Nice Bomb, and other terrifying objects. All of these stories ingeniously resolve into a novel. Terry's Evil Inventor even deploys Search Engines – actual engines who search for people. All of which was testament to his eager grasp of the fledgling world of the internet and emails and even a Twitter account @PythonJones. As such Terry was ideal as the spokesman for Unbound. A publisher with a fresh idea. That of putting the power of reading back in the hands of the reader – books would be sponsored by those people who wanted to read them, rather than the publisher taking a punt on the books they thought people would want to read. Unbound's titles relied on a readership pledging financial support and being printed once enough money had been raised. Like communism this was a great idea in principle, though it was later less successful in practice. However, *Forgotten Heroes of Comedy* did emerge, although sadly Terry didn't live to see the completed book. He knew it was happening, though, and saw some of the proof pages. The fact that our authors' residuals would not even cover a pint, let alone a celebratory, slap-up dinner, was and is a moot one. The book was the thing. Writing was the thing. Swapping ideas, working together over pints in his favourite pub and having a jolly good time – that was most certainly the thing.

# CHAPTER FOURTEEN
## PRESSING THE RESET BUTTON

*It doesn't worry me what anyone says,*
*except when publicity hurts others.*

TERRY was a wonderful friend and cherished those he loved deeply, but being close to him was not without its challenges and those in his intimate circle could find their patience tested. Certainly, ever uncompromising as he was, Terry was prone to making choices that would make his own life difficult, as well as vexing or even hurting those around him.

Some struggled with his forthright honesty and his need to be open about almost everything. For Michael Palin, who had been a close friend of Alison and Terry as a couple ever since they had got together, it could become awkward: 'Terry used to talk a lot about sex and I used to find it a bit much after a while, to be honest. Terry had this need to be honest about everything. I would say: "Oh come on!" It all got a bit boring . . . Anyway, he loved Al and that was that. They were a great couple and Helen and I had many good times with them, but there were definitely other people who Terry would become fond of. Terry's little dalliances.'

Both Terry and Alison were candid about the openness of their relationship. Terry much more so than Alison, although conversations about the arrangement would take place with close friends, including Annabel Leventon: 'It was fairly common knowledge. I could never quite understand it myself, but Terry told me this had been the understanding before they got married and carried on after they got married. Alison certainly seemed more reticent about it than Terry was. I remember once having dinner with them and Terry was preparing to go off on a book tour of Australia. Quite innocently, I said to Alison, "Oh, are you going too?" And she said: "No, no I'm not!" I said, "Why not?", and Alison, quite coy, said, "Well, he's taking a little friend with him!"'

There were quite a few little friends along the way – and then one who became much more than that. Swedish-born Anna Söderström had come to England, in 2002, as a nineteen-year-old to study modern language at Hertford College, Oxford. Terry had just turned sixty when they met, as Anna remembers: 'It was my second year at Oxford and Terry came to Cherwell College to give his *Who Murdered Chaucer?* talk. We met at the book signing afterwards.' Anna was beautiful and intelligent, and they were in Oxford, the place where, forty years earlier, Terry had been beautiful and intelligent. Terry rediscovered his lost youth.

According to Michael Palin: 'How can I say it? Terry had quite a number of physical relationships and, of course, with Terry, he was a nice bloke and I think those physical relationships turned into something a little more complex if he was not careful. And that's what happened when he met Anna.'

Annabel Leventon reflects: 'Anna wanted a father figure . . . and got Terry. She was quite open about it. She had been so in love with Monty Python. She would have been happy with any one of them! Terry was the one.'

One day, Terry asked Michael to meet Anna over lunch. This was very unusual and Michael was not comfortable with the situation: 'Anna was clearly a fan and the atmosphere changed slightly, as it has to do when someone from outside comes in. You are just that little bit more guarded about what you say.' Terry was obviously in a much more serious kind of relationship than Michael had ever seen before: 'Basically, Anna had moved in and wasn't going to move out of Terry's life.' Michael personally felt that Terry acted a bit irresponsibly. He should have said 'No' to certain things that Anna wanted him to do. Michael honestly didn't think Terry wanted to leave Alison. He describes how Terry was always quite vague. He would say, 'Oh, Mike, I still love Alison but it's how it is!', but it got to a certain point when the relationship with Anna became so all-encompassing that Alison was getting squeezed out.

Before Anna, it had been a case of Alison turning a blind eye. And, at the very beginning, Anna was perceived as just another one of Terry's 'little friends'. Still, as Michael says: 'it increasingly became an exclusive relationship. Terry's affair with Anna grew and grew. There was an intensity there that, one knew, would end up meaning one side or the other was going to suffer.' It was Alison in the end. When it got to the stage when Terry decided he was going to move out of the family home, Michael couldn't believe it: 'It was so unlike Terry. But that relationship with Anna was in a different league and once he moved out it was inevitable that his relationship with Alison would completely break down.' Terry left Grove Park in April 2005, clutching his most precious books and personal effects, and moved into rented accommodation at the little 'White House', in Highgate. At the time, Anna was still at Oxford.

As with the break-up of any couple of many years' standing, it proved sad and troublesome for the circle of friends they shared. For Michael Palin: 'I absolutely didn't want to lose contact with Alison, and there was no reason why we should.' Michael's wife, Helen, was a good friend of Alison's, often getting together with her and Maggie Gilliam. For most, there was no question of suddenly withdrawing oneself in favour of an allegiance to Terry, or putting that friendship with Alison aside. Michael knew Terry didn't really want that, in any case. This was the complicated thing. Terry became a bit lost in the middle. At the same time, Terry was Michael's friend and Michael could never say, 'Well, I don't want to meet this woman who you are moving in with.' So Michael always kept both doors open.

Michael would provide a bridge between Terry and his past, as would Alison's sister Kate Hepburn, who kept in touch with Terry. Both Michael and Kate would be frequent dinner guests at the new home that Terry had bought in 2005. A little over a year later, in 2006, Terry and Anna moved into the house known as the Hexagon, in Highgate, a 1960s design wonder by architect Leonard Michaels. Michael Palin explains that: 'I was still extremely fond of Terry. He had taken a certain course, and as a good friend I had to try and understand that. And try to understand what the reasons were for it, and, to a certain extent, go along with it, but at the same time making sure that I was somehow sticking up for Alison. It was all very complicated.'

Walking such a tightrope in order to keep everybody happy was indeed difficult, and sometimes painful. With hindsight, the increased argumentativeness; the harking back to his halcyon days at Oxford; that forgetfulness and food envy; and the oversharing of personal, even intimate information are all pointers to the dementia that would plague Terry's last few years. He had always been open with friends about his lifestyle, and it was very much in keeping with the way he had approached everything, but now he would often take complete strangers into his confidence. If he was having an affair, he was quite intense about it. During the party for Michael Palin's sixtieth birthday in 2003, there was a good mix of showbiz people and Helen's friends, one of whom was called Bernadette. Her husband was a very nice man who made pool tables. During the party, he said to Michael: 'I went to the loo and Terry Jones was there next to me and he went off for about ten minutes telling me all about this affair he was having and how difficult it was becoming for him. And what sort of situation he was in!' Quite reasonably, he didn't quite know what to say. He had never spoken to Terry before – about anything – and this was Terry's opening gambit! Terry needed to unload himself. Like everything else he did, he wanted to be honest with people. He would be honestly angry. He would be honestly happy. He would be honestly honest.

As Annabel Leventon says: 'In a perfect world, your actions wouldn't affect the legacy, or the family or anything, but we all have weak spots. And Terry's weak spot was a pretty face.'

There was also a lot of the student about Anna. Not only was she attractive and young, she was also fiercely intelligent. Terry would often compare his own intellect, unfavourably, with Anna's: 'We debate about everything all the time. And I can never win. Anna is the most perceptive and incisive of companions.' More importantly still, for Terry, Anna would be a partner who would, on occasions, work alongside him as an equal collaborator. Each would have their own creative projects, but the most ambitious they did together was *Evil Machines*, a nightmarish musical comedy based upon the book that was, at the time, languishing in his bottom drawer, waiting for the right publisher. In this theatrical reimagining of *Evil Machines*, a vacuum cleaner – 'there's no one meaner!' – and parking meters from hell sang opera . . . in Portuguese. The stage presentation of *Evil Machines* was a 2007 collaboration with Lisbon composer Luís Tinoco and a sixty-piece orchestra. Terry and Anna wrote the book for the performance, and journeyed to Portugal to oversee the production, which Terry directed. *Evil Machines* premiered in January 2008.

However, Terry and Anna's most precious collaboration would come in September 2009 when, as proof of his vitality and satisfaction of her desire to become a mother, their daughter, Siri, was born. Their new family unit was complete. Terry was joyful and full of optimism. He was tremendously excited about becoming a father again, at the age of sixty-seven, but he was also very calm at the prospect. He had done it all before, after all. Siri was born in the University College Hospital, just after eight o'clock in the evening. Terry was present at the birth and afterwards promptly nipped round to Charlotte Street for a pint and a curry to celebrate. He got recognised by a group of lads out for a drink, and got talking with them. Terry explained that he had just become a father again, and the men enthusiastically wetted the baby's head. A unique and unorthodox dad, ten weeks later, while Anna was still in recovery, Terry would stride into his local pub, with Siri in his arms, and order his usual pint at the bar.

For Terry, family was important and work was vital. When he was diligently writing at his desk every day and Siri crawled in to see him, he would stop work, play with her, and eagerly show her his favourite live performances of the Beatles on YouTube. There would be trips to the zoo too, but family holidays would never be compromised to cater for a small child. Terry would want to treat Siri like everybody else: here is the world. Isn't it fabulous? Savour everything. While he was undoubtedly a loveable and loving man, Terry was six parts selfishness and six parts pacifist. He wanted life and his work on his own terms, but he really didn't want to hurt anybody's feelings either. That's a balance that is simply impossible a lot of the time.

Daughter Sally concludes: 'It took me years to realise that Dad was not an empathetic man. He had great sympathy for people in difficult situations. He was always giving money to homeless people. People like that would really tug at his heartstrings, but he could never put himself in other people's shoes. He couldn't seem to understand why somebody had a problem with something because he couldn't see the problem. He just couldn't understand it from their perspective. He could be sympathetic but he couldn't understand it and thus wouldn't do anything about it.'

Terry certainly didn't want to hurt the feelings of his family, but he was obviously aware of the rifts and arguments and brickbats that were flying around when he set up home with Anna and then had a baby. Anna, who was twenty-six at the time of Siri's birth, was a source of controversy in the media too, as Terry was fully aware. Not only because of the forty-year age gap but also because of the fact that he had left the family home he had set up with Alison forty years before. Terry wasn't hurt by comments in the newspapers but he was upset when those stories hurt people close to him – certainly, the estranged wife and family at the heart of the story. Terry himself faced criticism from the press with confidence and stoicism, even when he was being called out as selfish, particularly in light of having a new child as he fast approached seventy. Terry countered with heartfelt comments, such as: 'I honestly don't think people who have children are acting selfishly or unselfishly. Having a child who will be loved, to parents who love each other, is the most important thing.' And, 'I have a reasonable chance of living another twenty years, and really hope I do!' When annoyed by reporters in the past, Terry had generally always been able to muster the patience to give them a polite and firm answer. That filter was still in place – just about.

However, at one point Terry appeared to consider playing the tabloid journalists at their own game and making a few quid out of the situation too. After a few pints one evening, he seriously suggested I get in touch with one of my contacts at the *Sun* or the *Daily Mail* and leak some details about being a dad again. All from the reliable source of an 'inner circle friend'. 'We'll split the money and have a lovely lunch on them!' he chuckled. We soon thought better of it. To poke that particular beast and get in bed with that type of journalist would start something we might soon lose control of. That these foolish notions could pop into Terry's head and seriously sit there and permeate for an hour or two was part of his world getting a bit unfocused, a bit cloudy.

Even as forthright as he always was and with his inherent predisposition to send up authority, Terry's antics had usually stayed on the right side of amusing. However, even before the move to Highgate there were signs that some of the silliness was starting to get out of hand. Michael Foreman's wife, Louise, relished Terry's company, though she remembers that the playfulness would sometimes go a little too far: 'we had been to a film premiere one evening and Terry was literally fighting this bollard in the street. The police politely told him to put it down. He would do that sort of thing, though. Going against authority without a care in the world. Finding humour in everything.'

The other issue was that the older Terry got the more any mild criticism would make him very angry. Even while he was still living in Camberwell with Alison, the cracks had begun to show. Publisher Colin Webb remembers one of those dinners at Grove Park: 'There was a poor bloke, who I'd never met before, but Terry took great exception to whatever this chap was saying and became incredibly passionate – even standing on the dining room table to make his point!' Alison Telfer recalls that the dinner parties became more frequent, Terry keener than ever to socialise, and yet he 'would tend more and more to argue. There was one point when basically every dinner party would include one of these moments when he was so angry he would have to get up and leave the table. His chair would fall over backwards and he would have to go out of the house and walk round the block for a few minutes to calm down. It got to the point when I was thinking "Oh, just go!"'

This continued after Alison and Terry split up and Terry moved in with Anna. 'The dinner parties got out of hand,' Anna remembers. 'When Terry and I had Siri, I would long for a few evenings with just the three of us, as a family, but Terry would always greet me with a long list of people who were arriving for dinner. It wouldn't be an exaggeration to say we hosted literally thousands of dinner parties in that time. We were invited out to hundreds but only accepted five or six times over all that time. Terry was suspicious of other people's choices of wine and other people's home cooking.' Indeed, Terry was only keen to eat out when it was at one of his London clubs. The Groucho; Black's; or his absolute favourite, the Two Brydges. Terry even fast-tracked a membership for me. Like him, I was very much at ease in a cosy pub or a members' club. Anna remembers once taking Terry to a wine bar: 'He looked at me as if to say, "Why? We could host a dinner party at home ..." but he went along with it, for me. He put one foot inside this wine bar and his face dropped. He just looked so dejected; so lost. We left straight away.' Me and Terry did step out of our comfort zone once though, when we stepped out to go Zumba dancing. It was one of Anna's passions, and one evening Terry and I joined her. We all got very hot and very happy. Never again though! Even though Terry was too exhilarated to get very cross that evening.

Terry's increasingly strong opinions were best kept in print. He was safest and happiest when writing thoughts down to be published for a quick profit and a swift release of the safety valve. He had written a collection of articles for the *Young Guardian*, from April 1987 to May 1988, the age of American president Ronald Reagan and British prime minister Margaret Thatcher. In the articles, Terry pontificated on subjects ranging from the poll tax to nuclear energy. A selection of these would be published as the book *Attacks of Opinion*, while the similarly earnest *Terry Jones's War on the War on Terror* was published by Nation Books for Christmas 2004, nearly a year after the start of the second Gulf War. As if to prove that Terry had not mellowed but just got more angry, it recorded his forthright and fiery thoughts of such 'ludicrous concepts' as a War on Terror: 'How do you wage war on an abstract noun? How do you know when you've won? When you've got it removed from the *Oxford English Dictionary*?' His targets were the chief players in this theatre of war: American president George W. Bush and British prime minister Tony Blair. Indeed, Terry would go so far as to support the movement to impeach Blair in the aftermath of the Gulf War.

Newspaper articles and published anthologies were the perfect way to get his thoughts out in the open, and channel that frustration and anger away from guests at his dinner parties. The written word was the way to soothe Terry's volatile temper. A skilful way of turning his explosive crossness into creativity. Still, old friends, such as Michael Palin, rather enjoyed pressing Terry's buttons. It was getting easier and easier to get a reaction: 'I would just prompt Terry by saying, "I think the Americans have got it right . . ." and he would explode: "The Americans!!" And I would say: "Yeah, well you know it's a democracy . . ." "Mike! Democracy!! That's the worst fucking thing . . . Democracy is useless . . ." and on and on he would go. Terry would get terribly angry. And throw things about. It would amuse me. Then he would instantly calm down and say, "I'm sorry, Mike. I got rather over-excited there!" So he would fly off the handle very easily. About things he had no control over.' I dread to think what he would have been like if he had lived through Covid and Boris Johnson and all that.

The Hexagon, the house that Terry and Anna made their home in leafy Highgate, was threatened soon after they had moved in by local developers' plans. The pages of the *Ham & High* local newspaper were full of it. And so was Terry. Millamant, the Isle of Man-based property development company, had been granted permission to raze the houses on the eighteenth-century estate of Fitzroy Farm, in Fitzroy Park, to the ground and construct a neoclassical home, three times the size of the demolished property. The new construction would also include a two-storey basement, with swimming pool, and would radically change the look and feel of Fitzroy Park. This was Terry's new manor, and he joined pressure groups and campaign meetings to try to stop the development. Moreover, he would use it as a source of comedy. The inspiration to write. *Trouble on the Heath*, his final completed novel – and his only work of fiction for adults – was born out of this same frustration and anger.

It was published by Accent Press Limited, in February 2011, as

part of the Quick Reads initiative to encourage literacy in adults
– an initiative that, for all his faults, had been spearheaded by
Tony Blair. More importantly to Terry, it was sponsored by the
Books Council of Wales. *Trouble on the Heath*, as the blurb
reveals, is: 'a comedy of Russian gangsters, town planners and a
dog called Nigel.' Our hapless hero is Malcolm Thomas, who is
horrified to find that his favourite view, from his dog's favourite
tree on Hampstead Heath, is about to be blocked and ruined by
– yes, you guessed it, the demolition of a property and the erec-
tion of a massive new house. His decision to take action creates
multiple comic complications as he encounters characters such
as corrupt town planners, violent gangsters and a kidnapped
concert pianist. The back cover copy promises a 'hilarious story'
that 'will make you laugh out loud', and is very much Terry
following the advice that you should always write about something you know. Well, apart from the violent gangsters and the
kidnapped concert pianist, of course. That was all from Terry's
fantastic, fevered imagination. Still, the character of Malcolm –
married to Angela, with a young son, Freddie – is very much
Terry himself. Malcolm is even a medieval historian – he rifles
through his knowledge of the Siege of Syracuse, the Siege of
Alexandria and the Siege of Troy to save the day. Terry's dog was
called Nancy rather than the nod to Terry's dead brother, Nigel,
but he certainly walked her on the Heath. And she was very
partial to the home-made sausage rolls in one of Terry's locals,
the Red Lion & Sun.

In the year that Monty Python turned forty, and Terry became
a dad again, he made what would be the first of three series of a
kids' show, *The Legend of Dick and Dom*, with popular slapstick
children's presenters Richard McCourt and Dominic Wood. This
was medieval history sliced up and served to children, to teach
them about the past and make them laugh. It was perfect for Terry
and he was absolutely aware of why he was cast as the wise but

sardonic narrator: 'They are great comics, those two, but Steve Ryde, the producer, wanted something or somebody who could link it all to *Monty Python and the Holy Grail*. And I was available. Great fun to do, though.'

The spectre of Python was never far away. Indeed, there often comes a time in the life of a prominent person when you become a character in a biographical film, and for Terry this time came in 2011. *Holy Flying Circus* was made for the BBC and written by Tony Roche, who also worked on the BBC comedy *The Thick of It* and would go on to write for *Succession*, HBO's smash hit. The one-off, ninety-minute TV film *Holy Flying Circus* is the story of the Pythons, though mainly centred around the controversy of *Life of Brian*, and the fraught appearance of John Cleese and Michael Palin (played by Darren Boyd and Charles Edwards) on the BBC2 discussion panel show *Friday Night, Saturday Morning*. *Holy Flying Circus* is anarchic and silly. Asking questions about free speech and whether people have the right not to be 'offended' by what they are shown, it uses plenty of comedic and dramatic devices that pay homage to the style of Monty Python.

Terry had been sent a preview disc to watch shortly before it aired on TV but decided to wait for a scheduled dinner date with me. This just so happened to be the day it was to be broadcast on television – Wednesday 19 October 2011, to be precise. We watched it, a few hours ahead of the BBC transmission, in order to be able to nip out for a few real ales and a bite to eat and to discuss it in convivial circumstances while the nation tuned in to watch it at home. There was much to discuss, in particular the performance of Rufus Jones as Terry. For Rufus, it was an 'awesome responsibility and the job of a lifetime to enter that booby-trap-filled Pythonic space. Terry's unique gumbo of intellectualism, sexiness, silliness and Welsh passion was an absolute performance playground to be in.' Not only was it brilliant throughout, there was a wonderfully cheeky moment where the characters of Michael and Helen Palin share a bedroom conversation. As was Terry's wont, this scene cast Rufus – in drag – as Helen. Not only was it a wonderful nod to Terry's penchant for playing women, it was awfully perceptive. For Michael and Terry's writing relationship and friendship was very much like a marriage. However, rather than pondering that deep dive into his bond with Palin, at this moment the real Terry paused the DVD player, squinted his eyes, then turned to me and said: 'That *is* me, isn't it?' Rufus was that good, that uncannily like the real Terry. Particularly in drag!

Over pints and dinner, Terry asked me if I could arrange a meeting with Rufus. A summit between Jones and Jones. I didn't know Rufus at the time, but we had exchanged a few comments on Twitter, so I direct-messaged him to say I was with Terry and that we had just seen *Holy Flying Circus*. This was something like an hour before the transmission on television. Rufus was initially petrified about Terry's reaction. I reassured him that Terry had loved it, and a meeting was arranged. Rufus recalls Terry being 'so sweet about my performance – generous, engaged, effusive.' Barry Cryer came along too, and much Grolsch beer was consumed. It was quite the comedy conclave. For Rufus, 'a warmer, more drunken and gossipy night in Highgate I could never have imagined.'

Terry also returned to the world of opera in 2011, collaborating with Oscar-winning composer Anne Dudley for a Royal Opera commission. Terry's contribution was a musical presentation of 'The Doctor's Tale', based upon 'The Good Doctor', his favourite story about the medical dog from his collection of children's stories, *Animal Tales*. The Royal Opera was delighted and so, the following year, Terry was asked to work with Anne Dudley once more, on an operatic staging of Edward Lear's *The Owl and the Pussycat*. Rather than adapting the original, Terry wrote an origins story: 'What interested me was how they got together,' he said. 'There must have been *some* tension.' At the end of the piece they did indeed jump into that famous pea-green boat, but the bulk of the opera dealt with the couple's exile from society, how everyone condemned their bizarre, cross-species love affair. The performance was staged as part of *Secrets*, a Hidden London project under the direction of opera theatre-maker Martin Constantine, which had the aim of putting on free shows that anyone could access and enjoy, outdoors and away from more formal performance spaces. An approach and ethos that appealed to Terry very much. Terry's opera was staged at the end of July 2012, along London's waterways, at Little Venice, Graham Street Gardens and Mile End.

That February, Terry had turned seventy years of age. It was also the year that his separation from Alison became final, in a divorce arrangement. Almost immediately afterwards, he married Anna, in a very quiet ceremony attended only by his new family and his new next-door neighbours. But 2012 was also the year that something very odd seemed to be happening to Terry.

His vagueness, affability and absent-mindedness had been part of his cerebral make-up for decades, but now not only did his temper seem ever more fragile, so did his memory. One evening, before Terry and I wandered off to the pub, Anna gave me a notepad. The pub we were going to was the Red Lion & Sun, where we had jotted down all those hundreds of names for the *Forgotten Heroes of Comedy* book. And the notepad was pretty much identical too. But this was no fun project. Anna and Terry were both concerned. He had started increasingly to lose track of conversations, to forget the names of the most everyday of objects. My mission, that evening, was to record any moments where Terry struggled for a word or a thought. Over a few pints, this happened once, maybe twice, and I duly jotted it down.

Over the following months, it got worse. Family and friends noticed it, of course, but it wasn't until that major Monty Python reunion, at the O2 in 2014, that the public started to become aware. Terry was thrilled to be an active Python again. Just so long as he could remember the words to 'Crunchy Frog' . . . The sketch's intricate list of confectionery ingredients had always been something of a minefield and a mouthful. Now, it was getting further and further out of Terry's reach. So much so that he wrote down his dialogue on the inside lid of the chocolate box. A comedy prop that John Cleese would, on occasions, take great delight in throwing across the stage mid-sketch. Not out of malice but sheer playfulness. Terry didn't see the joke.

It wasn't the only routine that was troubling Terry. After the initial hoo-hah of actually seeing the five surviving Pythons together again on stage, which even featured a moment for the audience to take photographs as the team posed, the O2 concerts really kicked off with the 'Four Yorkshiremen' sketch. Now, as any student of comedy knows, this classic deconstruction of northern one-upmanship is not a Monty Python original. It was written, it's true, by Graham Chapman and John Cleese, but also by Marty Feldman and Tim Brooke-Taylor, and originally performed for the 1967 television sketch series *At Last the 1948 Show*. But the sketch had long been considered a Monty Python property, much to the annoyance of Tim Brooke-Taylor, who would be present and justifiably lauded at the last night of the O2 run. Suffice to say, Terry had performed the 'Four Yorkshiremen' sketch many times on stage. Now, however, it was a skit that just refused to stay firmly in his brain.

In between the first five performances and the last five performances of the run there was a ten-day gap (necessitated, much to director Eric Idle's chagrin, by the fact that Robbie Williams had booked the venue for a string of gigs). This break was a blessed relief for Terry, who needed a breather. It gave him a moment to pause, to reflect, to analyse. He asked if I could meet up and talk about his concerns.

For once, I arrived at the pub before Terry, but within minutes the familiar dapper figure ambled in and placed a hand on my shoulder. We started going over the lines: me giving him the three feeds that, on the O2 stage, would come from John, Eric and Michael. The words were there, in Terry's head. It was just that they were coming out wrong. From out of a fog or, worse still, not coming out at all. Terry's anxiety was heightened because, he said, now *all* the sketches in the show were getting fuzzy. He had always been a quick study on lines of dialogue. No longer.

The obvious solution was to write certain long speeches on idiot boards over the heads of the audience in the auditorium, or on scraps of paper, even, concealed in pockets and folds of skirts (Terry was occasionally in drag again for the O2 shows). He could then just look out into the crowd or look down, and simply read out loud. But Terry was determined not to do that. He didn't want them as a reassuring backup either. He didn't want them at all. He wanted to learn the lines. Or re-learn them.

Terry's reaction to his failing memory, that afternoon in the pub, was not anger but frustration. He was struggling to come to terms with the fact that the words simply were not there. For they weren't. He closed his eyes. Tight. Scrunched up the fist of his right hand and tapped, rather than banged, his forehead. 'I know it,' he said. 'I know it. I know it.' Three times he said it, then he opened his eyes and asked the question: 'Don't I?'

The first line of defence for dementia is, sadly, denial. It's all you have. At first. In an attempt to gee him up, and foolishly thinking I might magically bring the words back to him, I said: 'Of course you know it, Terry. You know it. You know you do!'

He smiled ruefully and muttered, 'I know I know it, but, Rob, you don't understand. Every time I try to say those words, I look out to see twenty thousand faces looking back at me. Twenty thousand people who know them better than I do!'

In the end, it was those very people, those fabulous Python fans, who got Terry through those concerts, on a wave of nostalgia and pure love. The Python team too – Terry's fellow four survivors and the ever-glamorous Carol Cleveland – now, after the break from performance, fully aware something was wrong, rallied round and supported Terry through those last five shows. Despite the concerns for Terry, they had a whale of a time working together again. You could just tell. The Pythons never lost that spirit of being funny in each other's company. They still haven't. There is a tangible joy when they hang out. Terry's tiredness and confusion notwithstanding, he revelled in the riot of fun, the company of old cohorts and that colossal sea of comedy connoisseurs.

Though he was unable fully to enjoy the experience, as David Wood testifies: 'My wife Jackie and I had been invited by Terry to go over to Highgate for lunch. One or two of his emails of late had just begun to be a bit odd. This was a Sunday and we arrived and Terry came to the door and apologised for the fact that Anna wasn't there because she was doing a stall selling the loom-knitted scarves and children's clothes she was making. Terry had forgotten that she was doing it, so he was doing the meal. A few other people then came and he did very well. Then afterwards, he said let's go for a walk. It was during that walk on Hampstead Health that we two were separated from the rest of the party. When we were alone, Terry suddenly sighed and said: "Oh David, David, David! Oh David, David, David, David . . ." I tried to get him to chat and said, "So, how was the O2?" because that had only been a few weeks before. He said: "Oh, all right. I couldn't remember things and the more I couldn't remember the more they laughed! The more they enjoyed it." This really bothered him. He reflected that maybe they shouldn't have done it. The reputation of Python meant so much to him. And, going all the way back to Oxford, he had always been so serious and so passionate about his work. He was worried and upset but he wanted to work. He could feel himself losing hold of the reins of what he was doing. It was terribly sad.'

Hot on the heels of the O2 reunion came plans for the fortieth anniversary of *Monty Python and the Holy Grail*. The film was to enjoy a limited re-release in cinemas and a new trailer was put together for the occasion. André Jacquemin was, of course, in the recording studio: 'That promo was the last thing we did together. We had a session booked but Terry wasn't performing terribly well. His comedy wasn't happening quite how it should have been. I knew, intimately, how Terry would work and what he was capable of in the studio . . . and this was well below his standards, for sure. The guys I was working with were quite happy with it, but I said: "No! It's not good enough." I knew Terry wouldn't be happy with it and, as a result, I wasn't happy with it. I said: "I can't have this going out like this." It was a bit embarrassing . . . to my ear. People – the diehard fans – would have thought: "What's the matter with Terry?" In the end, I edited together a few bits that Terry had done really well and then I asked Mike Palin to come in and fill in the bits that Terry had not sounded right on. Mike, of course, under-stood completely and happily came in, and it worked out well. That was the unspoken bond between those two. I remember saying to Mike: "Look, if we have anything that we need to do, we have to do it now. It's not going to get any better." Basically, we would have to write off Terry, and new Python stuff, from that point. I knew it, and Mike knew it. Mike, being lovely as always, didn't want to put Terry through any more stress than was neces-sary, so that was that. Terry's last little bit of Python. I'm just so pleased that between the three of us we cobbled it together and it sounds really good. It's a lovely farewell from Terry, with a little help from his best friend and me.'

Whatever was happening in his brain, though, Terry was still determined to work. Moreover, there was panic and a need to earn money. He had a young family to support. With a little more help from his friends he could both capitalise on the popularity of Monty Python and keep his and the brand's integrity. Kim 'Howard' Johnson recalls that: 'Terry would try to get over to the annual Medieval Festival in Michigan, so I suggested we do some shows. We would screen *Monty Python and the Holy Grail*, and I would interview Terry after the screening. There would be a long line of people wanting autographs and Terry could make some good money. We did that several times. In New York too. Talking about his writing of comedy, performing a few scenes from the Python films. They proved very successful.' Although it was inevitably increasingly difficult, what with Terry's ever-worsening condition.

His desire to be creative, that palpable need to write – and the buzz he got from collaboration – saw him embark on one final project. It was an extant biography I'd written that inspired what would prove to be that final burst of creativity. Terry had read my book on Marty Feldman with interest – I had also interviewed him for it – and surmised that there was much more to say about the profound relationship between Marty and his power-behind-the-comedy-throne wife Lauretta. My favoured title for the autobiography had always been *Jeepers Creepers*, like the song, with its lyrics asking, 'Where'd you get those eyes?' Those eyes that had proved Marty's unique selling point in comedy. Lacking the dogged stubbornness of Terry, I abandoned that title when the publisher didn't like it. Terry, however, loved the title. He said: 'You should write a play. Just about Marty and Lauretta. Call it *Jeepers Creepers*. And I'll direct it!' So, the seed was sown. Martin Witts, of the Leicester Square Theatre, agreed to produce and all was set.

Terry's ability to nail down those thoughts in his head were getting worse and worse, though, and it could no longer be ignored. An NHS appointment was made and Terry's case was assigned to Professor Nick Fox, who remembers the referral letter very well: 'I've never had a referral letter like it before or since. It said: "Would you see this much-loved Python . . ." Having loved Terry's work, and their work, I felt it was a tremendous privilege and a huge responsibility to try and do the best for him. It is subtle and insidious. It is a steady decline. That agony of not knowing.

Just that something isn't right. The way Terry described it to me was that he was "empty of thoughts". Anna explained that he was finding it difficult to start sentences and then, once he had started, he found it difficult to find the words to finish them.'

Professor Fox gave Terry a brain scan, although he already had his suspicions of what the problem might be, but: 'I try not to be presumptuous about the information the patient may want. Terry was reticent to hear my initial thoughts and wanted to wait and see what the tests showed.'

Anna recalls: 'I went with Terry to see the neurologist. I remember the date. How could I forget it? Monday 14 September 2015. Terry was diagnosed with frontotemporal dementia. At that time, they could give no indication of what to expect, other than it was a progressive condition. It was only going to get worse. Typically, Terry was quite cheerful. He was always optimistic about the future. He did get very sad at the thought of not being able to direct *Jeepers Creepers*. We talked about it a lot. He so liked the play, and he so wanted to direct it.'

The decision was made that Martin Witts would take Terry, Anna and me to lunch. Terry's favoured way of addressing an issue. The plan was to ascertain whether Terry was match-fit for the job, so we asked him whether he still wanted to direct *Jeepers Creepers* and whether he thought he could. Terry was upbeat and firm: 'I want to direct this play, Martin. And I know I can.' Hands were shaken, contracts were signed. We were on. Bangor-born Meurig Wyn Jones, better known as writer and actor David Barry, who played Frankie Abbott in the sitcoms *Please Sir!* and *The Fenn Street Gang*, was also signed up as an assistant director and a safeguard. 'I was there just to help Terry along. He was clearly unwell, but he was still an incisive, and clever, director,' David remembers. 'He would spark with comedy ideas and, although he wasn't at the top of his game any more, there were still flashes of brilliance. One would just sit back and marvel. The entire company loved him.'

Indeed, Terry was the most generous and affable of company leaders. He remained positive and charming throughout, joined the cast and crew in the pub practically every night, and coaxed and reassured the actors through the ups and downs of rehearsal and performance.

*Jeepers Creepers*, a two-hander starring David Boyle as Marty and Rebecca Vaughan as Lauretta, was staged in the studio space at the Leicester Square Theatre, for a limited four-week run from 18 January 2016. Michael Palin was on board to record a cameo as a radio announcer, reporting on the death of Marty Feldman at the end of the play: 'I had a lot of respect for Marty. And Terry, of course. That horrible dementia was beginning to mess him around though. He was becoming more and more cross and bitter about it.'

Terry's diagnosis had now been clarified, to the more specific primary progressive aphasia, one of the rarer forms of dementia. As Professor Nick Fox remarks: 'True to form, Terry didn't have a common-or-garden variant. But let me break down that doctor-speak. Progressive is obvious. It was only going to get worse and there was nothing we could do about that. The aphasia bit means it was affecting Terry's ability to use language. It is not forgetfulness but more the thought process of communication. The damaged cells were in that part of the brain that controls speech and language. The cells in that area were dying, and eventually it would affect his powers of planning and judgement.' Ultimately, clinical suspicions were confirmed: Terry's dementia was caused by damage to the tau protein in the part of the brain that affects the apparatus of language. It is one of the most neglected forms of dementia. If only it had neglected Terry.

Terry now knew that this rare form of dementia would ultimately kill him but, before that, it was going to eventually rob him of the ability to communicate, to process words and, yes, to write. That was, perhaps, the cruellest blow of all. The man who had written and spoken so many hilarious, insightful, clever words was being deprived of his incredible abilities, the things that made Terry Terry, in front of our eyes. A friend of mine with medical experience told me to prepare for it getting increasingly hard to watch a friend deteriorate and, most chillingly of all, said: 'You will lose him twice: once when the ability to communicate goes completely, and again when he passes away.' But, she assured me, 'if he is enjoying life and enjoying the challenge of work, cultivate that; enjoy it with him; be positive. It's the best thing to do.'

Terry was proud of the play and he loyally attended every single performance. Even on his seventy-fourth birthday. But already, he could no longer write. During rehearsals, he had been asked to write a piece about his friendship and admiration of Marty Feldman for the *Independent*. He quietly asked me if I could write it for him, from the many hours of interviews we had conducted for the Marty book. I agreed, but it was to be Terry's name on the byline. On the day after publication, someone in the rehearsal room said to Terry: 'I read the article, Terry. It was wonderful.' And without a blink, he said: 'No, Rob wrote that. Wasn't it great?' Bless him. I whispered: 'No . . . you are not supposed to tell people that!' Honest, to a fault.

Terry would not sanction an official press release about his diagnosis until after the run of *Jeepers Creepers*. Besides, he had a few more of his closest friends to tell first. Annabel Leventon remembers when he gave her the news: 'Terry was always so open. He looked so intensely at me and said: "Look, this is really bad news. I've got dementia and I can't write any more. I don't know what I'm going to do." I was so shocked. It was heartbreaking. I didn't know what he was going to do either. I just took his hand and reassured him that we would all be there for him.'

Although he was being asked to write and perform and direct, and offers for more theatre productions were already on the table, *Jeepers Creepers* was Terry's final professional engagement. Now, the truth had to be faced with dignity and honesty. It was the only way Terry could deal with it.

# CHAPTER FIFTEEN

## THE SILENT WORLD OF TERRY JONES

*One day my chair will be empty,*
*And the pen that I wag will be still,*
*And unless something big can prevent me,*
*I'll be under – not over – the hill.*

I T'S Tuesday afternoon. Lunchtime in a north London pub. An elderly man sits alone at a corner table, nursing a half pint of good ale. He's still got his Abercrombie & Fitch overcoat on – there are cold north-easterly winds blowing relentlessly outside – and he sports a natty silk paisley scarf. The grey hair is still curly and well cut. This is a gentleman. A man of distinction.

The handful of other drinkers may know him by sight. Some will have undoubtedly recognised him. He still looks like someone who is familiar to many from his decades-long television career. Still, no one bothers this elderly man. He looks a little lost.

This, now, is Terry Jones, internationally acclaimed founding member of the Monty Python team. It's the final act of a long and prolific life, following the cruellest twist. Like those north-easterly winds, the dementia is relentless, and has largely robbed him of speech. This most erudite and free-thinking of men is trapped within his own thoughts. And what thoughts: political debate, historical theory, comic genius . . .

It was into this scene that I walked. I had done it a hundred times or more. A rustic, welcoming boozer in town. With a chum in it. The most rustic and welcoming and intelligent and generous

347

person in my life. But the Terry Jones I knew had almost completely gone. No more the cheery greeting, the proffered drink, the off-centre grin, and the promise of an evening of good food and even better conversation.

That old Terry Jones was still there though, deep behind those vacant eyes and that bewildered expression. As I approached his table, Terry looked up. For a moment, the clouds parted. A reassuring spark of recognition was ignited in his doleful eyes. He opened his mouth to speak. Nothing came out, but the movement became a beaming smile, accompanied by an outstretched hand. Then it was gone. The elderly man with the lost look was back. The greatest prize of all had been there, though. Just for a moment. Terry had been pleased to see me and had been able to demonstrate that pleasure.

The close community of publicans and stall-owners and inhabitants of Highgate Village had taken Terry to their hearts. Each and every one of them looked out for him and looked after him. It was a tangible manifestation of something Terry had felt from the moment he had moved into the area a decade or so before: 'in a way it makes the world smaller, it makes it like a village. It's really how I felt the world always ought to be, where you feel you know people and people are interested in you. So, it's like a retreat into childhood really – when you're a baby everybody's interested in you and it's rather the same thing.'

The official statement had come in September 2016. And, with some sort of a sense of relief, Terry could now openly say to the press and anybody who seemed concerned, 'I've got dementia, you know. My frontal brain lobe has absconded!' That was the statement. Clean and simple, with a hint of resigned comedy about it. For Professor Nick Fox: 'the press release was just amazing. It was marvellous. Terry was a marvel. It showed that wit, even in that situation, and if he hadn't done it in that way, if he had said everything was all just so awful, he knew it would have damaged his unique position to do something positive for dementia patients and their loved ones.' So, if Terry had to face this condition, he was going to do it with resolve and determination and a smile on his face. For as long as possible, at least. And he was determined to be open about it. He wanted people to talk about dementia. He felt that if he could help, just a little bit, to dispel any mystery or stigma that surrounded the condition, it was the very least he could do. Nick Fox explains that: 'Terry was very clear about that, and I thought that was very admirable. There are many people who are famous, who for very understandable reasons would not want it to be known that they had any problems. He was very keen to raise awareness but also that there should be more research in this area. It was impressive that he thought beyond his own situation. He wanted to make it clear that not all dementia is the same, and it isn't a disease that exclusively affects the very old.'

Terry was keen to dispel this myth that dementia is just about getting a little forgetful. He wanted to get people talking about it, and everybody who knew him was impressed by his willingness to be open and try to help. If he had dementia and was coping with it, as best he could, then it might make other people think they could too. Terry knew that it is dementia's greatest strength. That fear of talking about it only makes the situation worse for everyone involved. Nick Fox was certainly impressed: 'Terry's openness about his condition was so very, very important. It was almost coming from a simpler place which is – these are bad things, what can I do to help? If I can raise awareness, if I can help with research, I will. It wasn't as complex or selfish as wanting to know more about it for himself. He wanted to know more about it so that others could know more about it.'

None more so than his youngest daughter, Siri, who was just turning seven. For Terry, it was a way to allow her to understand the impossible – that her beloved daddy would, invariably, fade further and further away. Terry's ever-increasing state of confusion could be worrying and distressing. And very unfair.

Terry became apt to do the most outrageous and unpredictable things: he would be struck by ridiculous thoughts in the middle of the night and fire off accusatory emails; while cooking he would forget the flame on the cooker hob was hot and could hurt you. This was all part of his slow dance with dementia, of course, and it was something that his many friends got used to. We even expected it. As his dearest friend Michael Palin puts it: 'Frontotemporal dementia may cause loss of inhibition, but Terry was never very inhibited in the first place!' That was a necessary humorous spin on the situation. A little Pythonesque reasoning from a fellow Python. Some of Terry's behaviour behind closed doors would have appeared very odd, even disturbing, to those not within that inner sanctum.

The love and devotion to Anna and Siri was paramount but, naturally, Terry also had Alison and Sally and Bill. Within his heart and soul Terry had that profound fondness and concern, although his frequent emails had now got far less frequent, and when they did come they were strained and disjointed. Bill recalls Terry: 'answering emails from four years ago . . . as if it was now.' As the condition worsened Alison recalls: 'I was working in Paris and, to be honest, Terry and I were barely speaking at that point. One of our mutual friends said: "You must see Terry! While he can still communicate." It was clearly getting more and more serious, so I sent him an email saying: "Would you like to meet up?"'

Terry was clearly thrilled. He fired out a reply immediately: 'Yes. Let's have lunch in the pub!' Alison remembers: 'Terry was sat there with a drink when I arrived, and the first clue that some-thing was very wrong was that, when I entered the restaurant, he didn't order me a drink!' That was completely unlike Terry. He ordered himself another beer and Alison had to go and order her own drink. Then Terry picked up the menu. When he ordered, he read precisely what was written down: 'I'll have the pâté with a little bit of parsley, cherry tomatoes and a slice of buttered bread.

And the lamb cutlet with new potatoes and green beans served with a mint sauce.' Well, you don't say that. You say: 'I'll have the pâté followed by the lamb.'

Daughter Sally had also spotted this precise manner of talking, the great concentration it seemed to take for Terry to communicate. At the dinner parties in Highgate: 'Dad just started talking less and less and less. Usually it had been Dad who started the conversations and kept them going. Increasingly, the other people round the table would do all the talking, and he just started to disappear a bit. He was answering or repeating what other people said.'

Nick Fox appreciates that this: 'non-frequency of language can embarrass people. It hurts to listen to them speak, because you feel for the effort they are making. You want to help them when they stop in mid-sentence. You feel it in your heart because it is painful. You want to help them out of their struggle but even this could make Terry frustrated or angry because you may offer the word you thought he was struggling for, and it would be the wrong word. Then he's completely stuffed because you have put him off track. Eventually the grammatical structure is gone, and Terry would be talking and writing in telegraphese – just short, terse, single words.' One of Terry's last emails to Alison read: 'I don't rest the times are broken.'

By the time the condition was affecting Terry's judgement it was, naturally enough, making his driving rather erratic. Sally remembers Terry driving her up to the pub one day, and, although he was driving perfectly well, she could feel that it was a bit reckless; there was just no hesitation, and Sally thought, 'Bloody hell! I'm not sure about this . . .' Shortly after that, Terry relinquished his driving licence.

In May 2013, Terry had introduced the BAFTA Fellowship and presented it to Michael Palin. At the time, Terry was suffering from a sore throat and Michael, while thanking him for the very kind words, joked that they sounded like they may be his final words.

On Sunday 2 October 2016, Mike was on hand to return the favour when Terry was honoured at the BAFTA Cymru Awards. It was in recognition of Terry's unique contribution to film and television, but this was clearly something of a farewell performance. Dressed in his finest black-tie regalia and looking fit and healthy, his frustrating struggle to communicate was clear to all, even if his smile could have lit a path from the venue to Chester. His son Bill accompanied him on stage. Sally recalls: 'Dad was going on stage and he indicated to me to go up with him too and I mouthed, "No, thanks!" Bill did a beautiful job.' He held Terry's hand, and acknowledged the standing ovation of the audience. From deep within his silent world, all Terry could say was 'Quiet down!' as the crowd refused to stop applauding. The twinkle was still there, even if the words were not. Bill, through the natural tears of such an emotional tribute, spoke on behalf of Terry, saying: 'We would like to thank everyone. I know it's a great honour for Dad to win this award.' Reflecting on the evening now, Bill, with his dad's twinkle and art of irreverence, jokes through his emotion that: 'I was a bit annoyed about that. I was looking at these wonderful Welsh BAFTAs they were giving out. The BAFTA Cymru. Beautiful. Then Dad, getting the lifetime achievement, got a normal BAFTA. I felt a bit short-changed! It was a terrific honour though.'

It was an honour from his people too. Terry knew he was home. Wales would give him great joy in those final months and years. Sally recalls taking him back on several occasions, when they did all the usual walks. It was a place of such familiarity to him, of course, but even through the dementia Terry knew where he was. Thankfully, at first it wasn't a form of dementia that resulted in a loss of your memory and your sense of self. He was still there and the memory was still there. He just couldn't retrieve the information or express himself.

Certainly, when Sally took Terry back to the cottage for the first time after the diagnosis and his clear deterioration, she was concerned that he would have forgotten the gloriously quirky layout of the place. Everybody new to the cottage is warned to duck their heads as they navigate the corridor to the loo. As she watched him walk down the corridor, Sally saw that Terry remembered to duck. She says, 'I can't tell you how happy that made us. He remembered. It's a very basic place. You spend all your time boiling water and stoking the fire, but Dad loved it.'

As the dementia took hold, Terry's emotions were heightened too. At Christmas 2016, when Terry heard the news of the death of actress Carrie Fisher, Sally recalls that he 'cried and cried. Uncontrollably. He was so upset. He was inconsolable. It was very sad, of course, but Dad was so affected by it. Disproportionately so. They hadn't been personal friends. It was just that his emotions were out of control.' So much so that the death of a family member in Wales was kept from him. Sally explains, 'We all felt it was something that Dad didn't need to know. We didn't want to upset him unnecessarily.'

It was not long before Terry was completely robbed of his powers of speech. He could acknowledge only with whimpers and whines. The words would not form but the emotions were there. Like a mime artist. A silent comedy hero. Terry's comedy legacy and comedy roots. It made his obsessive rewatching of his favourite silent comedians all the more profound. There he would sit, in his screening room at home at the Hexagon, playing masterworks like *The Gold Rush*, *Long Pants*, *Safety Last!* and *The General*. Chaplin, Langdon, Lloyd and Keaton as unable to speak in those comedy films as Terry was unable to speak in life. Terry's own facial expression became more and more of a 'Great Stoneface', unable to express the emotions that were playing out in that locked-up brain of his. Often, the only person who could make him crack a smile was the real Great Stoneface, his ultimate comedy hero Buster Keaton.

One would sit with him, gazing up at these flickering shadows, these comedic ghosts from a century before. Terry's hand would take yours and gently squeeze at a moment he felt was particularly moving or particularly mirthful. His eyes would fill with tears – of sadness or joy or simply because he could not vocalise the fun he was having. His face would light up in silent rapture. To enter the silent world of Terry Jones was a privilege. But a heartbreaking one.

Anna sent out the call to his friends to provide fresh entertainment. She remembers, 'Terry was watching a lot of films at home and was going through our DVD library so quickly! You, Rob, were top of my list. You came round to have a good look at our film collection and see what we were missing. I knew you were the expert on Terry's taste, and it meant so much to his quality of life to have films he would love.'

To that end, I went armed with old films. Comedies and musicals were what was required. And I had thousands of those. In the end, though, what Terry wanted was familiarity. The same film over and over again. Like a child who only wants to watch the same Walt Disney film or hear the same bedtime story each and every night; the same fairy tale. Maybe even one of those tales that Terry had written for Sally. Alison put aside any pain or discomfort she may have felt at visiting Anna and Terry's home at the Hexagon and would go there to see him: 'I would shout, "Hello, Terry, I've come to visit you . . . hope you don't mind if I turn the film off!" There was always a film on.'

As Annabel Leventon recalls, 'Mike Palin and I started going round together to see Terry because it was really quite hard on your own. Terry lost the ability to speak, and he lost the ability to swallow properly, and he lost the ability to do anything but eat mashed food. It got horribly difficult but Mike and I would go round regularly together, and sit and have a bit of lunch with Terry.' Mike and Annabel would start reminding him about what they had done together, retelling jokes from the shows. Annabel would hold hands with Terry while she and Mike swapped memories. Terry was able to laugh along even after he couldn't speak. It delighted Mike that Terry would laugh at the jokes that Terry had written, not those that Mike had written!

Sociable to the last, Terry loved conversation to be taking place around him, even if he couldn't join in. And, in a reverse of those stories he had read to Sally, Sally enjoyed reading the diaries of Samuel Pepys aloud to her dad. 'He had lost the ability to read by then. Dad always loved to read the newspaper but he just couldn't. He still liked to sit there, with the newspaper in his hand, and while he had his coffee he would turn the pages. He couldn't read it but he liked to go through the actions of it.' Sally loved to get a reaction from him: 'Those moments when you get a flicker of a smile, or a single eyebrow would go up. That was very precious.'

Terry's routine became very rigid. He had to have his meals at regular times and then he had to watch *Guys and Dolls*. Eventually, it would become the only film he wanted to watch. It took Annabel Leventon right back to those Oxford days of Michael Rudman's acting workshop. Michael was obsessed with *Guys and Dolls*. People weren't welcome in the group unless they loved *Guys and Dolls*, and here were Terry and Annabel watching *Guys and Dolls* together. Nearly sixty years later.

In 2019, it was the fifty-fifth anniversary of *Hang Down Your Head and Die*, the play about capital punishment that Terry had starred in while in his third year at Oxford. David Wood was planning a reunion party. He remembers: 'I rang Mike Palin and said: "Should we invite Terry?" Mike knew how bad the condition had become by that stage and wasn't sure whether Anna would want him to go. Mike said he would speak to Alison, who said she would love to come – as she knew them all and had loved the show – and it was Alison who got Terry there. She told me that she had got permission from Anna to bring Terry along. It was all arranged.'

In order to put Terry at his ease, Michael Palin was seated on one side of him and Alison on the other. It made this round reunion table one of safety and familiarity. For David Wood, the whole day was 'incredibly moving. People were going up to Terry and saying "Hello" and he seemed aware and able to acknowledge people. Everyone said how lovely it was to have him there. Terry just sat there throughout. Quite expressionless.' David remembers thinking at the time that he was back to that amazing mime. That face of starkly white, clown-like lack of expression that he had brought to the play all those years before. *Hang Down Your Head* contained a beautiful song about this poor man who is about to go to the scaffold. At the reunion, those assembled sang it together, quite softly, and for the first time that day there was a flicker on Terry's face: 'It was a very touching look of recognition,' says David. 'Breaking through that fug of his memory. The song clearly rang some distant bell with him. Some of us found it very difficult to carry on singing but we did because we felt maybe in a very small way it was helping Terry, or certainly connecting with him. One last time.'

Nick Fox confirms that Terry would absolutely have been aware of what was going on: 'It wasn't a form of dementia that caused memory loss. It was almost as if there was a broken bit in the road between his thought process and communicating those thoughts. The brain stores a huge amount of information. Like a tree with lots of branches, which, in a split second, allows us to process what we are seeing and make the connections. Terry could process what he was seeing and hearing. Those memories of happy and familiar things would register with him.'

Even more familiar was Grove Park, Terry's old home, which Alison welcomed him back to on many occasions. The routine would be the same, though – old films. Over and over again. Alison remembers that, 'He watched some films so many times the centre of the DVD boxes fell apart. We had to buy brand new copies of *Guys and Dolls, Some Like it Hot, Holiday Inn, Way Out West* with Laurel and Hardy.' It was still old comedies and musicals. Comedies and musicals. The last firm favourite was the 1935 Fred Astaire and Ginger Rogers film musical *Top Hat*. Glamour. Dancing. Those glorious Irving Berlin songs. Bill remembers those final months with touching honesty: 'I was watching a film with Dad and when it finished he was trying to tell me something and I just couldn't understand what he wanted. He just couldn't communicate, and I saw him just give up in front of me. That was heartbreaking.' But watching his films, with loved ones, was Terry's idea of heaven. He would sit and watch them in company, holding hands. At all hours.

Sally recalls: 'He had a touch of asthma and this would some-times wake him up. On occasions, he would wake up at four in the morning, unbeknown to any of us.' Terry's own routine would logically tell him that, as he was awake, he should get dressed. The logic would also tell him that it was pitch black outside, so he shouldn't go out. Instead, he would put the telly on. Really loudly. And watch his films. Sally recalls, 'He wouldn't want to go back to bed, but he would still like the company. He would still like to hold a hand. On occasions, he would pinch your bum as well. So you had to watch it!' She laughs. He was playful to the end.

And pretty much to the end, just like Felix the Cat, he kept on walking. Sally explains, 'Dad was happy. Even if he couldn't tell you he was happy. Even with that slide through dementia he stayed mobile.' It was really important to him to keep walking every day. When they took him to Wales, he would always do the big walk back from the pub, along the ridge. Even if he couldn't put the brakes on, careering down those steep hills. And he would do a long walk on Hampstead Heath, every day.

Michael Palin, a frequent visitor, knew Terry's habits almost as well as Terry knew them. Mike would also invite old Oxford chums to come along and see Terry. For Nigel Pegram: 'The final time I saw him was at a lovely gathering of the last of *The Oxford Revue*. Mike, Terry, Annabel Leventon and I had lunch together.

Terry just grabbed my hand and all he could do was make those heartbreaking grunts and moans. He'd lost his speech completely by that time but he just held on to me. It was incredibly moving. And we then discovered that he'd picked up the tab! Generous to the very end. What a dear, dear friend he was. Annabel had to leave but then the three of us walked across Hampstead Heath with Terry charging ahead. In purple socks, with red and yellow spots on them! He then disappeared. Mike said, "I walk with him pretty much every day. This is what he does!"'

And Annabel Leventon remembers another unforgettable occasion. Barry Cryer had got in touch because, like Annabel and Mike Palin, he wanted to go and visit Terry. Annabel picked Barry up at Paddington and drove him over to the Hexagon. They had a lovely lunch. And then Terry wanted to go for his walk. Terry would slip on his big coat, put his shoes on . . . and be off, on a long, very brisk walk. Annabel knew exactly what was going to happen, because the routine was always the same. So Terry got ready for his walk and Barry said, 'I'll come with you. Are you going across the Heath?' Annabel says, 'I whispered: "Please, Barry. Don't go!", but he took no notice. Anyway, I sat there . . . and sat there . . . and they didn't come back! Finally I got a phone call from Barry. I said, "Are you all right?" and he said: "No, I'm not!"'

It transpired that Barry was sat on a bench outside Kenwood House with no idea how to get back. Annabel asked, 'Where's Terry?' and Barry replied, 'I don't know! I walked down this slope and I slipped in the mud, and Terry was already up the other side! He didn't stop. He didn't even look round! I cried out "Terry" several times, but I was stuck in the mud!' By the time Barry had got up, Terry was nowhere to be seen. He'd gone off into the woods, sticking to his daily course, head down, and just kept walking until he found his way home, as usual, homing pigeon-style.

Annabel laughs as she remembers having to try to work out

which bench, out of many, Barry was sat on: 'I told him, sit tight and I'll come and fetch you. Poor Barry was shaken to the core. Terry had got himself home. Safe and sound. It was the only time I ever saw Barry Cryer lose his sense of humour!' It was only in his last year that Terry stopped his daily walk across the Heath.

Family and friends would have to be Terry's voice, though his old sociability was still there. Sally explains, 'We wanted to take Dad out and to do fun things. To give him as much of his old life back as possible. He was back at Grove Park for the weekend and it was the wedding of a friend of mine. They ran a local pub, so I wanted to pop in and say hello, and I took Dad. Suddenly, he just dived into the crowd. I tried to follow him. He went up to this chap and tapped him on the shoulder. It was an old friend, from the Highgate allotments, who Dad had recognised and wanted to be with again. Dad's dementia never made him frightened of people. His faculties were still there. He just needed us to talk for him.'

At the very end, however, it was necessary to lock the door, even though the family felt terrible denying him his liberty. As Alison laments: 'We would lose him around Grove Park! He would wake up at four in the morning and get out of the house. Or he would walk off to get some wine from the shop. I had put this kind of satnav device on him, so we could track him.' One day, he was gone so long that Alison located him and found him stepping out into the middle of the road without looking. It was very difficult. Alison pulled up next to him and said, 'Terry, are you going to the shops? Would you like a lift?'

When the time came to celebrate fifty years of Monty Python, in October 2019, Terry was far too unwell to take an active part in the party. Instead, the decision was made to remaster and re-release and, slightly, rename 'I'm So Worried' as 'I'm (Still) So Worried'. As André Jacquemin remembers, the decision to do so was made by all four other Pythons. 'It was unanimous. The Python anniversary would be marked by Terry. From out of the dusty archives.' Terry personified the fearlessness and inventiveness of Python. He was never afraid to be a bit odd or embarrassing. Sometimes he would sing something that was so bad he would laugh his head off: 'He always saw the funny side of it if he was a bit rubbish! I can hear him now saying: "Oh God, we can't use that. That's terrible!" We thought the best way to mark Python at fifty was to have Terry singing, on behalf of all of us, and being just as silly as he always had been. Perfect.'

The end, when it came, was as nice as it could be.

It was at Christmas 2019 when the inevitable dark conversation had to take place. The family met with the palliative care team at the National Hospital for Neurology and Neurosurgery, in Queen Square, London. Sally remembers that they 'talked us through what the possible end might be. They said that, if the time came when Dad could not swallow his tablets, then he would have to go into hospital to receive antibiotics. There was absolutely no way he would want to be in hospital. We wanted to keep him out of hospital at all costs.'

That last Christmas was not good. At the start of the New Year, Terry was confined to bed for two weeks and was unconscious for several days, before rallying and waking up – very, very hungry!

Sally remembers the last time she saw him: 'I had made plans to take a week's holiday in Wales. I was uncertain whether to go but he was sat up in bed, enjoying his bowl of soup. I said: "OK, Dad, I'll see you." He gave me a big smile of recognition. He slipped back and went downhill very swiftly after that. He went into a coma. And that was that.'

Terry Jones died on Tuesday 21 January 2020 at the age of seventy-seven. His family issued a statement: 'to thank Terry's wonderful medical professionals and carers for making the past few years not only bearable but often joyful. We hope that this disease will one day be eradicated entirely. We ask that our privacy be respected at this sensitive time and give thanks that we lived in the presence of an extraordinarily talented, playful and happy man living a truly authentic life, in his words "Lovingly frosted with glucose."'

Terry's lasting personal legacy was the awareness he brought and still brings to dementia patients. In a final, tangible act, that multifaceted, incalculably inventive brain of his was donated to medical science. That extremely clever clump of grey matter that sang about Spam, ripped yarns, unpicked Chaucer, and laughed and loved and thoroughly enjoyed life might have let him down in the end. But ultimately, even that was doing some good. Helping to solve the ultimate riddle. For other people.

# THE EPILOGUE

## THE BRAIN OF TERRY JONES

*And it was gone! Like . . . that! And I was left behind.*
*I couldn't even wonder what I'd do without a mind.*

THAT Terry's brain is still doing so much good, in all sorts of
ways, is an incredible legacy. As Nick Fox says: 'it was an amazing brain and it is still an amazing brain. It was a decision made by
the family after Terry's death, but Terry was very well aware how
phenomenally important brain donations are. The brain really is
the final frontier. We really don't fully understand it. The only way
we can learn about it is through brain donation.'

In my capacity as comedy historian I often thank the heavens
for film and tape, preserving the work of great performers and
writers like Terry. It is a sort of immortality and, for Nick, 'it's a
rather lovely parallel. Terry's work is there for ever, and Terry's
brain is still tremendously important. That part of him is also sort
of immortalised now. It was flash frozen. Everything is kept and
when people request little bits of brain tissue, they will use Terry's
brain to test drugs; to assist in understanding the problems of
patients in need of care. Terry's brain will be helping others for
years and years to come.'

What a legacy; and what a comforting thought.

The personal recollections of my friendship with Terry Jones that
pepper this book are just a smidgeon of the hilarious, heartfelt and
just plain happy hours I spent with him. There were so many

wonderful moments that it's impossible to pick a favourite memory. Though there is one absolutely joyful, brief encounter that stands out and never fails to make me beam with delight.

Terry and I were working at a fan convention in Birmingham. You know the kind of thing – a huge aircraft hangar of a space, with various cult figures from *Doctor Who* and *Star Trek* pressing the flesh with a horde of adoring fans getting their prized 8x10 stills and film posters and tie-in annuals autographed by their heroes. I had been approached many, many times about whether Terry would be interested in attending one of these long weekends of relentless smiles and writer's cramp. He was sceptical, to put it mildly, almost in disbelief as he repeated back to me what I had just told him: 'I sit behind a table all day, just signing my name? Right! Why?' It was a fair question. With tongue in cheek, although not that far, I chuckled: 'The money, Terry! The money!' Once I had related the deal, which included lovely travel and accommodation, a few good meals out and a nice bottle or three of wine – plus a carrier bag or two of cash – Terry gave that off-kilter grin and said: 'What?! For just sitting behind a table all day and signing my name? Let's do it.' And so we did. Several times.

Fans were bowled over to get their Monty Python movie stills dedicated to them by the director. And I lost count of the number of coconuts devoted *Holy Grail* admirers got Terry to sign. For hours and hours, Terry didn't stop. Not even for a drink. He smiled and signed and shook hands and spoke – often at length – with each and every person who was in that elephantine, serpentine line. My duty was simple. To keep it all chugging along nicely and asking each person to whom they wanted the autograph made out, and spelling out anything that Terry would find helpful.

After a whole morning and much of the afternoon without a let-up, I looked up to see a young, handsome chap with wavy hair and a smile that could melt stone. It was Superman. Well, it was that charming actor from Iowa, Brandon Routh. This was the summer of 2006. *Superman Returns* had just hit cinemas and was well on the way to making nearly four hundred million dollars at the box office. Brandon Routh was pretty much the hottest young star in Hollywood at that precise moment. He was certainly the most bankable man in that cavernous signing hall. Terry, needless to say, had absolutely no idea who he was. People in neighbouring queues were craning their necks to hear the conversation for which I had a ringside seat.

Brandon Routh seemed lovely and was grinning with excitement. I was pretty excited too: 'Wow! Hello. Umm . . . Terry. This is Brandon Routh!'

Terry extended a hand, saying, 'Oh, a friend of Rob's . . . nice to see you.'

'No. No, Terry. This is Brandon Routh. He's Superman!'

Terry was nonplussed. Not unimpressed, just unaware: 'How nice,' he said. And he meant it. Terry thought this very personable chap was a super young man.

'You didn't queue, did you?' I asked.

'Oh, sure!' Brandon chuckled. 'I had an hour or so off and I wanted to meet Terry.'

Terry smiled again. Terry shook Brandon's hand again. Terry signed a photograph for Brandon and that was that. The couple of Monty Python fans behind Brandon were as spellbound and amazed as I was. 'Was that Superman?' they muttered. Terry smiled and said: 'Yes. What a lovely chap.' Taking the photograph proffered and extending a hand, he added: 'And so are you! Thanks so much for coming . . .'

When the crowd abated, a little later that afternoon, I tried again. 'You know, Terry, that was Superman. Superman actually queued up to get your autograph!'

Terry couldn't quite grasp why I was so impressed by that: 'Yeah! Lovely. What's that make me then? If Superman wanted my autograph?'

I said, 'Someone very, very special indeed.'

And he was. Wasn't he? Very, very special indeed.

Colin Webb talks of Terry 'as a pure life force. Not just a brilliant thinker and a provocative writer, but a true friend.' It is this power of loyal friendship that most sums up Terry. It is his superpower. Indeed, Michael Foreman expresses it beautifully when he says, 'Everyone who knew Terry remained friends with him.'

Professor Alan Ereira gets understandably emotional when he recalls his final meeting with Terry. 'He was already very ill and his last words to me were quite startling. Terry grabbed my hand and said: "I love you." It was a very close friendship.'

For Daphne Lambert and all involved with the Penrhos Brewery, it was simply that Terry wanted the world to be a kinder place: 'That was born of his generosity and his passion and his genuine inquisitiveness about people. Really genuine. You could watch him in the restaurant when he came in. He was genuinely interested in people and what they had to say. That is a wonderful quality.'

*Holy Flying Circus* actor Rufus Jones considers it 'the privilege of a career to be in Terry's shoes for a few weeks' and, warmly recalling their one and only meeting, 'a medieval blessing to be gathered up in a brotherly hug by that instinctual, polymath firebrand.'

With the spirit of Python in his soul, André Jacquemin chuckles when he says, 'Despite driving everybody nuts, Terry was an absolute genius. An absolute loveable genius. He would ask for the most impossible things but you ended up doing it, and making it work as best as you possibly could. Just for Terry. He had this passion and drive to just leap in and get things done. And he loved that quality in other people. He loved the need to create.'

André's lasting memory of Terry was after his final film, *Absolutely Anything*, was done and dusted. 'Terry took us out for some food at the Pizza Express in Soho. There was Bill, Ben, myself and Terry. He turned to us and said, "I just want to say thank you, guys. This film wouldn't have happened if not for you. I am so grateful that you are here with me." He was so appreciative. I was pretty touched by that. It meant a huge deal.'

For Annabel Leventon: 'Terry was the easiest-going, most companionable friend you could wish to have. He never, ever displayed a vestige of awareness of his very considerable prestige. He wore all his considerable talents so lightly that you tended to forget just how brilliant he was. He was a deeply serious man who just danced through life. Terry had a quality of enduring love. I am just so happy that he was part of my life for such a long time.'

Little wonder then that, just four days after what would have been Terry's seventy-eighth birthday, the Golders Green Crematorium was packed with those who loved him most. Annabel Leventon remembers, 'It was standing room only . . . even for friends like John Cleese, who stood head and shoulders above everybody else. It was a lovely service. All of us sang "Penny Lane". The order of service had a photo of Terry from his absolute peak, in the Seventies, and he looked absolutely beautiful. And irresistible.'

Nigel Pegram remembers that date of 5 February 2020 very well. 'It was simply the day we all waved goodbye to Terry. We all miss him. Always.'

The legacy of everything Terry achieved – and it was an awful lot – continues to bring joy in all sorts of ways. Perhaps the most pleasing happened at Annabel Leventon's eightieth birthday cabaret: 'Terry had gone by then, but Michael Palin came and performed the Bengal Tiger bit from *Bert Fegg*. The room was full of my great nieces and nephews, who were absolutely bewitched by this idea of "pass the Bengal tiger". You know, it's a bit like "pass the parcel". Except under the wrapping it's a Bengal tiger. The whole audience absolutely loved it but those children, in particular, loved it. In those words that they had written together, Mike brought Terry with him. It was a brilliant, beautiful thing for Mike to do.'

And those words of Terry remain. Just awaiting a fresh

audience to read them or recite them or listen to them. To laugh and cry and learn from them. The words were always the thing. And Wales, of course.

In a perfect bookend fashion, Wales called Terry back for one last good deed. One last celebration of all that talent. As a patron of the Victorian theatre, Theatr Colwyn, Terry was passionate about supporting and promoting the creative arts in his hometown. Now Colwyn Bay will have a bronze statue of Terry, sculpted by Llandudno-based sculptor Nick Elphick. Everybody close to Terry knew that he would baulk at anything too formal and serious. It would have to be silly. Seriously silly. So, the family decided that Terry should be immortalised as Monty Python's organist, with wild hair and an open smile. Stark naked, save for a neck-tie! As Terry Gilliam said, 'Now people can come from all over the world to rub Terry's bottom for good luck! He would love that more than anything.'

The Python on the Prom campaign for a statue of Terry Jones was supported by family, friends and admirers, including Steve Coogan, Emma Thompson and Suzy Eddie Izzard, who delight-fully pushed the appeal over its financial target. The excess and future monies raised will be donated equally between the Conwy Arts Trust and the National Brain Appeal, two charities very close to Terry's heart. 'Finally, Terry gets the recognition he deserves,' said Eric Idle. 'A statue no less. OK, so it's not an airport or a boule-vard, but a statue in Colwyn Bay is lovely and a wonderful way to remember this fabulous man.' Terry Gilliam agreed that 'the statue will make up for all the years that he wasn't here. I think he would have hated it, that's why we want it done. To punish him for all he did to us!' While John Cleese, comically and movingly, commented: 'I am so delighted that Terry is being immortalised in bronze, although I would have preferred that he be immortalised by not dying. Still, bronze is better than nothing.'

Fittingly, it was Michael Palin who spoke for all when he said, 'It will take care of Terry's "Welshness" because he was very keen on that and kept on about it! So with a statue he'd be stuck here for the rest of time!'

Colwyn Bay, the beautiful spot that saw the start of Terry's story, will be the eternal host for the end of Terry's story. Quite right too.

'Terry's greatest achievement was to live life so thoroughly,' concludes Michael Palin. 'That talent to enjoy life so very much. And to think about life so very much. To be so intense about everything he could do and everything he couldn't do. This was not somebody who just rambled through life. Terry always had an idea – a way it should be done – and everything he did was important. Everything Terry did, he had to do it well. Life with Terry was never, ever boring. He looked at life in a way that no one else did. Nobody saw things in quite the same way. You just couldn't sit back and relax. You had to get involved.'

And, speaking for myself, it was an unforgettable joy to get involved with Terry. Down the pub, our conversations would often turn back to words. I would invariably arrive to find Terry contently sitting at the bar, nose in the paper or, more often than not, a paperback novel. Once the pints were ordered the chat would bob and weave, as usual, tackling everything and nothing. On occasions, after the sparkling sting of one of his fascinating nuggets from the past, I would say, 'You know, Terry, you really need to write your autobiography.'

He would scrunch up his face in mock outrage. 'Oh, no. Who'd want to read that . . .?'

And before I could protest and yell, 'Loads of people!', Terry would shut down the line of enquiry with, 'Besides, I simply don't have the time. Tell you what, when I'm dead, you can write it for me.' So that's what I've done. And, dear Terry, I couldn't have done it without you.

# AFTERWORD

## BY TERRY GILLIAM

M Y final memory of Terry is of him walking on the Heath.
He looked fantastic. He had lost a little weight and was fitter and looked better than I had seen him in years. He was dressed immaculately. But there was no one at home. He was a shell. A beautiful shell.

He reminded me of somebody out of a children's story. Out of one of his children's stories. Or out of the children's literature he loved so much. Like the White Rabbit in Lewis Carroll's *Alice's Adventures in Wonderland*. Dressed so dapperly but in a state of anguish. He would be constantly taking his pocket watch out, checking the time and putting it back. Taking it out, looking at it and putting it back. As if he had somewhere he needed to be. Urgently. The sad fact was that he had nowhere to be. Nothing to get back to.

I like to think of him, head down, scurrying off quickly, and disappearing down the nearest rabbit hole, to find a permanent peace, a permanent happiness.

Terry Gilliam, Hampstead, May 2025

# ACKNOWLEDGEMENTS

A NNA Mrowiec, my brilliant and always-enthused commissioning editor, wise, fun and reassuring, who just got the tone of
Terry and the book immediately . . . and it wasn't just the sharing
of a bottle of his favourite Picpoul wine on that first meeting; Tom
Atkins, my assistant editor who was always there with an encouraging word and his vegan buns, which kept me going at many a
crucial moment; Liz Marvin, my pugnacious and upbeat editor
who was a comrade-in-arms throughout the hard and hilarious
whittling-down of my huge manuscript; Ella Watkins and Alice
Morley for publicity and marketing; Samantha Blake at The BBC
Written Archives Centre in Caversham for ferreting out the most
obscure contract or correspondence, particularly from Terry's
earliest days with the Corporation; Absana Rutherford and Jack
McMinn of The Oxford Comedy Archive; Catherine Mason and
Scott Smith at Doune Castle for kindness and enthusiasm equal to
Terry's own; Gemma Ross for everything really, but in particular
getting the proposal of this biography up to scratch, and being
terrier-like in placing it with the exact right people and the exact
right publisher; Terry's many friends and family who shared candid
and comic memories that brought Terry vividly back to life. For the
record, and in alphabetical order, here's the roll-call, alongside the
dates the interview was conducted. A comedy historian to the end!

Carolyn Allen, 17 October 2024; David Barry, 23 May 2025;
Carol Cleveland, 17 June 2025; Professor Alan Ereira, 27 September
2024; Louise and Michael Foreman, 25 November 2024; Professor

Nick Fox, 20 June 2025; Graeme Garden MBE, 23 May 2025; Terry Gilliam, 17 May 2025; Eric Idle, 16 May 2025; André Jacquemin, 10 October 2024; Kim 'Howard' Johnson, 6 March 2025; Bill Jones, 14 May 2025; Rufus Jones, 31 July 2025; Sally Jones, 21 February 2025; Daphne Lambert, 28 November 2024; Annabel Leventon, 3 October 2024; Sir Michael Palin, 3 July 2024; Nigel Pegram, 7 October 2024; Anna Söderström, 22 May 2025; Imogen Stubbs, 6 March 2025; Doctor Alison Telfer, 21 February 2025; Colin Webb, 11 October 2024; David Wood OBE, 25 September 2024.

Finally, an extra special mention to Alison, Sally and Bill who were always on hand for one final thought, one final rummage through Terry's archive, one final word of encouragement. And to Sir Michael Palin, Eric Idle and Terry Gilliam for their fore, middle, and after words. Pythons reunited. The most fitting of tributes. All for, as Eric refers to it, 'the big book about Terry'.

# PICTURE ACKNOWLEDGEMENTS

**Inset 1:**

Pages 1, 2, top, 3, top, 4, bottom, 5, bottom, 6, and 8: © John Sims and Terry Jones' personal collection

Page 2, bottom: © Nigel Pegram

Pages 3, bottom, and 7: © Trinity Mirror/Mirrorpix/Alamy.com

Page 4, top, and 5, top: ©Rolf Adlercreutz/Alamy.com

**Inset 2:**

Pages 2, top, and 8, bottom: © John Sims and Terry Jones' personal collection

Page 1: © Trinity Mirror/Mirrorpix/Alamy.com

Page 2, bottom: © Slapstick Festival, 2012. Photographer Adam Johnson.

Page 3, top: © PA Images/Alamy.com

Page 3, bottom: © RGR Collection/Alamy.com

Page 4, top: © Kim 'Howard' Johnson

Page 4, bottom: © Everett Collection Inc./Alamy.com

Page 5: © Associated Press/Alamy.com

Page 6, top: © Author's personal collection. Photographer Robert Ross.

Page 6, bottom: © WENN Rights Ltd/Alamy.com

Page 7, top: © ZUMA Press, Inc./Alamy.com

Page 7, bottom: © Author's personal collection. Photographer Justin Pollard.

Page 8, top: © Jon Furniss

# TERRYOGRAPHY

For a lengthy chronological listing of Terry's exhaustive professional achievements, please scan the QR code.

So prolific was Terry that this is completely incomplete, so, if you spot an omission, do drop us a line and we'll add it, to form an ever-evolving source of reference.

And why not leave a comment – either silly or serious or Spam. Enjoy.

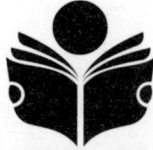

# RAISING READERS
## Books Build Bright Futures

Dear Reader,

We'd love your attention for one more page to tell you about the crisis in children's reading, and what we can all do.

Studies have shown that reading for fun is the **single biggest predictor of a child's future life chances** – more than family circumstance, parents' educational background or income. It improves academic results, mental health, wealth, communication skills, ambition and happiness.[1]

The number of children reading for fun is in rapid decline. Young people have a lot of competition for their time. In 2024, 1 in 10 children and young people in the UK aged 5 to 18 did not own a single book at home.[2]

Hachette works extensively with schools, libraries and literacy charities, but here are some ways we can all raise more readers:

- Reading to children for just 10 minutes a day makes a difference
- Don't give up if children aren't regular readers – there will be books for them!
- Visit bookshops and libraries to get recommendations
- Encourage them to listen to audiobooks
- Support school libraries
- Give books as gifts

There's a lot more information about how to encourage children to read on our website: **www.RaisingReaders.co.uk**

Thank you for reading.

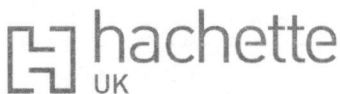
hachette UK

---

[1] National Literacy Trust, Book Ownership in 2024, November 2024
https://nlt.cdn.ngo/media/documents/Book_ownership_in_2024

[2] OECD. 2021. 21st-century readers: developing literacy skills in a digital world. Paris, France: OECD Publishing.
https://www.oecd.org/en/publications/21st-century-readers_a83d84cb-en.html